KU-262-273

Nasal Systemic
Drug Delivery

DRUGS AND THE PHARMACEUTICAL SCIENCES

A Series of Textbooks and Monographs

Edited by

James Swarbrick
School of Pharmacy
University of North Carolina
Chapel Hill, North Carolina

Nasal Systemic Drug Delivery

YIE W. CHIEN

Controlled Drug-Delivery Research Center
College of Pharmacy, Rutgers University
Piscataway, New Jersey

KENNETH S. E. SU

Pharmaceutical Research Department
Eli Lilly and Company
Indianapolis, Indiana

SHYI-FEU CHANG

Department of Pharmaceutics/Drug Delivery
Amgen Incorporated
Thousand Oaks, California

MARCEL DEKKER, INC.   New York • Basel

Library of Congress Cataloging-in-Publication Data

Nasal systemic drug delivery / [edited by] Yie W. Chien, Kenneth S. E.
  Su, Shyi-Feu Chang.
        p.   cm. -- (Drugs and the pharmaceutical sciences ; v. 39)
    Includes bibliographies and index.
    ISBN 0-8247-8093-0 (alk. paper)
    1. Intranasal medication. I. Chien, Yie W.   II. Su,
  Kenneth S. E.   III. Chang, Shyi-Feu   IV. Series.
  RM160.N37   1989
  615'.6--dc20   89-12007
                                                                CIP

This book is printed on acid-free paper.

Copyright © 1989 by MARCEL DEKKER, INC.   All Rights Reserved

Neither this book nor any part may be reproduced or transmitted in any form
or by any means, electronic or mechanical, including photocopying, micro-
filming, and recording, or by any information storage and retrieval system,
without permission in writing from the publisher.

MARCEL DEKKER, INC.
270 Madison Avenue, New York, New York 10016

Current printing (last digit).
10 9 8 7 6 5 4 3 2 1

PRINTED IN THE UNITED STATES OF AMERICA

Preface

Continuous intravenous infusion of drug at a programmed rate has been recognized as a superior mode of delivery. It is capable of bypassing gastro-intestinal incompatibility and hepatic "first-pass" metabolism, as well as achieving a constant, prolonged plasma drug level within a therapeutically effective range required for treatment. However, such mode of drug delivery entails certain potential risks and, therefore, necessitates hospitalization of the patient for close medical supervision of the medication (1).

Recently, there has been a growing awareness that the benefits of intra-venous drug infusion can be closely duplicated, without its potential hazards, by continuous drug delivery through the intact skin. Even though transder-mal delivery has been demonstrated to be very useful for controlled admini-stration of highly potent, lipophilic drugs to maintain a sustained plasma drug level within a therapeutically effective range, it often requires a time lag of several hours or longer to reach therapeutic levels, and the skin per-meation rate of hydrophilic and/or large drug molecules is often too low to be therapeutically useful (2).

Transnasal delivery has the advantages of providing direct entry of drug into the systemic circulation, as well as ease of administration. The nasal mucosa, unlike the skin, is not constructed from the highly keratinized stra-tum corneum, but from numerous microvilli underlined with rich vascularity. The nasal route, therefore, appears to be ideally suited for nonparenteral administration of drugs intended for systemic medication.

Historically, the use of the nasal route for drug delivery has received the attention of mankind since ancient times. Nasal therapy, also called "Nasaya Karma," has been a recognized form of treatment in the Ayurvedic system of Indian medicine. Psychotropic drugs and hallucinogens have been used, as nose snuff, by the Indians of South America. In more recent years, many drugs have been shown to achieve a better systemic bioavailability by self-medication through the nasal route than by oral administration. Some of them have been shown to duplicate the plasma profile as i.v. administration (3).

To assist readers who are interested in the potential of nasal drug delivery for systemic medication, the authors have conducted an extensive literature review of more than 750 scientific articles. The result of this extensive review has yielded a critical insight into this potential field of biomedical research, which forms the foundation of this book. To provide a better understanding of the sciences behind the development of various nasal drug delivery approaches, the book is organized into six chapters: It begins with the analysis of nasal anatomy and physiology (Chapter 1), animal models (Chapter 2), and physicochemical, biopharmaceutical, and toxicophysiological aspects (Chapter 3) important to nasal drug delivery. The book subsequently discusses the intranasal delivery of peptide/protein drugs (Chapter 4), nonpeptide molecules (Chapter 5), and diagnostic drugs (Chapter 6).

It is our intention in this book to provide all the scientific information published to date that a biomedical researcher/pharmaceutical scientist needs to know about the nasal delivery of systemic drugs.

The authors wish to express their appreciation for the excellent assistance provided by Ms. L. F. Chien in the preparation of this book.

REFERENCES

1. Chien, Y. W. *Novel Drug Delivery Systems*, Marcel Dekker, New York (1982).
2. Chien, Y. W. *Transdermal Controlled Systemic Medications*, Marcel Dekker, New York (1987).
3. Chien, Y. W. *Transnasal Systemic Medication*, Elsevier, Amsterdam (1985).

Yie W. Chien
Kenneth S. E. Su
Shyi-Feu Chang

Contents

Nasal Systemic
Drug Delivery

1
Anatomy and Physiology of the Nose

The bioavailability of a drug and hence its therapeutic effectiveness are often influenced by the route selected for administration. For a medication to achieve its maximal efficacy, a drug should be able to be administered easily so better patient compliance can be achieved; and it should be capable of being absorbed efficiently so greater bioavailability can be accomplished. The nasal route appears to be an ideal alternative to the parenterals for administering drugs intended for systemic effect in view of the rich vascularity of the nasal membranes and the ease of intranasal administration.

Several advantages can be achieved from delivering drugs intranasally: (a) avoidance of hepatic "first-pass" elimination, gut wall metabolism, and/or destruction in gastrointestinal tracts; (b) the rate and extent of absorption and the plasma concentration vs. time profile are relatively comparable to that obtained by intravenous medication; and (c) the existence of a rich vasculature and a highly permeable structure in the nasal membranes for absorption. These advantages have made the nasal mucosa a feasible and desirable site for systemic drug delivery.

However, there are some factors that should also be considered for optimizing the intranasal adminstration of drugs: (a) methods and techniques of administration; (b) the site of disposition; (c) the rate of clearance; and (d) the existence of any pathological conditions which may affect the nasal functions. These factors could potentially influence the efficiency of nasal absorption of drugs.

To study the intranasal delivery of drugs for systemic medication, it is important to first gain some fundamental understanding of the anatomy and physiology of the nose.

1.1 NASAL PASSAGE

The upper respiratory tract is constantly influenced by the inspired air. The nasal modification of the inspired air by filtration, humidification, and/ or warming are considered to be prime functions of the nose in man (1). To carry out its functions, the nose must control the rate of air flow, remove noxious agents, and introduce large quantities of fluid into the air stream.

The nasal passage which runs from the nasal vestibule (i.e., nasal valve) to the nasopharynx has a depth of approximately 12-14 cm (2) (Figure 1.1). In this passage, the nasal cellular apparatus is in close contact with mucus which protects the mucosa from the inspired air. There are three distinct functional zones in the nasal cavities (3,4); namely, vestibular, respiratory, and olfactory areas, which are arranged anteroposteriorly in this sequence of order (Figure 1.2). (a) The vestibular area serves as a baffle system, and its surface is covered by a common pseudostratified epithelium where the long hairs may provide the function of filtering airborne particles. (b) The respiratory area has a surface lined by a pseudostratified columnar epithelium, and is normally covered by a dense layer of mucus that is constantly moving toward the posterior apertures of the nasal cavity by a powerful system of motile cilia. (c) The olfactory region is about 10 cm^2, as compared to 170 cm^2 in the German shepherd dog. The olfactory airway lies above the middle turbinate between the nasal septum and the lateral wall of the main nasal passage. The airway here is only about 1-2 mm wide and is contiguous to the cribriform plate above. This region is generally free of inspiratory air flow.

The nasal passage is composed of a horizontally skin-lined vestibule with the passages being directed upward and backward, and is separated by a cartilaginous, bony nasal septum (5). The lateral wall is convoluted with strategically placed turbinates that mold the air stream to their configurations and changing dimensions.

The anterior nares mark the beginning of the double nasal airway, which extends from the entrance at the nostrils to the beginning of ciliated mucosa at the anterior ends of the nasal septum and turbinates (5,6). The main

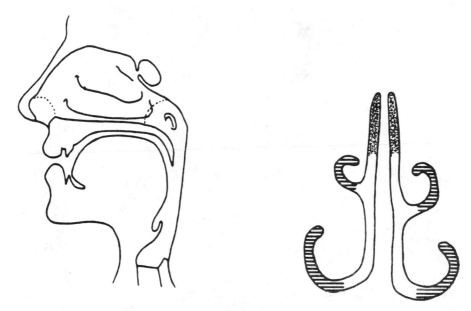

Figure 1.1 (Left) The upper airways seen from the midline. The dashed line just beyond the nostril marks the beginning of the nasal valve, whereas the dotted line shows approximately the beginning of the ciliated epithelium region. The dashed line near the nasopharynx indicates the posterior termination of the nasal septum. (Right) Section through the main nasal passage showing the nasal septum, folds of the turbinates, and airway. The stippled area indicates the olfactory region, which is generally free of inspiratory air flow. The hatched areas mark the meatal spaces, through which there is very little air flow, but in which there exist the communications with the paranasal sinuses and nasolacrimal duct. The clear areas represent the main nasal airway for inspiratory airflow and the region lined with richly vascular erectile tissue. This is the site primarily reached by the medications applied intranasally as nose drops or fine aerosol sprays. (From Ref. 1, reproduced with permission of Elsevier.)

nasal passage extends backward by approximately 6-8 cm to the posterior ends of the turbinates and the arch of the septum. Its cross section is large, but the width of the convoluted air stream is narrow. The lining is ciliated, highly vascular, and rich in mucous glands and goblet cells. The septum ends at the nasopharynx and the airways merge into one (7).

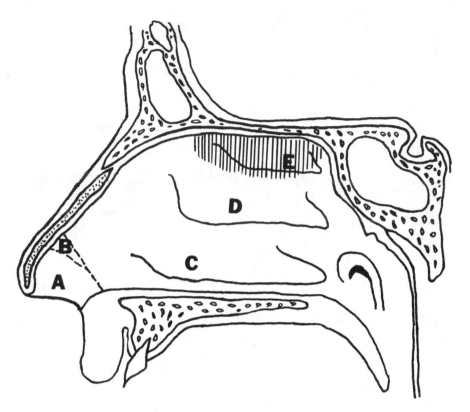

Figure 1.2 Diagram showing the lateral wall of the nasal cavity. A, nasal vestibule, B, internal ostium, C, inferior turbinate; D, middle turbinate, E, superior turbinate. The hatched areas indicate the olfactory region. (From Ref. 3, reproduced with permission of Elsevier.)

1.2 NASAL EPITHELIUM

The nasal membrane can be classified into olfactory and nonolfactory epithelia (5). The olfactory epithelium is a pseudostratified columna in type, and consists of specialized olfactory cells, supporting cells, and both serous and mucous glands, whereas the nonolfactory epithelium is a highly vascular tissue covered by a ciliated pseudostratified columnar epithelium (Figure 1.3). The olfactory cells are bipolar neurons and act as peripheral receptors and first-order ganglion cells.

There are two types of mucus covering the surface of the mucous membrane: one adheres to the tips of cilia, and the other fills the space among the

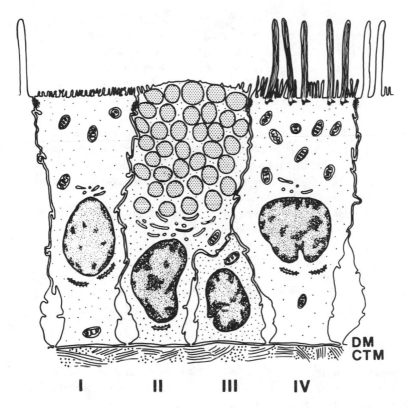

Figure 1.3 Transmission electron microscopic view of various cell types in
the nasal epithelium. I, nonciliated columnar cell with microvilli, II, goblet
cell with mucous granules and Golgi apparatus, III, basal cell, IV, ciliated
columnar cell with mitochondria in the apical part, DM, double membrane,
CTM, connective tissue membrane. (From Ref. 125, reproduced with permission of Blackwell.)

cilia. Numerous groups of microvilli can be seen microscopically among the
groups of cilia. All microvilli are of short clublike appearance and there are
approximately 500 microvilli on the surface of each ciliated cell. These cells
with microvilli are called goblet cell. Another type of epithelial cell is observed in the free surface of the mucous membrane. They are rounded or
elonged in shape and rough on the surface. These cells are defined as squa-
mous cells. However, some polygonal or elonged cells apparently have

numerous microvillilike processes on their outer surface. These basal cells of the lining epithelium have a looser intercellular connection and a wider intercellular space than in the ciliated cells. Furthermore, the subepithelial layer is seen to be packed with fibrils and covered with a homogeneous gelatinlike substance. The individual fine fibrils form bundles, but they are separated from each other with branches connecting the adjacent fibril to form networks.

Adequate moisture is required to maintain the normal functions of the nasal mucosa (8). Dehydration of the mucous blanket increases the viscosity of the secretions and reduces the ciliary activity. Thus, the recovery of heat and moisture from the expired air by the nasal membranes is of fundamental importance for retaining its normal functions.

In many animal species, including man, pronounced respiratory and cardiovascular responses associated with primary reflex from the nose can be elicited by appropriate stimulation of the nasal mucous membrane (9). Histamine has been detected in the nasal mucosa and also in the nasal secretions of allergic rhinitis (10). Another smooth muscle-stimulating substance, probably an unsaturated acid, has also been found in the nasal mucosa of the dog and sheep.

1.3 NASAL SECRETIONS

The composition of nasal secretions is complex and consists of a mixture of secretory materials from the goblet cells, nasal glands, and lacrimal glands and a transudate from plasma (11,12).

In a clean, noninfected, nonallergic, and nonirritated nose, the mucosa is covered by a thin layer of clear mucus which is secreted from the mucous and serous glands in the nasal mucosa and submucosa (13). This mucous blanket is moved posteriorly by the ciliary beat at a rate of about 1 cm/min, so that the nasal mucus is renewed approximately every 10 min. A total of approximately 1500-2000 ml of mucus is produced daily, which contains 90-95% water, 1-2% salt, and 2-3% mucin. The mucus has a two-layer composition: The watery (sol) layer is located immediately adjacent to the mucosal surface, and the mucous (gel) layer, which is more superficial. Normal nasal secretions contain about 150 mEq/L of sodium, 40 mEq/L of potassium, and 8 mEq/L of calcium as well as about 600 mg% of proteins, including 57 mg% of albumins and 133 and 50 mg% of immunoglobulins A (IgA) and G (IgG), respectively (14).

In addition to mucous glycoproteins, nasal secretions contain a variety of other proteins: lysozymes (15,16), enzymes (17), IgA, IgE, IgG, and albumins (14-18); kallikrein-like substance (19), protease inhibitor (20,21), prostaglandins (22-24), reagenic and antibacterial antibody (25), influenza virus-neutralizing activity, and hemagglutination-inhibiting activity (16,26) as well as serum proteins like gamma A-globulin, gamma G-globulin, albumin, and siderophilin (27,28).

The functions of mucus include: (a) acts as a retainer for the substances in the nasal duct; (b) behaves as an adhesive; (c) has water-holding capacity; (d) transports particulate matter; (e) exhibits surface electrical activity; (f) protects the mucosa; (g) acts as a mesh with permeability; and (h) allows heat transfer (13). Both experimentally and clinically, it has been reported that the nasal epithelium may be altered to produce excess mucus by different agents, including gases, viruses, bacteria, and certain diseases, such as allergic rhinitis (11). In addition, parasympathetic stimulation from methacholin, histamine, or SRS-A (slow-reacting substance of anaphylaxis) will also stimulate the secretion of mucous glycoproteins.

1.4 NASAL MUCOCILIARY CLEARANCE

Nasal ciliary clearance is one of the most important physiological defense mechanisms of the respiratory tract to protect the body against any noxious materials inhaled. There are approximately five ciliated cells for each mucous cell, with an average of 200 cilia extending from every ciliated cell on the surface of psuedostratified columnar epithelium. An individual cilium is approximately 5 μ in length and 0.2 μ in diameter (29), which moves at a frequency of about 20 beats/sec (30). The fine structure of the cilium consists of a ring of nine outer doublets surrounding a central pair (31) (Figure 1.4). Each doublet contains an A and B subfibril with both an inner and an outer dynein (a complex protein with adenosine triphosphatase [ATPase] activity) arm located on the A subfibril with a radial spoke extending toward the central doublet. The microtubules are surrounded by a cell membrane which is an extension from the body of the respiratory epithelial cell. Cilia beat in a synchronized fashion in a highly complicated manner. The motion of the cilia is dependent upon the microtubules sliding past one another with the dynein providing the needed ATPase activity. The bending of the cilia is thought to be caused by the radial spokes detaching and reattaching onto the central microtubules (32). Their coordination may be associated with neutral innervation, chemical pacemaking stimulation from hormones (e.g., epinephrine, serotonin), and the effects of ions (e.g., calcium, potassium) (33).

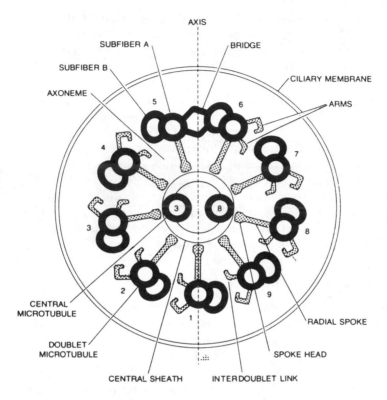

Figure 1.4 Diagram of cilium cross section, viewed from base toward tip. A ring of nine doublet microtubules surrounds two single central microtubules. Each doublet microtubule has two subfibers, A and B: Dynein arms project from subfiber A toward the next microtubule's subfiber B. (From Ref. 126, reproduced with permission of *Sci. Am.*)

In general nasal mucociliary clearance carries the airway secretions backward to the nasopharynx (34). This material is dispatched by a wiping action of the palate to the stomach periodically through swallowing. However, there is an area in the anterior nares of the inferior turbinate from which mucociliary clearance moves material forward, and this provides a clearance of deposited foreign materials from the body by nose blowing and wiping (35). Nasal clearance proceeds at an average rate of about 5-6 mm/min (36-39).

The nasal mucociliary function can be impaired by certain air pollutants, but not be relative humidity or temperature of the ambient air (36,37,40-42).

In patients with pathological conditions, their mucociliary function may be impaired. Slow mucociliary clearance is associated with nasal polyposis, or an injury to the nasal mucosa as a result of viral infections and other environmental insults occurring during childhood (37). Drying of the nasal mucous membrane will cause the cessation of ciliary activity, whereas prompt moistening will restore its normal activity (42). The optimum temperature range for mucociliary activity is 28-30°C. Hypotonic saline solutions tend to inhibit mucociliary activity, whereas hypertonic saline solutions will cause it to stop. A highly significant correlation between nasal ciliary beat frequency and log MTT (mucus transport time) was recently established in human volunteers. The data suggest that nasal ciliary beat frequency is the main factor in the nasal mucociliary clearance in healthy volunteers (43). The transport times, as measured by saccharin sodium, ranged from 2.5 to 20.0 min.

The arrest of ciliary mobility by drugs has been studied. The nasal administration of propranolol solution (0.1%) was reported to arrest the ciliary movement of both human adenoids and chicken embryo tracheas within 20 min (44) (Table 1.1). Cocaine solution yielded an immediate and complete paralysis of cilia at 10%, caused the arrest of ciliary activity after 2-3 min at 5%, and stopped ciliary activity at 2.5% after 1 h of continuous application (45). However, a 25% cocaine paste is an effective and safe local anesthetic, since sufficient cilia escape direct contact with cocaine crystals, allowing the mucous blanket to continue to be swept backward. Lidocaine and pontocaine were studied as to their effect on the mucus clearance ability of the human nasal ciliated epithelium (46). Lidocaine at the concentration of 4% did not impair mucus flow, whereas 2% pontocaine caused an immedi-

Table 1.1 The Decreasing Effect of Propranolol on the Ciliary Beat Frequency of Chicken Embryo Tracheal Epithelium and Human Adenoid Epithelium

Compound	Concentration	Species	Frequency[a] (%) Time (min)		
			2	10	20
Propranolol HCl	1%	Chicken	0	0	0
	0.1%	Chicken	70	8	0
	0.1%	Human	77	25	0

[a]Frequency as a percentage of the initial frequency.
Source: From Ref. 44, used with permission.

ate and complete cessation of both ciliary activity and mucus flow. Xylometazoline was also reported to diminish the mucociliary transport significantly (47). In another study, the use of xylometazoline at the concentration of 1 mg/ml over a 6-week period did not induce any major functional and structural changes in normal nasal mucosa (48). In subjects with common colds, a prolonged recovery in the mucociliary transport time was observed during the continued use of nose drops. A very diluted solution of adrenocorticotropic hormone (ACTH) esterase inhibitors was found to accelerate the nasal ciliary movement, whereas higher concentration slowed it down (49). Atropine was observed to slow the cilia beat, whereas morphine inhibited it. All of these effects are reversible. Tween 20 was reported to facilitate the nasal mucociliary clearance in the frog, which may be due to the reduction in adhesiveness caused by the surface-active agent (50).

Normal mucociliary transport is dependent upon the optimal interaction between the cilia and mucus, which was reportedly influenced by the ingredients in hair spray (51). The depression was significant at 15-60 min after exposure and did not regain normal values until 1.5 hr later. The alcohol content of the hair spray may also have affected the rheological properties of the mucus.

It has been reported that a gas which rapidly affects ciliary activity at low concentration and is relatively resorbed in the nasal cavity will be more toxic than a gas which is not resorbed in the nose and has little influence on the cilia.

1.5 NASAL BLOOD FLOW

The blood vessels in the nasal mucosa are of importance in the functions of the nose for thermal regulation and humidification of the inhaled air, and for controlling the lumen of the nasal passage.

The nasal mucosa is highly vascular. The surface of epithelium is supplied with a dense network of erectile carvernous tissue, which is particularly well developed over the turbinates and septum (52,53). The vascular bed provides a rich surface for drug absorption. Constriction of the blood vessels would decrease blood flow and blood content in the nasal mucosa, whereas vasodilation would yield the opposite response. The penetration of drug through the sinus mucosa is partly influenced by the blood flow in the region under normal and pathological conditions.

The arterial supply to the nose is derived from both the external and the internal carotid arteries. The terminal branch of the maxillary artery, which is a branch of the external carotid, supplies the sphenopalatine artery, which in turn supplies blood to the lateral and medial wall of the nasal chamber (54). On the other hand, the anterior and posterior ethmoid branches from the ophthalmic artery, which is a branch of the internal carotid artery. These vessels supply the anterior portion of the nose. The porosity of the endothelial basement membrane seems to facilitate the exposure of the contractile elements in the blood wall to agents carried by the blood. The nasal vascular bed is so designed that rapid exchange can be made for fluid and dissolved substances between the blood vessels and the nasal tissues (55). The capillary flow in the nasal mucosa was reported to be about 0.5 ml/g/min, whereas the anteriovenous shunt flow was found to be 60% of the total blood flow in the cat. Sympathetic stimulation was reported to produce a greater reduction in shunt flow than in capillary flow (56).

Many different factors, both local and general, have been identified to affect the vasomotor reaction of the nose. The local factors include the changes in the ambient temperature and humidity, the nasal administration of vasoactive drugs, the external compression of large veins in the neck, trauma, and inflammation (52). The general factors that affect nasal blood flow include emotion, fear, frustration, humiliation, anxiety, changes in environmental temperature, hyperventilation, and exercise (57,58). Nasal airway resistance was reported to increase at rest in the supine position and to decrease during exercise owing to some changes in the thickness of nasal mucosa as regulated by the capacitance vessels (58). The data suggest that the blood flow and the blood content of the human nasal mucosa are not affected in the same way by exercise.

The blood flow in the maxillary sinus mucosa in humans was reported to be in the range of 0.58-1.25 ml/g/min, as measured by microspheres (59-61), 0.09-0.77 ml/g/min, as measured by the R_b [86] Cl technique (62), or 34-44 ml/min, as measured by [133] Xe technique (63).

Nasal mucosal blood vessels are surrounded by adrenergic nerves, in which alpha-adrenoceptors show a functional predominance. Stimulation of these receptors produces a decrease in both blood content and blood flow in the nasal mucosa of both animals (64-66) and humans, (67,68).

The nasal blood flow is very sensitive to a variety of agents applied topically or systemically. The drugs that were reported to increase the blood flow in humans included histamine (63), fenoterol (69,70), isoproterenol (71), phenylephrine (72), and albuterol (72). The administration of oxymetazoline (63,73) or clonidine (73) in humans was found to decrease the nasal blood flow.

Table 1.2 Response of the Nasal Airway to Some Vasoactive Agents

Increased patency	Decreased patency
Alpha agonists, e.g.,	Beta agonists, e.g.,
Norepinephrine	Isoproterenol
Epinephrine	Nylidrin
Methoxamine	
Phenylephrine	Alpha antagonists, e.g.,
Serotonin	Phenoxybenzamine
Dopamine	Phentolamine
Prostaglandins	
Cocaine	Acetylcholine
Antihistamines	Histamine
Tyramine	Papaverine
Vasopressin	Aminophylline
	Reserpine
	K^+

Source: From Ref. 74, reproduced with permission.

Prostaglandins (PGE_1, PGE_2, PGA, and PGF_{1a}) are generally considered to be vasodilating agents. However, they were observed to induce a constriction of the nasal blood vessels in the dog (74). While PGE_1 and PGE_2 were found to be equipotent to epinephrine, their duration of action was observed to last more than seven times longer in normal human subjects (75). A partial list of drugs and their general effect on nasal patency is shown in Table 1.2.

1.6 NASAL NERVE SUPPLY

The nasal blood vessels and glands have a rich nerve supply both from the autonomic system and from the somatic system. The nasal mucous membrane derives its sensory supply from the cranial nerve and contains sympathetic and parasympathetic fibers of the autonomic nervous system (76). Figure 1.5 shows the origin of the autonomic innervation of the nose.

The autonomic innervation of about three-quarters of the nasal mucous membrane reaches the nose via the vidian nerve and follows the distribution of the second division of the trigeminal nerve to the nose (77,78). The vidian nerve may consist of parasympathetic and also sympathetic cholinergic fibers (78). The capillary vessels (or resistance vessels) receive the primary alpha-adrenergic sympathetic fibers (constrictor), but may also

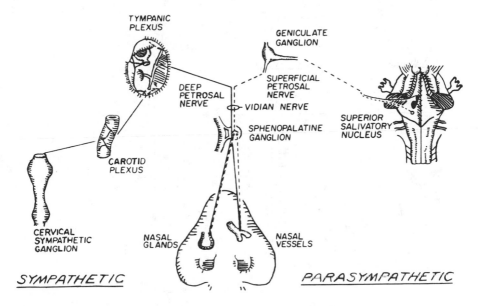

Figure 1.5 Autonomic nasal innervation. Origin of sympathetic and parasympathetic fibers to the nasal mucosa. (From Ref. 76, reproduced with permission of the *Ear Nose Throat J.*)

receive a small beta-adrenergic innervation (dilators). There is a rich parasympathetic innervation of the glands. Nervous stimulation of the glandular cholinoceptors causes a significant hypersecretion and vasodilation (Figures 1.6 and 1.7). When the cholinergic nerve is stimulated, the arterioles in the concha dilate, permeability through the capillary wall changes, the uptake of serum constituents through the basement membranes into the gland increases, and secretion is formed and then squeezed out of the nasal gland (79). Therefore, the cholinergic innervation is dominant in the functioning of the nasal glands, whereas adrenergic innervation is predominant in the functioning of the vascular system of the nasal mucosa. Stimulation of the vidian nerve in the case for 3 min was noted to induce nasal secretions, whereas stimulation for 15 sec produced a vasoconstriction in the nasal cavity.

While the arterioles of the inferior concha are richly endowed with adrenergic nerves, the nasal gland is almost devoid of adrenergic nerve fibers (79). Electrical stimulation of the sympathetic nerves, using lower impulse

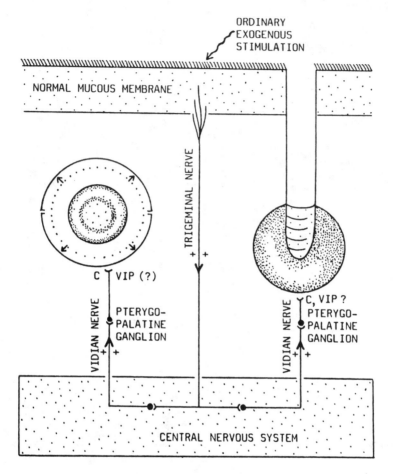

Figure 1.6 Stimulation of sensory nerves, e.g., by the unconditioned inhaled air, initiates parasympathetic reflexes, which cause significant hypersecretion, and slight, transient vasodilation. C, cholinoceptor, VIP, vasoactive intestinal polypeptide. (From Ref. 127, reproduced with permission of *J. Allergy Clin. Immunol.*)

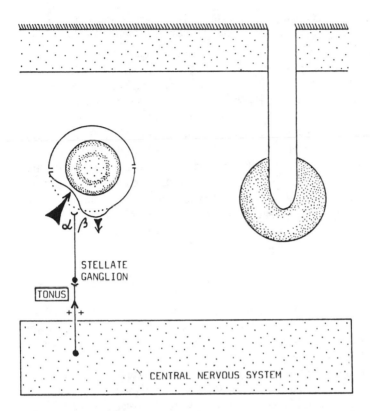

Figure 1.7 Sympathetic innervation of blood vessels. There is a continuous impulse traffic in efferent sympathetic fibers to the blood vessels, keeping them partially constricted. Action on alpha-1-adrenoceptors causes marked vasoconstriction, and stimulation of beta-2-adrenoceptors causes slight vaso-dilation. (From Ref. 127, reproduced with permission of *J. Allergy Clin. Immunol.*)

frequencies, was reported to affect mainly the capacitance vessels (80). At minimal effective frequency of 2-5 Hz, the sympathetic activity-induced stimulation of vidian nerve was noted to increase nasal secretion and also induce vasoconstriction in the nasal cavity (81).

The adrenergic transmitter, norepinephrine, , was found to be present in the typical nasal adrenergic nerve terminals (82). In all studies with mammals, the nasal mucosa of the inferior concha was observed to be dominated by a rich adrenergic plexus surrounded by a thin muscle layer of the wide veins of the erectile tissue. This adrenergic plexus is considered to be of great importance in regulating the blood flow through the nasal mucosa. The alpha-1, beta, and muscarinic receptors were reported to be present in human mucosa (83). Both isoprenaline and terbutaline, beta-receptor-stimulating agents, were found to decrease nasal blood flow resistance and nasal potency; i.e., dilation of resistance and capacitance vessels (84). However, propranolol, a beta-receptor-blocking agent, was noted to reduce the effect of isoprenaline and terbutaline on the resistance vessels. Therefore, it is evident that the effects of isoprenaline and terbutaline in the nasal vascular bed of the cat are mediated via beta-adrenergic receptors, at least in the resistance vessels (85).

It has been suggested that vasomotor rhinitis is a result of increased parasympathetic activity in the nasal mucosa (78). Following parasympathetic stimulation of the nasal mucosa in the cat, the secretory and vascular responses were reportedly blocked by atropine (86,87).

1.7 NASAL ENZYMES

Many enzymes exist in nasal secretions. These are cytochrome P-450-dependent monooxygenases (88-92); lactate-dehydrogenase (93); oxidoreductases (94); hydrolases, acid phosphatase and esterase (95), NAD^+-dependent formaldehyde dehydrogenase and aldehyde dehydrogenase (96); leucine aminopeptidase (97); phosphoglucomutase, glucose-6-phosphate dehydrogenase, aldolase, lactic dehydrogenase, isocitric dehydrogenase, malic enzymes, glutamic oxaloacetic transaminase, glutamic pyruvic transaminase (98); NAD^+-dependent 15-hydroxyprostaglandin dehydrogenase (99); carboxylesterase (100), lysosomal proteinases and their inhibitors (101); β-glucosidase, α-fucosidase, and α-galactosidase (102); succinic dehydrogenase (103); lysozyme (104); and steroid hydroxylases (105).

Cytochrome P-450-dependent monooxygenase has been reported to catalyze the metabolism of different xenobiotics (88-93). It has also been observed to metabolize many compounds in the nasal mucosa, such as nasal decongestants, nicotine, and cocaine (89); phenacetin (106); N-nitroso-diethylamine (107,108); N-nitrosonornicotine (109); nitrosoamine (110); aminopyrine (111); and progesterone (112).

Insulin (zinc-free) was found to be hydrolyzed slowly by leucine aminopeptidase (97). The amino acids, released from zinc-free insulin in the in vitro studies, were estimated by ion-exchange chromatography. The results are shown in Table 1.3. Prostaglandins of the E series were observed to be inactivated by the nasal mucosal 15-hydroxyprostaglandin dehydrogenase

Table 1.3 Amino Acids Released from Insulin By Leucine Aminopeptidase

Amino acid	Moles/Mole insulin	Amino acid	Moles/Mole insulin	Amino acid	Moles/Mole insulin
Phe	0.72	His	0.99	Ser + AspNH$_2$	1.36
Val	1.63	Leu	1.43	Cys-S-Cy	a
Ileu	0.40	Ala	0.48	Arg	0.0
Gly	1.09	Glu	1.24	GluNH$_2$	a

[a]Not determined.

(99). Progesterone and testosterone were metabolized by several steroid hydroxylases in the nasal mucosa of rats (105). Carbon-14-labeled progesterone (or testosterone) was observed to be selectively taken up in the mucosa covering the olfactory region of the nasal cavity.

1.8 NASAL pH

The normal pH of the nasal secretions in the adult ranges approximately from 5.5 to 6.5, whereas in infants and young children it ranges from 5.0 to 6.7 (113-115). During acute rhinitis, acute sinusitis, and in the more acute phases of allergic rhinitis, the pH of nasal secretions was found to be on the alkaline side and then shifted back to acidity when the stage of clinical resolution was reached. The course of nasal pH can be altered by the influence of cold or heat: Cold air produces a drift toward alkalinity, whereas heat yields a drift toward acidity. The pH of the nasal secretions also varies with sleep, rest, the ingestion of food, emotion, and infection. A nasal pH of 6.5 or below has been believed to be critical for preventing the growth of pathogenic bacteria in the nasal passage (116,117).

Lysozyme (MW = 14,000) is a substance found in various body tissues and secretions, including nasal secretions, and has the ability of dissolving certain bacteria. As a result, it is responsible for maintaining an antiseptic nostril (118-120). The activity of lysozyme is influenced by the hydrogen ion concentration in the nasal secretion with the optimum pH in the slightly acidic region, and its activity was reported to be sharply diminished in alkaline secretions (121), which often occur with the acute common cold. If the nasal pH becomes alkaline, the enzyme is inactivated and the protective barrier is largely removed, which in turn increased the susceptibility of nasal tissue to microbial infection.

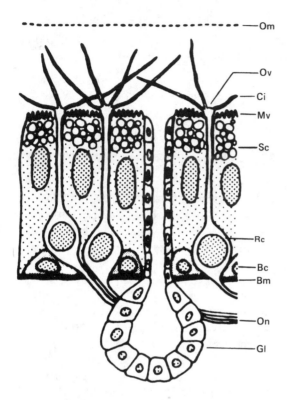

Figure 1.8 A schematic diagram of olfactory epithelium. Om, surface of the olfactory mucus, Ov, olfactory vesicle, Ci, olfactory cilia, Mv, microvili, Sc, supporting cell (secretory granules inside the cell are indicated), Rc, olfactory (receptor) cell, Bc, basal cell, Bm, basement membrane, On, olfactory nerve, Gl, olfactory gland. (From Ref. 128, reproduced with permission of Academic Press.)

1.9 NASAL OLFACTORY REGION

The olfactory region, a small patch of tissue containing the smell receptors, is located at the very top of the nasal cavity near the inner end of the upper throat. The patch has a yellowish tinge, in contrast to its surrounding pink tissue, and consists of several million tiny endings of the olfactory nerve whose bundles pass through the cribriform plate and enter the farthest forward extension of the brain. A schematic diagram of the olfactory epithelium is shown in Figure 1.8. The possibility that drugs, absorbed nasally via the olfactory mucosa, enter through the olfactory neurons and the supporting cells directly into the brain as well as into the systemic circulation in monkeys was reported (122).

1.10 NASAL PATHOPHYSIOLOGY

The nose is an important reservoir for infectious agents, especially the respiratory viruses and microorganisms, which cause diseases in humans. The common cold and related symptoms are the most frequent human infections. Allergic nasal diseases are also commonly known to affect normal nasal conditions. Although surprisingly little is known about the effects of nasal conditions on nasal absorption, some data have been reported. For example, nasal polyposis, atrophic rhinitis, and severe vasomotor rhinitis can reduce the capacity of nasal absorption (123). In some subjects with a severe nasal allergy, an excessive response of the secretory system to irritants could wash away the drug solution administered into the nasal cavity before the drug is absorbed by the nasal membrane.

The common cold or any pathological conditions involving mucociliary dysfunction can greatly affect the rate of nasal clearance and, subsequently, the therapeutic efficacy of the drugs administered nasally. It was reported that the insufflation of cerulein, an active decapeptide, to three subjects with nasal congestion or chronic rhinitis was found to produce no pharmacological responses (124).

REFERENCES

1. Proctor, D. F. The upper aiways. I. Nasal physiology and defense of the lungs, *Am. Rev. Respir. Dis., 115*:97 (1977).
2. Maron, Z., Shelhamer, J., and Kaliner, M. Nasal mucus secretion, *Ear Nose Throat J., 63*:36 (1984).
3. Proctor, D. F., and Anderson, I. *The Nose, Upper Airway Physiology and the Atmospheric Environment*, Elsevier, Amsterdam (1982).
4. Graziadei, P. P. C. The mucus membrane of the nose, *Ann. Otol. Rhinol. Laryngol., 79*:433 (1970).
5. Geurkink, N. Nasal anatomy, physiology and function, *J. Allergy Clin. Immunol., 72*:123 (1983).
6. Scott, W. R., Taulbee, D. B., and Yu, C. P. Theoretical study of nasal deposition, *Bull. Math. Biol., 40*:581 (1978).
7. Negus, V. E. *The Comparative Anatomy and Physiology of the Nose and Paranasal Sinuses*, Livingstone, Edinburgh (1958).
8. Ingelstedt, S. Humidifying capacity of the nose, *Ann. Otol., 79*:475 (1975).

9. Allison, D. J., and Porvis, D. A. Adrenal catecholamine secretion during stimulation of the nasal mucous membrane in the rabbit, *J. Physiol.* (*Lond.*), *217*:327 (1971).

10. Toh, C. C., and Mohiuddin, A. Vasoactive substances in the nasal mucosa, *Br. J. Pharmacol.*, *13*:113 (1958).

11. Marom, Z., Shelhamer, J., and Kaliner, M. Nasal mucus secretion, *Ear Nose Throat J.*, *63*:36 (1984).

12. Kuijpers, W., Kiaassen, A. B. M., Jap, P. H. K., and Tonnaer, E. Secretory characteristics of the rat nasal glands, *Acta Otolaryngol.* (*Stockh.*), *95*:676 (1983).

13. Taylor, M. The origin and functions of nasal mucus, *Laryngoscope, 84*: 612 (1974).

14. Lorin, M. I., Gaerlan, P. F., and Mandel, I. D. Quantitative composition of nasal secretions in normal subjects, *J. Lab. Clin. Med.*, *80*:275 (1972).

15. Ogawa, H., Kami, K., Suzuki, T., and Mitsui, T. An immunohistochemical study of lysozyme in the human nasal mucosa, *Keio J. Med.*, *28*:73 (1979).

16. Rosen, R. D., Alford, R. H., Butler, W. T., and Vannier, W. E. The separation and characterization of proteins intrinsic to nasal secretion, *Eur. J. Immunol.*, *97*:369 (1966).

17. Schorn, K., and Hochstrasser, K. Biochemical investigations of nasal secretions, *Acta Otorhinolaryngol. Bel.*, *33*:603 (1979).

18. Shelhamer, J., Maron, Z., and Kaliner, M. The constituents of nasal secretion, *Ear Nose Throat J.*, *63*:31 (1984).

19. Eccles, R., and Wilson, H. A kallikrein-like substance in cat nasal secretion, *Br. J. Pharmacol.*, *49*:712 (1973).

20. Hochstrasser, K., Haendle, H., Reichert, R., and Werle, E. Uber vorkommen und eigenschaften eines proteasenin ibito in menschlichem masensekret, *Hoppe Seylers Z. Physiol. Chem.*, *352*:954 (1971).

21. Reichert, R., Hochstrasser, K., and Werle, E. der proteaseninhibitorspiegel in menschlichem masensekret unter physiologischen und pathophysiologischen Bedingungen, *Klin. Wochenschr.*, *49*:1234 (1971).

22. Karim, S. M. M., Adaikan, P. G., and Kunaratnam, N. Effect of tropical prostaglandins on nasal patency in man, *Prostaglandins, 15*:457 (1978).

23. Okazaki, T., Reisman, R. E., and Arbesman, C. E. Prostaglandin E in the secretion of allergic rhinitis, *Prostaglandins, 13*:681 (1977).

24. Bedwani, J. R., Eccles, R., and Jones, A. S. A study of the synthesis and inactivation of prostaglandin E by pig nasal mucosa, *Acta Otolaryngol.* (*Stockh.*), *98*:308 (1984).

25. Remington, J. S., Vosti, K. L., Lietze, A., and Zimmerman, A. L. Serum proteins and antibody activity in human nasal secretions, *J. Clin. Invest.*, *43*:1613 (1964).

26. Powell, K. R., Shorr, R., Cherry, J. D., and Hendley, J. O. Improved method for collection of nasal mucus, *J. Infect. Dis., 136*:109 (1977).

27. Rossen, R. D., Butler, W. T., Cate, T. R., Szwed, C. F., and Couch, R. B. Protein composition of nasal secretion during respiratory virus infection, *Proc. Soc. Exp. Biol., 119*:1169 (1965).

28. Rossen, R. D., Schade, A. L., Butler, W. T., and Kasel, J. A. The proteins in nasal secretion: A longitudinal study of the A-globulin, G-globulin, albumin, siderophilin and total protein concentrations in nasal washings from adult male volunteers, *J. Clin. Invest., 45*:768 (1966).

29. Ewert, G. On the mucus flow rate in the human nose, *Acta Otolaryngol. (Stockh.), (Suppl.), 200*:1 (1965).

30. Laurenzi, G. A. The mucociliary stream, *J. Occup. Med., 15*:174 (1973).

31. Herzon, F. S. Nasal ciliary structural pathology, *Laryngoscope, 93*:63 (1983).

32. Warner, F. D., and Satir, P. The structural basis of ciliary bend formation, *J. Cell. Biol., 63*:35 (1974).

33. Gosselin, R. E. Physiologic regulators of ciliary motion. Presented at *Duke University Medical Center Symposium on "Structure, Function and Measurement of Respiratory Cilia"*, Durham, North Carolina, Feb. 18-19, (1965).

34. Proctor, D. F. The upper airways. I. Nasal physiology and defense of the lungs, *Am. Rev. Respir. Dis., 115*:97 (1977).

35. Hounam, R. F. The removal of particles from the nasopharynx (NP) compartment of the respiratory tract by nose blowing and swabbing, *Health Phys., 28*:743 (1975).

36. Proctor, D. F., Anderson, I. B., and Lundqvist, G. Clearance of inhaled particles from the human nose, *Arch. Intern. Med., 131*:132 (1973).

37. Proctor, D. F. Nasal mucous transport and our ambient air, *Laryngoscope, 93*:58 (1983).

38. Proctor, D. F., and Wagner, H. N. Clearance of particles from the human nose, *Arch. Environ. Health, 11*:366 (1965).

39. Sakakura, Y., Ukai, K., Majima, Y., Murai, S., Harada, T., and Miyoshi, Y. Nasal mucociliary clearance under various conditions, *Acta Otolaryngol., 96*:167 (1983).

40. Andersen, I. B., Lundqvist, G., and Proctor, D. F. Human nasal mucosal function under four controlled humidities, *Am. Rev. Respir. Dis., 106*: 438 (1972).

41. Anderson, I. B., Lundqvist, G. R., Denmark, A., and Proctor, D. F. Human nasal mucosal function in a controlled climate, *Arch. Environ. Health, 23*:408 (1971).

42. Geurkink, N. Nasal anatomy, physiology and function, *J. Allergy Clin. Immunol., 72*:123 (1983).

43. Duchateau, G. S. M. J. E., Graamans, K., Zuidema, J., and Merkus, F F. W. H. M. Correlation between nasal ciliary beat frequency and mucus transport rate in volunteers, *Laryngoscope, 95*:854 (1985).

44. Donk, H. J. M., and Merkus, F. W. H. M. Decreases in ciliary beat frequency due to intranasal administration of propranolol, *J. Pharm. Sci.*, *71*:595 (1982).

45. Barton, R. P. E., and Gray, R. F. E. The transport of crystalline cocaine in the nasal mucous blanket, *J. Laryngol. Otol.*, *93*:1201 (1979).

46. Ewert, G. The effect of two topical anesthetic drugs on the mucus flow in the respiratory tract, *Ann. Otol.*, *76*:359 (1967).

47. Simon, H., Drettner, B., and Jung, B. Messung des schleimhaut-transportes in menschlichen Nase mit ^{51}Cr markierten harzkugelchen, *Acta Otolaryngol. (Stockh.)*, *83*:378 (1977).

48. Petruson, B., and Hansson, H. A. Function and structure of the nasal mucosa after 6 weeks use of nose-drops, *Acta Otolaryngol. (Stockh.)*, *94*: 563 (1982).

49. Burn, J. H. Acetylcholine as a local hormone for ciliary movement and the heart, *Pharmacol. Rev.*, *6*:107 (1954).

50. Ryde, C. The effect of a surface-active agent ("Tween 20") on speed of transportation by the frog's ciliated mucous membrane, *Acta Pharmacol. Toxicol.*, *18*:153 (1961).

51. Borum, P., Holton, A., and Loekkegaard, N. Depression of nasal mucociliary transport by an aerosol hair-spray, *Scand. J. Respir. Dis.*, *60*:253 (1979).

52. Cuana, N. Blood and nerve supply of the nasal lining, in *The Nose: Upper Airway Physiology and the Atmosphere Environment* (D. F. Proctor and I. Anderson, Eds.), Elsevier, Amsterdam (1982), pp. 45-66.

53. Dawes, J. D. K., and Prichard, M. M. L. Studies of the vascular arrangements of the nose, *J. Anat.*, *87*:311 (1953).

54. Geurkink, N. Nasal anatomy, physiology and function, *J. Allergy Clin. Immunol.*, *72*:123 (1983).

55. Cauna, N., and Hinderer, K. H. Fine structure of the blood vessels of the human nasal respiratory mucosa, *Ann. Otol. Rhinol. Laryngol.*, *78*:865 (1969).

56. Ånggård, A. Capillary and shunt blood flow in the nasal mucosa of the cat, *Acta Otolaryngol. (Stockh.)*, *78*:418 (1974).

57. Olson, P., and Bende, M. Influence of environmental temperature on human nasal mucosa, *Ann. Otol. Rhinol. Laryngol.*, *94*:153 (1985).

58. Paulsson, B., Bende, M., and Ohlin, P. Nasal mucosal blood flow at rest and during exercise, *Acta Otolaryngol. (Stockh.)*, *99*:140 (1985).

59. Drettner, B., and Aust, R. Plethysmographic studies of the blood flow in the mucosa of the human maxillar sinus, *Acta Otolaryngol. (Stockh.)*, *78*:259 (1974).

60. Drettner, B., Aust, R., Backlund, L., Falk, B., and Jung, B. Comparative measurements of the mucosal blood flow in the human maxillary sinus by plethysmography and by xenon, *Acta Otolaryngol. (Stockh.)*, *85*:111 (1978).

61. Loring, S. H., and Tenney, S. M. Gas absorption from frontal sinus, *Arch. Otolaryngol. (Stockh.)*, 97:470 (1973).

62. Kunlien, J. A., Schiratzki, H., and Drettner, B. Blood flow in the rabbit maxillary sinus mucosa, *Acta Otolaryngol. (Stockh.)*, 99:144 (1985).

63. Bende, M., Flisberg, K., Larsson, I., Ohlin, P., and Olsson, P. A method for determination of blood flow with ^{133}Xe in human nasal mucosa, *Acta Otolaryngol. (Stockh.)*, 96:277 (1983).

64. Hall, L. J., and Jackson, R. T. Effects of alpha- and beta-adrenergic agonists on nasal blood flow, *Ann. Otol.*, 77:1120 (1968).

65. Malm, L. Responses of resistance and capacitance vessels in feline nasal mucosa to vasoactive agents, *Acta Otolaryngol. (Stockh.)*, 78:90 (1974).

66. Anggard, A., and Edwall, L. The effects of sympathetic nerve stimulation on the tracer disappearance rate and local blood content in the nasal mucosa of the cat, *Acta Otolaryngol. (Stockh.)*, 77:131 (1974).

67. Richerson, H. B., and Seebohm, P. M. Nasal airway response to exercise, *J. Allergy*, 41:269 (1968).

68. Bende, M. The effect of topical decongestant on blood flow in normal and infected nasal mucosa, *Acta Otolaryngol. (Stockh.)*, 96:523 (1983).

69. Borum, P., and Mygind, N. Inhibition of the immediate allergic reaction in the nose by beta-2-adrenostimulant fenoterol, *J. Allergy Clin. Immunol.*, 66:25 (1980).

70. Schumacher, M. J. Effect of a beta-adrengergic agonist, fenoterol, on nasal sensitivity to allergen, *J. Allergy Clin. Immunol.*, 66:33 (1980).

71. McLean, J. A., Mathews, K. P., Ciarkowski, A. A., Brayton, P. R., and Solomon, W. R. The effects of topical saline and isoproterenol on nasal airway resistance, *J. Allergy*, 58:563 (1976).

72. Lung, M. A. K. Y., and Wang, J. C. C. Nasal blood flow and airway resistance: Canine study, *Ann. Otol. Rhinol. Laryngol.*, 94:198 (1985).

73. Anderson, K. E. Adrenoceptors in the control of human nasal mucosal blood flow, *Ann. Otol. Rhinol. Laryngol.*, 93:179 (1984).

74. Stovall, R., and Jackson, R. T. Prostaglandins and nasal blood flow, *Ann. Otol. Rhinol. Laryngol.*, 76:1051 (1967).

75. Jackson, R. T. Prostaglandin E_1 as a nasal constrictor in normal human volunteers, *Curr. Ther. Res.*, 12:711 (1970).

76. Babin, R. W. A review of the autonomic control of nasal function, *Ear Nose Throat J.*, 56:443 (1977).

77. Krajina, Z., and Poljak, Z. Relationship between the vegetative innervation and the sensibility of the nasal mucosa, *Acta Otolaryngol. (Stockh)*, 79:172 (1975).

78. Malcomson, K. G. The vasomotor activities of the nasal mucous membrane, *J. Laryngol. Otol.*, 73:73 (1959).

79. Nomura, Y., and Matsura, T. Distribution and clinical significance of the autonomic nervous system in the human nasal mucosa, *Acta Otolaryngol. (Stockh.)*, 73:493 (1972).

80. Malm, L. Sympathetic influence on the nasal mucosa, *Acta Otolaryngol.* (*Stockh.*), *83*:20 (1977).
81. Wilson, H., and Yates, M. S. The role of sympathetic nerves in nasal secretion in the cat, *Acta Otolaryngol.* (*Stockh.*), *85*:426 (1978).
82. Dahlstrom, A., and Fuxe, K. Adrenergic innervation of the nasal mucosa of certain mammals, *Acta Otolaryngol.* (*Stockh.*), *59*:65 (1965).
83. Ishibe, T., Yamashita, T., Kumazawa, T., and Tanaka, C. Adrenergic and cholinergic receptors in human nasal mucosa in case of nasal allergy, *Arch. Otorhinolaryngol.*, *238*:167 (1983).
84. Ishii, T. The cholinergic innervation of the human nasal mucosa: A histochemical study, *Pract. Otorhinolaryngol.*, *32*:153 (1970).
85. Malm, L. β-Adrenergic receptors in the vessels of the cat nasal mucosa, *Acta Otolaryngol.* (*Stockh.*), *78*:242 (1974).
86. Änggård, A. The effect of parasympathetic nerve stimualtion on the microcirculation and secretion in the nasal mucosa of the cat, *Acta Otolaryngol.* (*Stockh.*), *78*:98 (1974).
87. Änggård, A. Parasympathetic influence on the nasal mucosa, *Acta Otolaryngol.* (*Stockh.*), *83*:22 (1977).
88. Dahl, A. R. The inhibition of rat nasal cytochrome P-450-dependent mono-oxygenase by the esssence heliotropin (piperonal), *Drug Metab. Dispos.*, *10*:553 (1982).
89. Dahl, A. R., and Hadley, W. M. Formaldehyde production promoted by rat nasal cytochrome P-450-dependent mono-oxygenase with nasal decongestants, essences, solvents, air pollutants, nicotine, and cocaine as substrates, *Toxicol. Appl. Pharmacol.*, *67*:200 (1983).
90. Hadley, W. M., and Dahl, A. R. Cytochrome P-450-dependent mono-oxygenase activity in rat nasal epithelial membranes, *Toxicol. Lett.*, *10*:417 (1982).
91. Dahl, A. R., Hadley, W. M., Hahn, F. F., Benson, J. M., and McClellan, R. O. Cytochrome P-450-dependent mono-oxygenase in olfactory epithelium of dogs: Possible role in tumorigenicity, *Science*, *216*:57 (1982).
92. Hadley, W. M., and Dahl, A. R. Cytochrome P-450-dependent mono-oxygenase activity in nasal membranes of six species, *Drug. Metab. Dipos.*, *11*:275 (1983).
93. Schorn, K., and KochstraBer, K. Das Isoenzymmuster der laktatdehydrogenase im nasensekret, *Laryngol. Rhinol.*, *55*:961 (1976).
94. Werner, E., and Meyer, P. Lokalisation von kohlenhydraten und einigen oxydoreduktasen in der regio respiratoria der normalen nasenschleimhaut des menschen, *Acta Histochem. Bd.*, *33*:S179 (1969).
95. Werner, E., and Meyer, P. Lokalisation von lipiden und hydrolasen in der regio respiratoria der normalen nasenschleimhaut des menschen, *Acta Histochem. Bd.*, *35*:S61 (1970).

96. Casanova-Schmitr, M., David, R. M., and Heck, H. D'A. Oxidation of formaldehyde and acetaldehyde by NAD^+-dependent dehydrogenases in rat nasal mucosa homogenates, *Biochem. Pharmacol., 33*:1137 (1984).

97. Smith, E. L., Hill, R. L., and Borman, A. Activity of insulin degraded by leucine aminopeptidase, *Biochim. Biophys. Acta, 29*:207 (1958).

98. McFarland, L. Z., Martin, K. D., and Freedland, R. A. The activity of soluble enzymes in the avian nasal salt gland, *J. Cell. and Comp. Physiol., 65*:237 (1965).

99. Bedwani, J. R., Eccles, R., and Jones, A. S. A study of the synthesis and activation of prostaglandin E by pig nasal mucosa, *Acta Otolaryngol. (Stockh.), 98*:308 (1984).

100. Scott, W. T., and McKenna, M. J. Hydrolysis of several glycol ether acetates and acrylate esters by nasal mucosal carboxylesterase in vitro, *Fund. Appl. Toxicol., 5*:399 (1985).

101. HochestraBe, K. Proteinases and their inhibitors in human nasal mucus, *Rhinology, 21*:217 (1983).

102. Schorn, K., and Hochestrasser, K. Biochemical investigations of nasal secretions, *Acta Otol. Rhinol. Laryngol., 33*:603 (1979).

103. Taylor, M. The origin and functions of nasal mucus, *Laryngoscope, 84*: 612 (1974).

104. Ogawa, H., Kami, K., Suzuki, T., and Mitsui, T. An immunohistochemical study of lysozyme in the human nasal mucosa, *Keio J. Med., 28*:73 (1979).

105. Brittebo, E. G., and Rafter, J. J. Steroid metabolism by rat nasal mucosa: Studies on progesterone and testosterone, *Steroid Biochem., 20*: 1147 (1984).

106. Brittebo, E. B., and Ahlman, M. Nasal mucosa from rat fetuses and neonates metabolizes the nasal carcinogens phenacetin, *Toxicol. Lett., 23*: 279 (1984).

107. Brittebo, E. B., Lindgren, A., and Tjalve, H. Foetal distribution and metabolism of N-nitrosodiethylamine in mice, *Acta Pharmacol. Toxicol., 48*:355 (1981).

108. Lofberg, B., and Tjalve, H. The disposition and metabolism of N-nitrosodiethylamine in adult, infant and foetal tissues of Syrian golden hamsters, *Acta Pharmacol. Toxicol., 54*:104 (1984).

109. Lofberg, B., Brittebo, E. B., and Tjalve, H. Localization and binding of N-nitrosonornicotine metabolites in the nasal region and in some other tissues of Sprague-Dawley rats, *Cancer Res., 42*:2877 (1982).

110. Brittebo, E. B., Castonguay, A., Furuya, K., and Hecht, S. S. Metabolism of tobacco-specific nitrosoamines by cultured rat nasal mucosa, *Cancer Res., 43*:4343 (1983).

111. Brittebo, E. B. N-Demethylation of aminopyrine by the nasal mucosa in mice and rats, *Acta. Pharmacol. Toxicol., 51*:227 (1982).
112. Brittebo, E. B. Metabolism of progesterone by the nasal mucosa in mice and rats, *Acta. Pharmacol. Toxicol., 51*:44 (1982).
113. Fabricant, N. D. Significance of the pH of nasal secretions in situ, *Arch. Otolaryngol., 34*:150 (1941).
114. Fabricant, N. D. Effect of progressively buffered solution of ephedrine on nasal mucosa, *J.A.M.A., 151*:21 (1953).
115. Fabricant, N. D. The pH of the throat, nose and ear, *Eye Ear Nose Throat Monthly, 43*:60 (1964).
116. Tweedie, A. R. Reaction of nasal mucus, *Acta Otolaryngol. (Stockh.), 24*:151 (1936).
117. Buhrmester, C. C. A study of the hydrogen ion concentration, nitrogen content and viscosity of nasal secretions, *Ann. Otol., 42*:1042 (1933).
118. Fabricant, N. D. Relation of the pH of nasal secretions in situ to the activity of lysozyme, *Arch. Otolaryngol., 41*:53 (1945).
119. Meyer, K. The relationship of lysozyme to avidin, *Science, 99*:391 (1944).
120. Thompson, R. Lysozyme and its relation to antibacterial properties of various tissues and secretions, *Arch. Pathol., 30*:1096 (1940).
121. Jackson, R. T., and Turner, J. S. Some observations on nasal pH, *Arch. Otolaryngol., 84*:446 (1966).
122. Gopinath, P. G., Gopinath, G., and Anand Kumar, T. C. Target site of intranasally-sprayed substances and their transport across the nasal mucosa: A new insight into the intranasal route of drug delivery, *Curr. Ther. Res., 23*:596 (1978).
123. Proctor, D. F. Nasal physiology in intranasal drug administrations, in *Transnasal Systemic Medications* (Y. W. Chien, Ed.), Elsevier, Amsterdam (1985), pp. 101-106.
124. Agosti, A., and Bertaccioni, G. Nasal absorption of Caerulein, *Lancet, 1*:580 (1969).
125. Mygind, N., *Nasal Allergy*, Blackwell Scientific Publications, London (1979), pp. 3-38.
126. Satir, P., How cilia move, *Sci. Am., 231*:45 (1974).
127. Mygind, N., Medication of nasal allergy, *J. Allergy Clin. Immunol., 70*:149 (1982).
128. Takagi, S. F., *Biophysics of Smell, Handbook of Perception*, VI(A), Academic Press, New York (1979), pp. 233.

2

Animal Models Used in Nasal Absorption Studies

In general, there are two types of animal models which can be used for nasal absorption studies; i.e., whole animal model and an isolated organ perfusion model.

2.1 IN VIVO NASAL ABSORPTION MODELS

2.1.1 Rat Model

The rat model used for studying the nasal delivery of drugs was first presented in the late 1970s and then reported in 1980 (1,2). The surgical preparation for in vivo nasal absorption is described as follows: The rat is anesthetized by intraperitoneal injection of sodium pentobarbital. After an incision is made in the neck, the trachea is cannulated with a polyethylene tube. Another tube is inserted through the esophagus toward the posterior part of the nasal cavity (Figure 2.1). The passage of the nasopalatine tract is sealed to prevent the drainage of the drug solution from the nasal cavity into the mouth. The drug solution is delivered to the nasal cavity through the nostril (2), or through the esophagus cannulation tubing, as reported elsewhere(3). The blood samples are then collected from the femoral vein.

Since all the possible outlets in this rat model are blocked after surgical preparation, the only possible passage for the drug to be absorbed and transported into the systemic circulation is penetration and/or diffusion through the nasal mucosa.

Rat Model

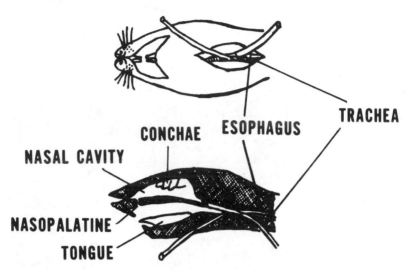

Figure 2.1 The top and side views of the cannulation arrangement for in vivo studies in the rats. (From Ref. 42, reproduced with permission of the copyright owner—Elsevier Science Publishers.)

Using the rat model described in Figure 2.1 or similar setup, the nasal absorption and permeability of the following drugs/compounds have been studied: propranolol (2,4); progesterone (5); testosterone (6); naloxone and buprenorphine (7); ergotamine tartate (8); sulbenicillin, cefazolin, cephacetrile, phenol red, salicyclic acid, aminopyrin, and bucolome (9); insulin (10-13,21); enkephalins (14); enviroxime (15); dobutamine (16,17); clofilium tosylate (3); glucagon (18); cyclo-(-Pro-phe-D-Trp-Lys-Thr-Phe) (i.e., SS-6) and horseradish peroxidase (19); sodium guaiazulene-3-sulfonate (20); calcitonin (21); secretin (22); nicardipine (23); substance P (24); and others.

2.1.2 Rabbit Model

The in vivo rabbit model for nasal drug delivery is outled as follows: Rabbits weighing approximately 3 kg are either anesthetized or maintained in the conscious state depending on the purpose of the experiment. The rabbit is anesthetized by an intramuscular injection of a combination of ketamine and xylazine. The drug solution is delivered by nasal spray into each nostil, while the rabbit's head is held in an upright position. During the study, the rabbit breathes normally through the nostrils, and body temperature is maintained at 37°C with the use of a heating pad. The blood samples are collected via an indwelling catheter in the marginal ear vein or artery according to the experimental protocol (25).

As an animal model for nasal absorption studies, the rabbit combines several advantages: whereas it is a laboratory animal as commonly accessible as the rat, rabbit permits pharmacokinetic studies as large animals, like the monkey. The rabbit is relatively inexpensive, readily available, and easily maintained in the laboratory setting. The blood volume of the rabbit is sufficiently large (approx. 300 ml) to permit frequent blood sampling (1-2 ml), and allow a full characterization of the absorption and determination of the pharmacokinetic profile of a drug.

The rabbit model described here has been used in studying the nasal absorption and nasal controlled delivery of progesterone (25) and its hydroxy derivatives (26). To avoid the interference of endogenous steroids in radioimmunoassay, the pharmacokinetic studies of these progestational steroids were conducted in ovariectomized rabbits.

2.1.3 Dog Model

The in vivo dog model for nasal absorption studies is briefly outlined as follows: The dog is either anesthetized or maintained in the conscious state depending upon the characteristics of the drug and the purpose of the study. In the anesthetized model, the dog is anesthetized by intravenous injection of sodium thiopental and maintained with sodium phenobarbital. A positive pressure pump provides ventilation through a cuffed endotracheal tube, and a heating pad keeps the body temperature at 37-38°C. The blood samples are collected from the jugular vein according to the experimental protocol (26).

This dog model has been used in studying the nasal absorption of propranolol (2), insulin (28-31), and other drugs/compounds.

2.1.4 Sheep Model

The in vivo sheep model for nasal drug delivery is basically similar to that described for the dog model. Male in-house bred sheep are selected for their lack of nasal infectious diseases.

Because of their larger nostril and body size compared to the rat model, rabbit, dog, and sheep models are suitable and practical for evaluating parameters involved in the nasal delivery of drug from a more sophisticated formulation. A kinetic study of the drug absorption profile within a single animal can be easily conducted.

The sheep model has been used in studying the nasal absorption of insulin (32,33), metkephamid (27), and other drugs/compounds.

2.1.5 Monkey Model

The in vivo monkey model for nasal absorption studies is outlined as follows: Monkeys weighing about 8 kg each are either tranquilized, anesthetized, or maintained in the conscious state depending upon the purpose of the experiment. The monkey is tranquilized by intramuscular injection of ketamine hydrochloride, or it is anesthetized by intravenous injection of sodium phenobarbital. The drug solution is delivered into each nostril, while the head of the monkey is held in an upright position. The monkey is then placed in a supine position in a metabolism chair for 5-10 min after nasal administration. During the entire course of the study, the monkey is breathing normally through the nostrils. The blood samples are collected via an indwelling catheter in the vein according to the experiment protocol (27).

The monkey model has been used in studying the nasal absorption of insulin (34), luteinizing hormone-releasing hormone (LHRH) analog (34,35), nicardipine (23), and other compounds.

In summary, the rat is small, low cost, easy to handle, and inexpensive to maintain. Undoubtedly, the rat model is the most often used animal for nasal drug delivery studies. Unfortunately, there are confined applications that can limit the biopharmacuetics and pharmacological studies of nasal drug absorption. The primate model continues to be useful even though it is expensive and has come under increased pressure from animal rights groups. As described previously, rabbit, dog, and sheep models are particularly useful for formulation studies. However, the constraint of an animal model and the difference in physiology/anatomy among the models (Table 2.1) are unavoidable. Nevertheless, the use of an animal model still plays an important role in the assessment of nasal delivery of drugs.

Table 2.1 Interspecies Comparison of Nasal Cavity Characteristics

	Rat	Rabbit[b]	Beagle dog	Rhesus monkey	Man
Weight	250 g	3 kg	10 kg	7 kg	~ 70 kg
Naris cross section	0.7 mm^2	3.1 mm^2	16.7 mm^2	22.9 mm^2	140 mm^2
Bend in naris	40°	38°	30°	30°	n.a.
Length	2.3 cm	4.7 cm	10 cm	5.3 cm	7–8 cm
Greatest vertical diameter	9.6 mm	25 mm	23 mm	27 mm	40–45 mm
Surface area[a] (both sides of nasal cavity)	10.4 cm^2	$\sim 90 \text{ cm}^2$	220.7 cm^2	61.6 cm^2	181 cm^2
Volume (both sides)[a]	0.4 cm^3	1.6 cm^3	20 cm^3	8 cm^3	$16–19 \text{ cm}^3$
Bend of nasopharynx	15°	45°	30°	80°	~ 90°
Turbinate complexity	Double scroll	Complex scroll	Membranous, branched	Simple scroll	Simple scroll
Sinuses	Maxillary recess frontal sinuses	Maxillary, ethmoid, frontal sinuses	Maxillary, sphenoid, frontal sinuses	Maxillary recess	Frontal, sphenoid maxillary, ethmoid sinuses

[a]Includes sinuses for rat, rabbit, beagle dog, and rhesus monkey. Does not include sinuses for man.
[b]Unpublished data from D. Corbo and M. Corbo; personal communication.

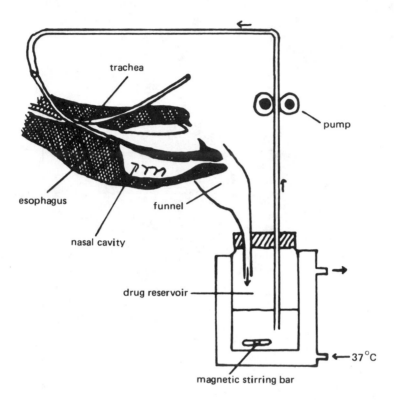

Figure 2.2 The experimental setup for ex-vivo nasal perfusion studies. (From Ref. 42, reproduced with permission of the copyright owner—Elsevier Science Publishers.)

2.2 EX VIVO NASAL PERFUSION MODEL

Figure 2.2 shows the experimental set-up for the in situ nasal perfusion studies (36). The same surgical preparation as that described previously in the in vivo rat model may be followed. During the perfusion studies, a funnel is provided between the nose and reservoir to minimize the loss of drug solution. The drug solution to be evaluated is placed in the reservoir, which is maintained at 37°C, and is circulated through the nasal cavity of the rat by means of a peristaltic pump. The perfusion solution passes out from the nostrils, through the funnel, and flows into the reservoir again. The drug solution in the reservoir is stirred constantly and the amount of drug ab-

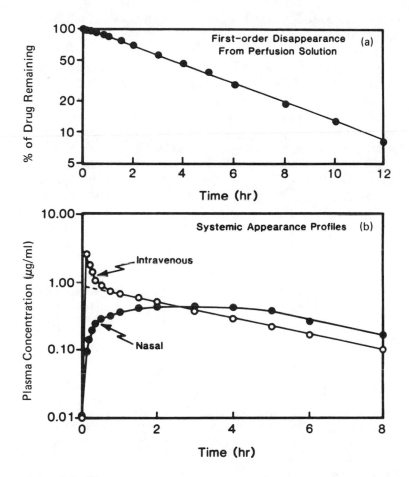

Figure 2.3 The ex-vivo nasal absorption study of hydromorphone in the rabbits ($n = 3$): (a) First-order disappearance of drug from the perfusion solution; (b) comparative plasma profiles of drug following nasal delivery and intravenous administration at same dose (5 mg/kg).

sorbed is then determined by measuring the drug concentration remaining in the perfusing solution. Because of the experimental condition, the possible loss of drug activity due to stability, such as the loss of peptides and proteins by proteolysis, aggregation, and other factors, must be considered.

The ex vivo nasal perfusion model described here has been performed in studying the nasal absorption of salicyclic acid, aminopyrin, and phenol red (8); leucin enkephalin (36), sodium benzoate, sodium barbital, sodium phenobarbital, sodium pentobarbital, sodium secobarbital, L-tyrosine, and propranolol hydrochloride (37,38); hydralazine (39); insulin and polethylene glycol 4000 (40), and other drugs/compounds.

Using rabbit as the animal model, the ex viv nasal perfusion model can also be used for studying the pharmacokinetics of drugs following nasal absorption (41). The experimental procedure is outlined as follows: The rabbit is anesthetized with parenteral urethane-acepromazine and a midline incision is made in the neck, and the trachea is cannulated with a polyethylene neonatal endotracheal tube. The esophagus is isolated and ligated. The distal end of the esophagus is closed with suture, and flexible Tygon tubing is inserted into the proximal end and advanced to the posterior part of the nasal cavity. The nasopalatine tract which connects the nasal cavity to the mouth is closed with an adhesive to prevent the drainage of drug solution from the nasal cavity. Drug-containing isotonic buffer solution is recirculated using a peristaltic pump. The kinetics of nasal absorption is monitored by simultaneous measurements of the disappearance of the drug from the perfusion solution and the appearance of the drug in the systemic circulation (Figure 2.3).

REFERENCES

1. Hirai, S., Yashiki, T., and Matsuzawa, T., Nasal absorption of drugs. Effect of surfactants on the nasal absorption of insulin in rats, presented at the 98th Annual Meeting of the Pharmaceutical Society of Japan, April 1978.
2. Hussain, A., Hirai, S., and Bawarshi, R., Nasal absorption of propranolol from different dosage forms by rats and dogs, J. Pharm. Sci., 69:1411 (1980).
3. Su, K. S. E., Campanale, K. M., and Gries, C. L., Nasal delivery system of a quaternary ammonium compound: Clofilium tosylate, J. Pharm. Sci., 73:1251 (1984).
4. Hussain, A., Hirai, S., and Bawarshi, R., Nasal absorption of propranolol in rats, J. Pharm. Sci., 68:1196 (1979).
5. Hussain, A., Hirai, S., and Bawarshi, R., Nasal absorption of natural contraceptive steroids in rats—Progesterone absorption, J. Pharm. Sci., 70:466 (1981).
6. Hussain, A., Kimura, R., and Huang, C. H., Nasal absorption of testosterone in rats, J. Pharm. Sci., 73:1300 (1984).

7. Hussain, A., Kimura, R., Huang, C. H., and Kashihara, T., Nasal absorption of naloxone and buprenorphine in rats, *Int. J. Pharm., 21*:233 (1984).
8. Hussain, A., Kimura, R., Huang, C. H., and Mustafa, R., Nasal absorption of ergotamine tartrate in rats, *Int. J. Pharm., 21*:289 (1984).
9. Hirai, S., Yashiki, T., Matsuzawa, T., and Mima, H., Absorption of drugs from the nasal mucosa of rat, *Int. J. Pharm., 7*:317 (1981).
10. Hirai, S., Yashiki, T., and Mima, H., Effect of surfactants on the nasal absorption of insulin in rats, *Int. J. Pharm., 9*:165 (1981).
11. Hirai, S., Yashike, T., and Mima, H., Mechanisms for the enhancement of the nasal absorption of insulin by surfactants, *Int. J. Pharm., 9*:173 (1981).
12. Su, K. D. E., Oeswein, J. Q., and Campanale, K. M., Intranasal administration of human zinc insulin in rats: Absorption and possible mechanisms, *APhA Acad. Pharm. Sci., 15*:89 (1985).
13. Su, K. S. E., Howey, D. C., Campanale, K. M., and Oeswein, J. Q., Intranasal adminstration of human sodium insulin in rats, dogs, and humans: Absorption and possible mechanisms, *Diabetes, 35*:A64 (1986).
14. Su, K. S. E., Campanale, K. M., Mendelsohn, L. G., Kerchner, G. A., and Gries, C. L., Nasal delivery of polypeptides, I: Nasal abosrption of enkephalins in rats, *J. Pharm. Sci. 74*:394 (1985).
15. Su, K. S. E., and Campanale, K. M., Simple animal model for assessing nasal delivery of an antirhinovirus compound, *APhA Acad. Pharm. Sci., 14*:174 (1984).
16. Su, K. S. E., Wilson, H. C., and Campanale, K. M., Recent advances in intranasal drug delivery systems, in *Drug Delivery Systems: Fundamentals and Techniques* (P. Johnson and J. G. Loyd-Jones, Eds.), Ellis Horwood, Chichester, England (1987), pp. 224-242.
17. Su, K. S. E., Campanale, K. M., and Gries, C. L., Intranasal administration of catecholamine in rats: Dobutamine hydrochloride, *APha Acad. Pharm. Sci., 15*:89 (1981).
18. Mishima, M., Wakika, Y., Nakano, M., Hirota, M., Ikei, S., and Akagi, M., Promotion of nasal absorption of glucagon in rats and a totally pancreatectomized patient, *J. Clin. Exp. Med., 140*:223 (1987).
19. McMartin, C., Hutchinson, L. E. F., Hyde, R., and Peters, G., Analysis of structural requirements for the absorption of drugs and macromolecules from the nasal cavity, *J. Pharm. Sci., 76*:535 (1987).
20. Mukai, H., Sugihara, K., and Sugiyama, M., Studies on the absorption of sodium guaiazulene-3-sulfonate, *J. Pharmacobiodyn., 8*:329 (1985).
21. Morimoto, K., Morisaka, K., and Kamada, A., Enhancement of nasal absorption of insulin and calcitonin using polyacrylic acid gel, *J. Pharm. Pharmacol., 37*:134 (1985).

22. Ohawaki, T., Ando, H., Watanabe, S., and Miyake, Y., Effect of dose, pH and osmolarity on nasal absorption of secretin in rats, *J. Pharm. Sci., 74*:550 (1985).

23. Visor, G. C., Schuessler, B., Thompson, J., and Ling, T., Nasal absorption of the calcium antagonists nicardipine in rats and rhesus monkeys, *Drug Dev. Indus. Pharm., 13*:1329 (1987).

24. Karasck, E., Rathsack, R., Fechner, K., and Grafenberg, M., Nasal absorption of substance P in rats, *Pharmazie, 41*:289 (1986).

25. Corbo, D. C., Huang, Y. C., and Chien, Y. W., Nasal delivery of progestational steroids in ovariectomized rabbits. I. Progesterone—comparison of pharmacokinetics with intravenous and oral administration, *Int. J. Pharm., 46*:133 (1988).

26. Chien, Y. W., Corbo, D. C., and Huang, Y. C., Nasal controlled delivery and pharmacokinetics of progestational steroids and effect of penetrant hydrophilicity, in *Proceedings of the 15th International Symposium on "Controlled Releaase of Bioactive Materials"* (J. Heller et al., Eds.), Controlled Release Society, Lincolnshire, Illinois (1988), pp. 191-192.

27. Su, K. S. E., and Campanale, K. M., Unpublished data.

28. Nagai, T., Nishimoto, Y., Nambu, N., Suzuki, Y., and Sekine, K., Powder dosage form of insulin for nasal administration, *J. Controlled Release 1*: 15 (1984).

29. Hirai, S., Ikenaga, T., and Matsuzawa, T., Nasal absorption of insulin in dogs, *Diabetes, 27*:296 (1978).

30. Su, K. S. E., and Campanale, K. M., Nasal delivery of insulin: Biopharmaceutical aspects and animal model choice, presented at the 3rd Annual Meeting of the American Association of Pharmaceutical Scientists, October, 1988.

31. Longenecker, J. P., Moses, A. C., Flier, J. S., Silver, R. D., Carey, M. C., and Dubovi, E., Effects of sodium tarodihydrofusidate on nasal absorption of insulin in sheep, *J. Pharm. Sci., 76*:351 (1987).

32. Su, K. S. E., and Campanale, K. M., Unpublished data.

33. Su, K. S. E., Campanale, K. M., and Layne, T. D., Unpublished data.

34. Anik, S. T., McRae, G., Nerenberg, C., Worden, A., Foreman, J., Huang, J., Kushinskey, S., Jones, R. E., and Vickery, B. H., Nasal abosrption of nafarelin acetate, the decapeptide [D-Na1(2)] LHRH, Rhesus Monkeys I, *J. Pharm. Sci., 73*:684 (1984).

35. Vickery, B. H., Anik, S., Chaplin, M., and Henzl, M., Intranasal administration of nefarelin acetate concentration and therapeutic applications, in *Transnasal Systemic Medication: Fundamentals, Developmental Concepts and Biomedical Assessments* (Y. W. Chien, Ed.), Elsevier, Amsterdam (1985), pp. 201-215.

36. Hussain, A., Faraj, J., Aramaki, Y., and Truelove, J. E., Hydrolysis of leucine enkephalin in the nasal cavity of the rat—A possible factor in

the low bioavailability of nasally administered peptides, *Biochem. Res. Comm., 133*:923 (1985).

37. Huang, C. H., Kimura, R., Barwarshi-Nassar, R., and Hussain, A., Mechanism of nasal absorption of drugs. I: Physicochemical parameters influencing the rate of in-situ nasal absorption of drugs, in rats, *J. Pharm. Sci., 74*:608 (1985).

38. Huang, C. H., Kimura, R., Barwarshi-Nassar, R., and Hussain, A., Mechanism of nasal absorption of drug. II: Absorption of L-tyrosine and the effect of structural modification on its absorption, *J. Pharm. Sci., 74*: 1298 (1985).

39. Kaneo, Y., Absorption from the nasal mucous membrane. I. Nasal absorption of hydralazine in rats, *Acta Pharm. Suec., 20*:379 (1983).

40. Kotani, A., Hayashi, M., and Awazu, S., Selection of volume indicator for the study of nasal drug absorption, *Chem. Pharm. Bull., 31*:1097 (1983).

41. Chang, S. F., Moore, L. C., and Chien, Y. W., Pharmacokinetics and bioavailability of hydromorphone; Effect of various routes of administration, *Pharm. Res., 5*:718 (1988).

42. Chien, Y. W., *Transnasal Systemic Medications*, Elsevier, Amsterdam/Oxford/New York/Tokyo (1985).

3
Physicochemical, Biopharmaceutical, and Toxicophysiological Considerations

3.1 PHYSICOCHEMICAL PROPERTIES OF DRUGS

As with the development of other dosage forms for a drug, preformulation studies have to be first carried out to assess the physical, chemical, and biopharmaceutical properties of the drug molecule before a nasal delivery system is developed. Whether the drug candidate is a traditional small organic molecule or a macromolecule developed from biotechnology, there are unique problems and challenges that need to be resolved at first. The physical, chemical, and biopharmaceutical properties of a drug molecule need to be evaluated and understood. The preformulation data form the basis for the subsequent development of a suitable nasal delivery system to achieve the maximum stability and optimum bioavailability of the drug to be delivered. The following basic physicochemical properties need to be determined in order to develop a successful formulation: (a) solubility, (b) compatibility, (c) polymorphism, and (d) stability (1).

3.2 PARAMETERS AFFECTING NASAL ABSORPTION

3.2.1 Effect of Perfusion Rate

The effect of perfusion on nasal absorption was examined using the in situ nasal perfusion technique (2). The results indicated that as the perfusion rate is increased, the rate of nasal absorption of phenobarbital first increases and then reaches a plateau level which is independent of the rate of perfusion ($\geqslant 2$ ml/min).

39

3.2.2 Effect of Perfusate Volume

As the volume of perfusion solution increases, the first-order rate of disappearance of phenobarbital has been observed to decrease (2) (Figure 3.1).

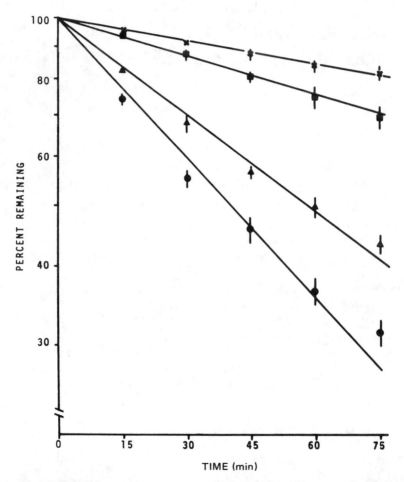

Figure 3.1 Time course for the percent (mean ± SEM, n = 3-5) of phenobarbital remaining in the in situ perfusing solution (at pH 6, 37°C) as a function of perfusion volume. (x) 20 ml; (■) 10 ml; (▲) 5 ml; (●) 3 ml. (From Ref. 2, used with permission.)

Table 3.1   Intrinsic Nasal Absorption Rate Constants (k_a)

Compound	k_a (ml/min)
Propranolol	0.054
Phenobarbital	0.048
L-Tyrosine	0.012
Phenol red	0.007

Source: From Ref. 2, used with permission.

The effect of perfusate volume on nasal absorption was also studied using drugs with various chemical structures (2). The results suggest that the intrinsic rate constant of nasal absorption varies from one drug to another (Table 3.1).

3.2.3   Effect of Solution pH

The effect of the pH of perfusion solution on the nasal absorption was examined using a water-soluble ionizable compound, like benzoic acid (pKa = 4.19), in the pH range of 2.0 to 7.1 (2). The extent of nasal absorption was found to be pH dependent (Figure 3.2). A greater nasal abosrption was achieved at pH lower than pKa, at which the penetrant molecule exists as a nonionic species. The rate of nasal absorption decreased as pH increased, owing to ionization of the penetrant molecule.

3.2.4   Effect of Drug Lipophilicity

The rate and the extent of absorption of a drug across a biological membrane are often influenced by its lipophilicity. The effect of lipophilicity on the extent of nasal absorption was studied using a series of barbiturates at pH 6, at which the barbiturates (pKa = 7.6) exist entirely in their nonionized form (2). A 40-fold difference in the partition coefficient was noted between pentobarbital and barbital, which, however produces only a fourfold change in the extent of nasal absorption (Table 3.2). Furthermore, it was also observed that the great difference in partition coefficients (n-octanol/pH 7.4) between propranolol and L-tyrosine (15.1 vs. 0.02) has resulted in only a very small variation in the rate constants of nasal absorption (0.054 ml/min vs. 0.012 ml/min) (see Table 3.1). Studies on the nasal delivery of a series of progestational steroids in ovariectomized rabbits (3) demonstrated that the

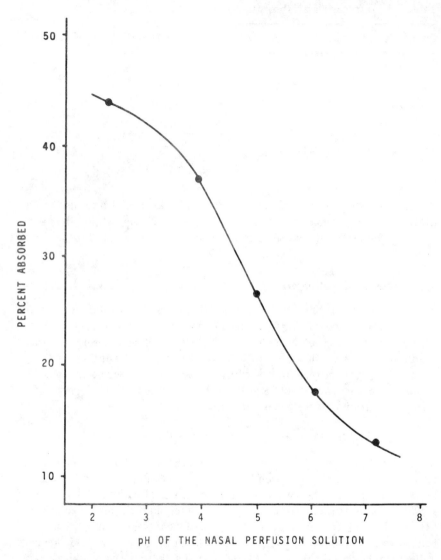

Figure 3.2 The extent of nasal absorption (in 60 min) of benzoic acid as a function of pH. (From Ref. 2, used with permission.)

Table 3.2 Relationship Between the Extent of Nasal Absorption and Partition Coefficient

Barbiturate	$(PC)_{CHC1_3/H_2O}$[b]	% Absorbed[a]	
		Nasal	Gastro-intestinal[b]
Barbital	0.7	5.0 (±3.0)[c]	12
Phenobarbital	4.8	10.6 (±3.9)[c]	20
Pentobarbital	28.0	20.3 (±4.7)[d]	30
Secobarbital	50.7	23.9 (±3.4)[c]	40

[a]In rats at pH 6 for 60 min.
[b]Shanker, L. S., *J. Med. Pharm. Chem.,* 2:343 (1960).
[c]Mean ± standard deviation ($n = 3$)
[d]Mean ± standard deviation ($n = 4$)
Source: From Ref. 2, used with permission.

(Octanol/H_2O) partition coefficient does not reflect the lipophilicity of progesterone and its hydroxy derivatives and predict their partitioning behavior in the nasal mucosa. The systemic bioavailability of the progesterone and its hydroxy derivatives following nasal administration is correlated well with (nasal mucosa/buffer) partition coefficient (Figure 3.3).

The results appear to suggest that the permeation of a drug molecule across the biological membranes, like nasal mucosa, is not only a function of the physicochemical properties of the drug, like lipophilicity, but also dependent upon its stereochemical conformation during membrane transport.

3.2.5 Effect of Initial Drug Concentration

The effect of variation in initial drug concentration in the perfusion solution on nasal absorption was studied by monitoring the disappearance of L-tyrosyl-L-tyrosine and the formation of L-tyrosine using the in situ method in the rat (2). It was observed that the concentration of L-tyrosine formed is dependent upon the initial concentration of L-tyrosyl-L-tyrosine (Table 3.3), suggesting that the nasal absorption of L-tyrosine is dependent upon the initial concentration.

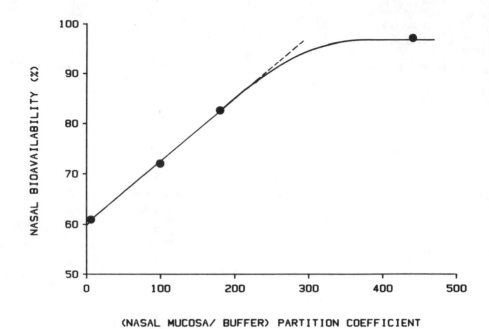

Figure 3.3 Progesterone levels in rabbit. Relationship between the systemic bioavailability of progesterone and its hydroxy derivatives following nasal spray administration and (nasal mucosa/buffer) partition coefficient. (From Corbo, D. C., and Chien, Y. W., Unpublished data.)

Table 3.3 Dependency of L-tyrosine Formation During the In Situ Nasal Absorption Studies on Initial Concentrations of L-tyrosyl-L-tyrosine[a]

Time (min)	Concentration of L-tyrosine Formed (mean ± SEM)		
	$1.18 \times 10^{-3} M$	$2.22 \times 10^{-3} M$	$4.89 \times 10^{-3} M$
2	—	0.032 (±0.003)	0.036 (±0.004)
15	0.104 (±0.042)	0.110 (±0.023)	0.148 (±0.029)
30	0.197 (±0.086)	0.220 (±0.055)	0.287 (±0.060)
45	0.297 (±0.122)	0.322 (±0.085)	0.444 (±0.087)
60	0.388 (±0.224)	0.412 (±0.113)	0.597 (±0.109)
N[b]	3	3	4

[a]Isotonic phosphate buffer (0.1M, pH 7.4) at 37°C.
[b]Number of rats studied.
Source: From Ref. 2, used with permission.

44

3.3 PATHWAYS FOR NASAL ABSORPTION

Some drugs with poor oral absorption, like insulin, and the drugs which are subjected to extensive hepatic first-pass metabolism, like propanolol, can be better absorbed through the nasal mucosa. The process of transport across the nasal membrane involves either diffusion of drug molecules through the pores in the nasal mucosa or participation of some nonpassive pathways before they reach the blood stream (4).

In addition, the olfactory epithelium is known to be a portal for substances to enter the central nervous system (CNS) and the peripheral circulation. However, the mechanism of transport still remains unknown. Moreover, the nasopharynx has been shown to act as the portal of entry for some of the most common viral diseases; i.e., measles, common cold, smallpox, chickenpox, and poliomyelitis (5,6). As early as 1900, the Chinese and Hindus had already practiced the spraying of a finely powdered virus into the nostriles to vaccinate against smallpox (7). Immunity to scarlet fever and diphtheria could be produced, respectively, by nasal application of the scarlet fever toxin (8) and the diphtheria toxin (9).

Whereas ephedrine, epinephrine, nicotine, and horse serum were found to be unable to pass through the nasal membrane, the nasal absorption of phenol red, penicillin, sulbenicillin, cefazoline, and cephacetrile was reported to produce a urinary excretion which was nearly one-half of that resulting from the intramuscular injection of an equivalent dose. Furthermore, the nasal delivery of propranolol, hydralazine, clofilium tosylate, ergotamine tartrate, disodium cromoglycate, progesterone, testosterone, buprenophine, naloxone, cocaine, hyoscine, atropine, or estradiol has reportedly achieved a rapid and complete absorption. However, the intranasal administration of polypeptide hormones has been often found to achieve only a very low bioavailability as compared to intravenous injection.

Therefore, it is important to investigate the pathways for nasal absorption. Hopefully, by gaining some fundamental understanding of the pathways for nasal absorption, the nasal delivery rate and the transnasal bioavailability of drugs can be improved and controlled. Evidence has been generated to demonstrate the potential existence of a communication between the subarachnoid space and the nasal cavities, and between the lymphatic plexus in the nasal mucosa and the subarachnoid space as well as between the perineural sheaths in the olfactory nerve filaments and the subarachnoid space (10). The potential pathways involved in the nasal absorption of drugs reported in the literature are summarized in Table 3.4.

Table 3.4 Potential Pathways for Nasal Absorption

Substances	Possible pathways
Albumin	
Albumin (73) (labeled with Evans blue and horseradish peroxidase)	Nasal mucosa → sensory nerve cells of olfactory epithelium → subarachnoid space → blood stream
Egg albumin (74)	Nasal mucosa → lymphatic stream
Serum albumin (75)	Nasal mucosa $\xrightarrow[\text{(occasionally)}]{}$ lymphatic stream
Amino Acids	
Amino acids (76) (arginine, glutamic acid, glycine, prolin, serin, γ-aminobutyric acid)	Nasal mucosa $\xrightarrow[\text{active transport}]{}$ blood vessel
Tritiated leucine (77)	Nasal mucosa → olfactory nerve fibers → CNS
Bacteria	
Rabbit virulent Type III pneumococci (78)	Nasopharyngeal epithelium → lymphatics → cervical lymphatic vessel → blood vessel
E. coli and staphyloccus (79)	Nasal mucosa → lymphatics → blood
Clofilium tosylate (80)	Nasal mucosa $\xrightarrow[\text{or diffusion}]{\text{absorption}}$ epithelial cells → systemic circulation
Dopamin (81)	Nasal mucous membrane → CSF and serum (detected within 15 min after administration)
Dyes	
T-1824 (82)	Nasal membrane → blood stream
Vital dyes, trypan blue, Evans blue (83)	Nasal mucous membrane → lymph
Potassium ferrocyanide (84)	Nasal mucous membrane → olfactory receptor nerve cells → lymphatic meshwork → retropharyngeal lymph nodes

Table 3.4 (Continued)

Substances	Possible pathways
Potassium ferrocyanide and iron ammonium citrate (84-86) filaments	Nasal membrane → perineural sheaths of the olfactory → cranial cavity → subarachnoid space and cervical lymph nodes
	Nasal membrane → olfactory sensory cells → subarachnoid space and pia-arachnoid membrane
	Nasal membrane → lymphatic vessels and olfactory nerve → olfactory bulb
Hormones Estradiol (81,87,88)	Nasal membrane → CSF (within 1 min)
	Nasal membrane → olfactory neurons → brain and CSF
Norethisterone (81,89)	Nasal membrane → olfactory dendrites → nervous system → supporting cells in the olfactory mucosa → submucosal blood vascular system
	Nasal membrane → peripheral circulation (high levels) and CSF (low levels) → CNS
Progesterone (81,87,88)	Nasal membrane → olfactory dendrites → nervous system → supporting cells in the olfactory mucosa → submucosal blood vascular system → CSF
	Nasal membrane → CSF (within 1 min)
Inorganic Substances Colloidal gold (90)	Nasal mucosa → olfactory mucosa → olfactory rods → supporting cells → blood vessels

Table 3.4   (Continued)

Substances	Possible pathways
Colloidal ^{198}Au suspension (91)	Mucous membrane of the olfactory region → CSF in the subarachnoid space at the anterior part of the brain
Colloidal silver (92)	Nasopharyngeal mucous membrane → olfactory nerve cells → systemic lymphatics
Lead carbonate (93)	Dissolved in nasal mucus and then absorbed as a true solution
Chloride salt (94) ($CsCl$, $SrCl_2$, $BaCl_2$, $CeCl_3$)	Nasal membrane → blood circulation
ThB (NO_3)$_2$ (thorium B) (95) and and $H_3P^{32}O_4$	Nasal septal mucosa → anterior scala → CSF → CNS
Penicillines (96)	Nasal membrane → blood stream
Virus	
Herpes virus encephalitis (97)	Nasal mucosa → peripheral and cranial nerves → CNS
Herpes virus simples (98)	Nasal mucosa → cranial nerve → CNS
Mouse-passage strain of herpes virus (99)	Nasal mucosa → trigeminal and olfactory pathways → CNS
Neurotropic virus (100,101)	Nasal mucosa → axis cylinders of the olfactory nerves → CNS
Poliomyelitis virus (102-105)	Nasal mucous membrane → olfactory nerve → CNS
Vaccina virus (106,107)	Nasal mucosa → submucous lymphatics → cervical lymphatic pathways → CNS
Water	
Distilled water (108)	Nasopharynx → cervical lymph

3.4 ENHANCEMENT OF NASAL DRUG ABSORPTION

Several methods have been used to facilitate the nasal absorption of drugs:

1. Structure modification. The chemical modification of a drug molecule has been commonly used to modify the physicochemical properties of a drug and could also be utilized to improve the nasal absorption of a drug.
2. Salt or ester formation. The drug could be converted to form a salt
   or an ester for better transnasal permeability. For example, nasal absorption could be improved significantly by forming a salt with increased solubility in nasal fluid (Table 3.5) (1) or an ester with enhanced uptake by nasal epithelium (Table 3.6) (2).
3. Formulation design. Proper selection of pharmaceutical excipients
   in the development of nasal formulation could enhance the formulation stability and/or the nasal bioavailability of a drug.
4. Surfactants. Incorporation of surfactants into nasal dosage forms
   could modify the permeability of nasal membranes, which may facilitate the nasal absorption of drugs.

Survey of the literature indicates that surfactants have been extensively
evaluated for the possibility of enhancing the nasal absorption of drugs, including peptide and protein drugs. A number of surfactants have been reported to enhance the absorption of drugs through the nasal mucosa to a
level sufficient to achieve their systemic effects. Mild surfactants at low
concentrations may only alter membrane structure and permeability (11),

Table 3.5 Comparison in Nasal Bioavailability of Compound ^{14}C-LY140091

Formulation	Route of administration	No. of animals	AUC^c (mcg · min/gm ± S.E.)	Bioavailability^d %
Solution^a	i.v.	3	142.98 (±45.13)	
Solution^a	Nasal	4	142.08 (±42.84)	99.4
Suspension^b	Nasal	3	50.03 (±14.71)	35.0

^{a}LY140091 sodium salt dissolved in saline.
^{b}LY140091 suspended in saline.
^{c}Calculated from 0 to 5 hr.
^{d}Calculated from the ratio of (AUC)$_{nasal}$ over (AUC)$_{iv}$.
Source: From Ref. 1, used with permission.

Table 3.6 Calculated Nasal Absorption Rate Constants[a] of L-Tyrosine Carboxylic Acid Esters and N-Acetyl-L-Tyrosine[b]

Compound	Apparent partition coefficient[c]	k_a (min^{-1})
L-Tyrosine methyl ester	1.97	0.0116
ethyl ester	5.20	0.0254
n-propyl ester	20.79	0.0230
t-butyl ester	62.50	0.0105
N-Acetyl-L-tyrosine	0.0256	0.0024

[a]Perfusate volume, 5 ml.
[b]At pH 7.4 and 37°C
[c]Octanol/pH 7.4
Source: From Ref. 2, used with permission.

whereas certain surfactants at high concentrations may disrupt and even dissolve biological membranes.

The nasal absorption of scarlet fever toxin was reportedly enhanced in the presence of 1% sodium taurocholate, which produces immunity (8). The nasal absorption of gentamicin (60 mg/ml in saline solution) in humans was observed to increase by the incorporation of 1% sodium glycocholate and peak serum levels were achieved in 30-60 min (12). Polyoxyethylene-9-lauryl ether (BL-9, 0.5%) in saline solution and sodium glycocholate (30 mM) were found to improve the nasal absorption of hydralazine in both in situ and in vivo nasal absorption studies in rats (4,13). Incorporation of sodium glycocholate and polyacrylic acid gel (Carbopol gel, 0.1 w/v) into nasal preparations of calcitonin was found to result in a rapid reduction of the plasma Ca^{2+} level (14,15). Polysorbate 80 (1%) in saline solution was observed to promote the nasal absorption of progesterone (16) and testosterone (17) in rats. The peak plasma concentrations were obtained within 6 min, with an almost 100% bioavailability as compared to intravenous administration. The nasal absorption of atropine and hyoscine from nasal spray or nose drops was observed to be more rapid, complete, and uniform with the addition of sodium lauryl sulfate (18,19).

Crystalline porcine insulin administered intranasally with 1% sodium glycocholate in saline solution (pH 7.6) to humans was found to yield a relatively prompt increase in the plasma levels of immunoreactive insulin (IRI) in a similar trend as that by intravenous injection (20). On the other hand, addition of other surfactants, like lysozyme, HCO-60, and BYCO-E, resulted in only a negligible absorption of insulin. It was rather surprising to note that incorporation of 1% sodium ursodeoxycholate in the nasal insulin solution does not reduce the blood glucose level in spite of the increase in plasma IRI concentration. However, the addition of 1% saponin, sodium glycocholate, or BL-9 in nasal solutions of crystalline porcine insulin enhanced significantly either the extent or the duration of hypoglycemia; and the blood glucose level in dogs was reduced by 25-100% within 1-2 hr after intranasal administration (21). The results indicated that the alteration of the nasal mucosa by surfactants increases the permeability of mucous membrane, which leads to enhancement in the nasal absorption of insulin. Coadministration of insulin with 1% surfactant (such as the surfactant of nonionic ether type, anionic or amphoteric-type, bile salts, saponin, and surfactin) in rats was noted to produce a reduction in blood glucose levels (22). The results suggested that the surfactants with an HLB value of 8-14 yield a greater reduction of blood glucose levels. It was hypothesized that the surfactant molecule increases the nasal permeability or reduces the proteolytic enzymes' activity in the nasal mucosa, and therefore promotes the nasal absorption of insulin. BL-9 was noted to produce a maximum hemolytic and protein-releasing effect on the biomembrane, whereas it yielded only a slight inhibition of the enzymatic degradation of insulin (23). On the contrary, sodium glycocholate produced a lesser extent of both hemolytic and protein-releasing effects, whereas it exhibited a marked inhibition of the leucine aminopeptidase activity.

Aerosol spray of insulin (500 U/ml) with 1% sodium deoxycholate resulted in a peak serum insulin concentration of 103 ($\pm$49) μU/ml within 10 min after nasal administration (24). The blood glucose level began to fall by 10 min and reached the nadir level of 54 ($\pm$14)% by 30 min. The nasal absorption of insulin was approximated to be 10-20% as efficient as intravenous administration.

Nagai et al. (25) reported that the nasal absorption of insulin in powder form is better than that in liquid form. The onset of nasal insulin absorption in dogs was found to be the fastest with the preparation containing microcrystalline cellulose (MCC). The nasal absorption of insulin was sustained in the preparation containing neutralized Carbopol 934 (CP-Na) added to the freeze-dried insulin powder. The powder dosage form of insulin with Carbopol 934 (CP), by freeze-dried, was observed to achieve greater enhancement in the nasal absorption of insulin. This powder dosage form successfully produced hypoglycemia to the extent which is one-third of that achieved by intravenous administration. The nasal absorption of insulin

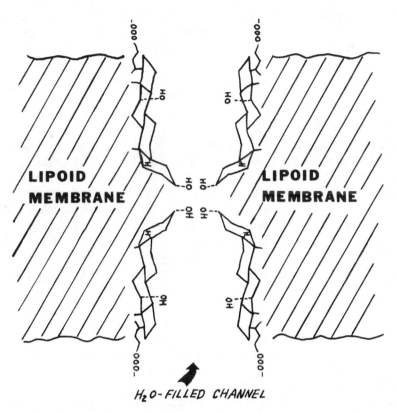

Figure 3.4 A schematic illustration of the molecule model for reverse micelle formation on cell membranes. Two pairs of sodium deoxycholate molecules are shown stacked end-to-end, spanning a lipid bilayer and forming an aqueous pore for the transport of insulin monomers from the extracellular space, where high concentrations of insulin monomers are solubilized in mixed bile salt and insulin micelles. (From Ref. 34, used with permission.)

(1 U/kg) in 0.1 and 1.0% polyacrylic acid gel produced the maximum hypoglycemic effect at 30 min and 1 hr, respectively, after administration (15).

Intranasal administration of aerosolized insulin (1 U/kg), which contains 1% laureth-9 as an enhancer, was found to produce a rapid absorption of insulin within 15 min, which lowers the blood glucose level by 50% in 45 min in fasting normal control subjects and in 120 min in fasting diabetics (26).

Studies on the retention time in the HPLC chromatogram suggested that the potency of adjuvant in enhancing the nasal absorption of insulin correlates positively with the increase in the hydrophobicity of the bile salts (27). The rank order of: deoxycholate > cholate > ursodeoxycholate was found for the enhancement of nasal insulin absorption. Using the bile salt at the level of 1%, all plasma insulin concentrations peaked at 10 (±1) min with a simultaneous falling in blood glucose levels. As high as 10-20% of the insulin dose administered was absorbed into the systemic circulation in the presence of 1% sodium deoxycholate. The nasal absorption of insulin occurred at the critical micellar concentration (CMC) of a bile salt in aqueous solution and reached the maximum as the micelle formation was well established.

As a result, it was hypothesized that bile salts act as the absorption adjuvants by (a) producing a high juxtamembrane concentration of insulin molecules via solubilization in the mixed bile salt micelles, and (b) forming a reverse micelle within the nasal membrane (Figure 3.4), through which the insulin molecules diffuse through the polar channels in the nasal membrane and get into the blood stream. It was concluded tht insulin, by coadministration with an appropriate bile salt, can be absorbed into the blood stream through the nasal mucosa with reproducible kinetics and good efficiency.

3.5 DRUG DISTRIBUTION IN THE NASAL CAVITY

The drug distribution in the nasal cavity is one of the important factors which affects the efficiency of nasal absorption. The mode of drug administration could affect the distribution of a drug in the nasal cavity, which in turn will determine the absorption efficiency of a drug. Using a cast of the human nose (Figure 3.5) (1), it was demonstrated that a significant difference in drug distribution was observed by comparing different types of nasal delivery systems, like nose drops, plastic bottle nebulizer, atomized pump, and metered-dose pressurized aerosol (28,29). The results indicated that the atomized pump is the best nasal delivery system because it gives a constant dose and a very good mucosal distribution (Figure 3.6). The results also suggest that the use of a large volume of a weak solution is preferable to a small volume of a concentrated solution. This may be of particular importance when vasoconstrictor is used locally (30).

A simulated nasal cavity made of acryl resin was developed for studying the distribution of beclomethasone diporpionate (BD) areosol particles in the nasal cavity (31). No significant difference was found among gas, liquid,

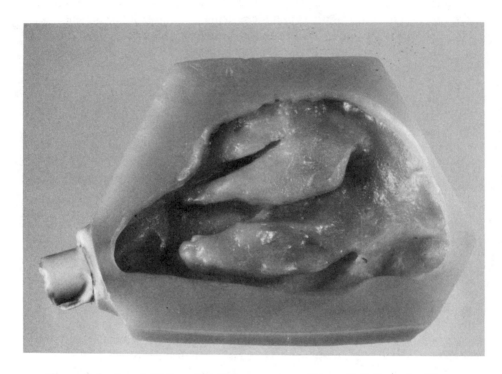

Figure 3.5 A cast of the artificial human nose. (From Ref. 2, used with permission.)

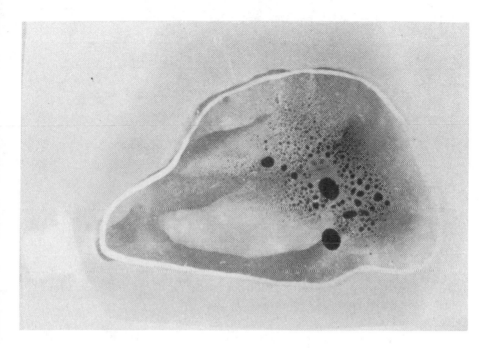

Figure 3.6 A simulated distribution of drops delivered from a nasal drop device. (From Mygind, 1979, reproduced with permission of the copyright owner—Elsevier Science Publishers.)

and powder preparations. The highest concentration of BD was usually found at the anterior portion of the middle turbinate.

3.6   DELIVERY SYSTEMS FOR INTRANASAL DRUG ADMINISTRATION

There are several types of drug delivery systems which have been long used for the delivery of drugs to the nasal cavity, such as nasal spray, nose drops, saturated cotton pledget, aerosol spray, and insufflator. Table 3.7 lists the drugs that have been administered intranasally for systemic medication and the type of drug delivery devices used.

Technetium-99m-labeled human serum albumin was administered into the human nose by a nasal spray or nose drops. The results showed that about 40% of the dose cleared rapidly with average halftimes ranging from 6 to 9

Table 3.7 Delivery Means and Devices for Intranasal Administration of Drugs

Drugs	Delivery devices
ACTH	Insufflator Nebulizer (De Vilbis No. 40)
ACTH-α 1-18	Pressurized insufflator Nebulizer flask Automatic dose-controlled nebulizer aerosol
Alsactide (ACTH 17)	Nasal spray
Adrenal corticosteroids	Nasal spray Nose drops Nasal jelly Insufflator Submucosal injection into the anterior tip of inferior turbinate Metered-dose aerosol
Angiotensin II-antagonist (1-N-Suc-5-Val-8-Phg) AII	Hamilton syringe with a polyethylene tube (PE-20)
Antihistamines	Nasal spray Nose drops
Atropine	Nasal spray Nose drops Nasal aerosol
Buprenorphine	Micropipet
Buserelin	Nasal spray Ointment formulation
Cerulein	Atomizer Nasal spray
Calcitonin	Nose drops
Clofilium tosylate	Drug solution delivered to nasal cavity through esophagus cannulation and syringe
Cocaine	Nasal spray Nose drops Cotton pledget Gauge packtail Insufflator Rubbing with cocaine mud

Table 3.7 (Continued)

Drugs	Delivery devices
Cromoglycate disodium	Nasal spray Insufflator Microsyringe
Dopamine	Nasal spray
DDAVP	Nasal spray Metered-dose nasal spray Calibrated plastic tube Rhynil (a graded nasal tube) Plastic (rhinyl) catheter
Enviroxime	Metered-dose nasal spray
Ergotamine tartrate	Micropipet
Estradiol-17β	Nasal spray Nose drops Microsyringe
Gentamicin	Nasal spray
Glucagon	Nose drops
Gonadotropin-releasing hormone (GnRH)	Nose drops Administered in a solution of natural plant gum which becomes gel in contact with nasal mucosa and remains in place
Hydralazine	Micropipet
Hyoscine (scopolamine)	Nasal spray Nose drops
Insulin	Metered-pump sprayer Metered-dose aerosolized spray Fixed-volume aerosol spray Nasal spray Nose drops Cotton pledget
Human interferon (HuIFN-α)	Nasal spray Nose drops Cotton pledget Aerosol spray Metered-pump sprayer
Interferon inducer (CP-20961)	Nasal spray emulsion Nasal suspension

Table 3.7   (Continued)

Drugs	Delivery devices
Ipratropium	Nasal spray
Isosorbide dinitrate	Nasal spray (IsoMack spray)
LHRH	Nasal spray Graded plastic nasal catheter (Rhynil, Ferring AB)
Lypressin	Nasal spray
Meclizine HCl	Nose drops
Methacholine	Nasal aerosol Nose drops
Nafarelin acetate	Nasal spray
Naloxone	Micropipet
Nicotine	Tobacco snuff Injected into dog's frontal sinus
Nitroglycerin	Metered-dose spray Instilled through Teflon i.v. catheter
Norethisterone	Glass atomizer
Oxytocin	Nasal spray Nose drops Cotton pledget Aerosol-activated spray Rhinyl (a plastic application tube) Graded polyethylene tube Direct instillation by tuberculin syringe and 25G needle
Penicillines	Nebulizer (DeVilbiss No. 40) Aerosol with intermittent negative pressure in the nasal passages and nasal accessory sinuses Aerosol with a balanced calibrated suction and pressure
Pentagastrin	Insufflator Snuff
Phenylephrine	Nose drops
Phenyl-p-guanidinibenzoate (PGB)	Nose drops

Table 3.7 (Continued)

Drugs	Delivery devices
Posterior pituitary extracts	Nose drops Cotton pledget Insufflator
Progesterone	Nasal spray by an atomizer connected to a respiratory pump Nasal spray by a glass atomizer Nasal solution administered by micropipet
Propranolol	Micropipet
Prostaglandins	Nose drops
Scarlet fever toxin	Nasal spray
Secretin	Microsyringe
Testosterone	Micropipet
Tetracosactrin ($\beta^{1\text{-}24}$-corticotropin)	Nasal insufflation (using a marvic inhaler)
Thyrotropin-releasing hormone (TRH)	Instilled through a polyethylene sheated cannula
Tramazoline	Metered-dose nasal spray (Tobispray)
Vaccines	Inhalation aerosol Nasal spray Nasal aerosol spray Nebulizer aerosol Nose drops
Vitamin B_{12}	Nose drops Insufflator
Xylometazoline	Nasal spray Nose drops

min (32). Following this initial rapid clearance phase, clearance of the spray was much slower than the drops, since most of the spray deposited on the nonciliated regions, whereas the solution from the nose drops spread more extensively over the nasal ciliated areas.

The metered-dose nebulizer is a recently introduced nasal drug delivery device which operates by mechanical actuation and delivers a predetermined volume of the formulation into the nasal cavity. The dose of active ingredient delivered intranasally depends upon its concentration in the formulation and the volume of solution delivered at each actuation. The metered-dose nebulizer has already been successfully utilized as the nasal delivery system for several topical drugs, such as corticosteroid (Extracort), beclomethasone dipropionate (Aldecin, Beconase, Becotide), flunisolide (Nasalide), tramazoline (Tobispray), and nasal decongestant (Rhinospray).

Recently, the feasibility of using the metered-dose nebulizer as the nasal delivery system for systemically effective drugs, like DDAVP ([1-desamino-8D-arginine] -vasopressin), enviroxime, insulin, and nitroglycerin, has been explored. The results suggested that intranasal administration of systemically effective drugs with sustained-release action might be feasible and desirable. The sustaiend-release formulations of propranolol, in which methylcellulose was incorporated, were administred intranasally in rats (33). A low initial but prolonged blood level was observed (Table 3.8). The systemic bioavailability of these sustained-release propranolol formulations was identical to that resulting from intravenous administration. Micorencapuslation of drugs by biodegradable or bioadhesive polymers may also be applied to develop a nasal sustained-release formulation.

A method for the physiological control of nasal mucosa using hydrogels like Carbopol 940 was established as early as in 1966 (34). The effect of pH and osmotic pressure of the hydrogels containing various adjuvants and medicinal substances and the influence of contact time of the nasal mucosa with the hydrogels were studied. A medicated hydrogel which can maintain the integrity of the nasal mucous membrane of the guinea pig was prepared (35). The results indicated that this hydrogel permits the achievement of a prolonged therapuetic effect without suppressing the ciliary functions during application. Hydrogels might be useful for preparing sustained-release nasal preparations to provide a long-term intimate contact of therapeutic agents with the nasal mucosa.

An inflatable nasal device walled with microporous membrane was developed (36) to provide a controlled release of drugs from a suspension formulation (Figure 3.7a). Following insertion into the rabbit nasal pas-

Table 3.8 Pharmacokinetic Parameters[a] Following Transnasal Delivery of Propranolol from Sustained-Release Dosage Forms[b]

Route	C_{max} (ng/ml)	t_{max} (min)	$AUC_{0-\infty}$ (ng hr/ml)	$\dfrac{AUC_{oral,nasal}}{AUC_{i.v.}}$
Intravenous			1033.8 (±30.8)	
Oral	96.9 (±18.6)	50.0	196.9 (±25.8)	0.190
Nasal solution	1161.4 (±29.0)	6.3	1033.0 (±48.7)	0.999
SR-A	949.0 (±46.5)	10.0	968.4 (±15.4)	0.936
SR-B	912.3 (±88.3)	13.3	1031.1 (±42.1)	0.997
SR-C	341.5 (±35.5)	71.2	1044.1 (±30.5)	1.009

[a]In rats (n = 3 or 4), C_{max} = peak plasma level, t_{max} = time to peak level, AUC = area under plasma concentration-time curve. The values stand for mean (± standard error).
[b]Sustained-release dosage forms: SR-A, SR-B, and SR-C.
Source: From Ref. 33, used with permission.

sage, the nasal device is inflated by filling with donor drug suspension. It conforms to the contour of the nasal passage, and it is left in place for prolonged duration (Figure 3.7b). Using progesterone as the model drug, the plasma profile of progesterone delivered by the controlled-release nasal device was compared to that attained by an immediate-release nasal spray in ovariectomized rabbits (36). The results (Figure 3.8) indicated that the nasal spray produces the peak plasma level of progesterone within 2 min, indicating a rapid absorption of progesterone by nasal mucosa. On the other hand, intranasal administration of progesterone by the nasal device has led to a gradual increase in the plasma concentration of progesterone, which reaches a plateau level within 20-30 min and remains elevated throughout the 6-hr insertion period. The systemic bioavailability of progesterone following intranasal administration by immediate-release spray formulation (82.5 ± 13.5%) and controlled-release nasal device (72.4 ± 25.7%) were not statistically different from one another, but were both significantly greater than that resulting from oral administration (7.9 ± 1.6%). The results suggest a nine- to 10-fold reduction in the extent of hepatic first-pass metabolism as well as a substantial prolongation of plasma drug level (from 10 to 300 min) by this nasal controlled drug delivery technique.

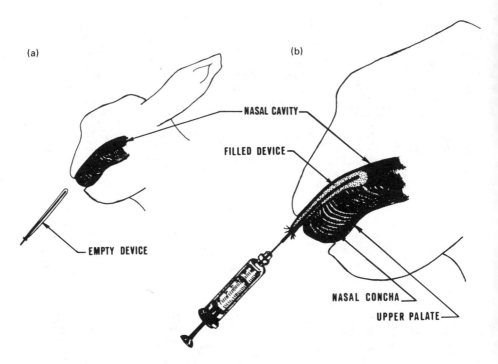

Figure 3.7 Diagrammatic illustration of the controlled-release nasal delivery device prior to insertion into the rabbit nasal passage (a), and the in situ filling of the nasal delivery device with the progesterone formulation in the nasal cavity (b). (From Ref. 3, used with permission.)

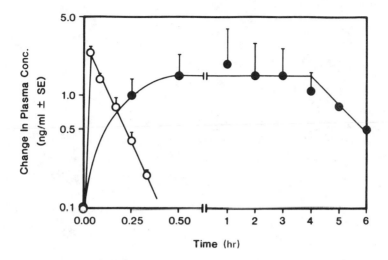

Figure 3.8 Time course for the change in the plasma concentration of progesterone after intranasal administration of progesterone in the ovariectomized rabbits ($n = 3$) by: (○) immediate-release nasal spray (2 μg/kg) and (●) controlled-release nasal device (60 μg/kg). (Modified from Ref. 3, used with permission.)

3.7 DRUG DEPOSITION IN THE NASAL CAVITY

Nasal deposition of particles is related to the individual's nasal resistance to air flow (Figure 3.9) (37). The high linear velocity and the bend in the air stream in the anterior nares results in impaction of a large proportion of particles that are small enough to enter the nasal airway (38). With nasal breathing, nearly all the particles with an aerodynamic size of 10-20 μm are so deposited. A significant fraction of the very small particles is also deposited in the nose, though many particles which are smaller than 2 μm pass with the inspired air into the lungs. The capacity of removal for the upper respiratory tract is 100% for particles with a size larger than 10 μm, and approximately 80% for particles of 5 μm (39). It drops progessively with further reduction in size and approaches zero for particles at 1-2 μm. Insoluble particles, which are deposited in the main nasal passage, are likely to be carried back by the ciliary movement and dispatched to the stomach (40). If the drug is introduced as a vapor or a soluble particle, it may readily pass into the lining secretions and then be absorbed from there into the blood.

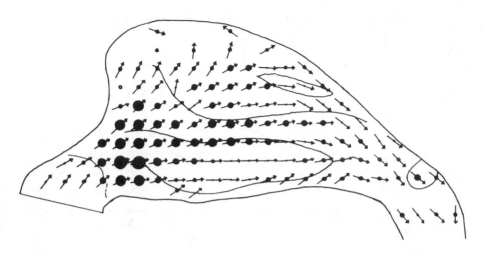

Figure 3.9 Diagram illustrating the linear velocity and direction of inspiratory air. Size of the dot indicates velocity. (From Ref. 52, used with permission.)

The deposition of aerosols in the respiratory tract is a function of particle size and respiratory patterns (41). The density, shape, and hygroscopicity of the particles and the pathological conditions in the nasal passage will influence the deposition of particles, whereas the particle size distribution will determine the site of deposition and affect the subsequent biological response in experimental animals and man. It was reported that 91.5 and 83.2% of the mass of the aerosol produced, respectively, by the jet and ultrasonic nebulizer were deposited in the upper respiratory tract of 15 normal adults (42). A uniform distribution of particles throughout the nasal mucosa could be achieved by delivering the particles from a new nasal spray using a pressurized gas propellant (43). A metered-dose delivery system developed for the nasal delivery of flunisolide, a synthetic fluorinated corticosteroid, was assessed to provide a consistent dose delivery and spray pattern which affects the deposition of droplets in the nasal cavity (44).

If the aerodynamic size distribution of an aerosol is known, respiratory tract deposition can be estimated from theoretical and experimental data relating deposition fraction to particle aerodynamic diameter (45). However, the estimation of deposition in the nasal cavity is complicated by the growth or shrinkage of particles resulting from water condensation or evaporation by humidity change (46). When exposed to an environment with increasing humidity, a hygroscopic particle responds and absorbs moisture to the extent of a few molecular layers at low relative humidities and becomes dissolved as humidity increases. It then becomes a saturated droplet, and at the same time its size undergoes an abrupt increase and it grows larger as humidity increases further or reduces as humidity decreases (47). The change in the particle size of aerosol depends on relative humidity: The greater the humidity, the larger the aerosol particle size (48).

The particle or droplet size of an aerosol is important for both efficacy and toxicity. For example, the metered-dose flunisolide solution discussed above requires that the majority of particles have a diameter of greater than 10 μm to achieve a localized delivery in the nasal cavity and to avoid any potential undesired effects resulting from any deposition of flunisolide aerosol in the lung (49). Numerous methods for sizing aerosol particles have been developed in the past. The most common ones are microscopy, light scattering, laser holography, and the cascade impactor method (49-51).

Of the three mechanisms usually considered for particle deposition in the respiratory tract, i.e., inertia, sedimentation, and diffusion, the inertial deposition is the dominant mechanism in the nasal deposition (42,52-54). Any particles with an aerodynamic diameter of 50 μm or greater do not enter the nasal passage. Several techniques, such as polydisperse (55) and monodisperse aerosols (56), have been employed to determine the regional and/or total deposition in the nasal passage. The results demonstrated a generally monotonic increase in percent total deposition when plotted against the parameter D_A^2O. This curve demonstrates the primary role of inertia, either in laminar or turbulent flow studied. The site of maximum deposition was found at 2-3 cm behind the tip of the nostrils (57).

The deposition site within the nasal cavity depends upon the type of delivery system used and the technique of administration applied (58). The deposition and clearance of solution with a relatively large volume of administration, as nasal spray and nose drops, were compared and the results indicated that following administration by the nose drops, a greater coverage of the nasal walls is achieved, which is independent of the volume administered over the range of 0.1-0.75 ml (59). The continuous air stream from the posterior outlet of the nose had only a little effect on the amount of the particles deposited at each region. The particles once deposited at the anterior region of the nasal cavity might be again conveyed posteriorly by the inhaled air, ciliary movement and/or diffusion in the mucous layer.

Experiments were undertaken to clarify the deposition of drug in the nasal cavity using the gas and powder sprays (60). A nose model molded from a

cadaver with some modifications to allow for postmortem shrinkage was
developed. Three types of nasal cavities were designed from the original
model, using dental compound and celluloid plate: (a) a straight septum with
normal turbinates, (b) a concave septum with hypertrophic turbinates, and
(c) a convex septum with atrophic turbinates. The inner surface of the cavity
except the anterior portion (corresponding to the vestibulum) was covered
with moistened filter paper. Beclomethasone dipropionate (BD) particles
were emitted into each nostril by fluorinated Freon propellant. Results indicated that the shape of the nasal cavity produces a greater effect on the
deposition of BD from the gas spray than from the powder spray. This
difference could probably be due to the spray angle and to the size and speed

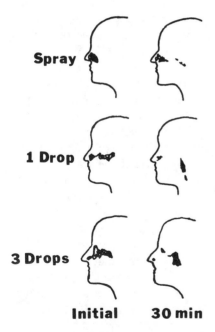

Figure 3.10 Diagram showing the sites of deposition and patterns of clearance following intranasal administration by nasal spray and nose drops. Each
pair of images is of the same subject, but the three pairs are of different subjects. (From Ref. 32, used with permission.)

of the aerosol particles. The particles from the spray container hit the localized area in the spray axis and thus were deposited there most densely. A
wider spray angle, therefore, more adequately advances the sprayed particles
beyond any obstacles, such as a deviated septum or hypertrophic turbinates.
The powder spray is, therefore, preferable with regard to the deposition
and distribution of drug particles in the nasal cavity, and improvement of the
delivery system and drug forms is necessary to achieve a better clinical effect
and easier manipulation by the patients.

The patterns of nasal deposition and the rates of clearance were studied
in normal subjects using nasal spray and nose drops of ^{99m}Tc-labeled human
serum albumin (HSA) (Figure 3.10) (32). The nasal spray deposited HSA
anteriorly in the nasal cavity, with little of the dose reaching the turbinates.
In contrast, the nose drops dispersed the dose throughout the length of the
nasal cavity, from the atrium to the nasopharynx, and the dosing with three
drops resulted in a greater coverage of the nasal walls compared with that
of a single drop. The solution deposited anteriorly in the nasal cavity was
slow to clear, especially with the spray administration. The nose drops
cleared more rapidly than the dose administered as a spray.

3.8 PHARMACOKINETICS OF NASAL ABSORPTION

Factors reported to affect the pharmacokinetic parameters following intranasal administration (61,62) are:

1. Physiology-related factors, such as
   a. Speed of mucus flow
   b. Presence of infection
   c. Atmospheric conditions
2. Dosage form-related factors, such as
   a. Concentration of active drug
   b. Physicochemical properties of active drug
   c. Density/viscosity properties of formulation
   d. pH/Toxicity of dosage form
   e. Pharmaceutical excipients used
3. Administration-related factors, such as
   a. Size of droplet
   b. Site of deposition
   c. Mechanical loss into the esophagus
   d. Mechanical loss to other regions in the nose
   e. Mechanical loss anteriorly from nose

The bioavailability of a drug after intranasal administration may be expressed in terms of absolute absorption, Ae, determined from the area under the curve (AUC) following the intravenous (i.v.) and intranasal (i.n.) dose.

$$Ae = \frac{(AUC)\,i.n.\,(Dose)\,i.v.}{(AUC)\,i.v.\,(Dose)\,i.n.} \tag{1}$$

where the AUC was extrapolated to an infinite time following the administration of a single intravenous or intranasal dose.

Ae can also be calculated from the urinary excretion data following intravenous and intranasal administration of a single dose of drug. It is determined from the total amount of drug excreted in the urine in the unmetabolized from (Au^{∞}):

$$Ae = \frac{(Au^{\infty})\,i.n.\,(dose)\,i.v.}{(Au^{\infty})\,i.v.\,(dose)\,i.n.} \tag{2}$$

Equation 2 is valid only when the fraction of drug dose absorbed and excreted in the urine is the same for both intravenous and intranasal routes. If the body is considered to act as a single compartment, the pharmacokinetic behavior of a drug administered by the intranasal route may be calculated according to the following model:

$$X_{IN} \xrightarrow{\text{absorption}} X_B, \quad V \xrightarrow{\text{elimination}} X_E$$

where X_{IN} represents the amount of drug administered to the nasal site, X_B represents the amount of drug in the central compartment, V is the apparent volume of distribution, and X_E is the amount of drug eliminated.

3.8.1 Zero-Order Transnasal Permeation Kinetics

In cases in which the absorption of drugs from the nasal site of administration follows zero-order kintics, e.g., a controlled delivery, the plasma profile of the drug may be described by

$$\frac{dX_B}{dt} = K_0 - K_e X_B \tag{3}$$

in which K_0 is the zero-order absorption rate constant, and K_e is the overall elimination rate constant. Then, the plasma concentration of drug may be expressed as

$$C_p = \frac{K_0}{Cl}\,(1 - e^{-K_e t}) \tag{4}$$

where Cl is the total body clearance, and t represents any specified time interval following the drug administration. The plasma drug level following a zero-order transnasal permeation of the drug would increase to a steady-state plateau level ($C_p{}^{ss}$) and then begin to decline exponentially after time t_p, which is the time when there is no more absorption of the drug from the nasal cavity.

3.8.2 First-Order Transnasal Permeation Kinetics

In cases where the absorption of drugs from the nasal site of administration follows first-order kinetics, the plasma profile of the drug can be described by

$$\frac{dX_B}{dt} = FX_{IN}K_a - K_eX_B \tag{5}$$

where K_a is the first-order absorption rate constant, F is the fraction of applied dose absorbed, X_{IN} is the amount of drug administered to the absorption site, X_B is the amount of drug in the central compartment, K_e is the overall elimination rate constant. Then, the plasma concentration of drug can be expressed as

$$C_p = \frac{FX^0{}_{IN}K_a}{V(K_a - K_e)} \left(e^{-K_et} - e^{-k_at}\right)$$

where $X^0{}_{IN}$ is the initial drug dose applied to the site of absorption at the time zero.

The pharmacokinetic data for the nasal absorption of drugs are listed in Table 3.9. The plasma concentration following intranasal administration shows a concentration profile which is more similar to the intravenous bolus injection than what can be achieved by other nonparenteral routes. The rate of transnasal permeation is very rapid and it takes a very short period of time to reach the peak plasma level. Drugs with poor oral absorption (e.e., insulin, sulbenicillin, cephacetrile, cefazoline, phenol red, and disodium cromoglycate) and drugs with extensive hepatic first-pass metabolism (e.g., progesterone, estradiol, testosterone, hydralazine, propranolol, cocaine, buprenorphine, naloxone, and nitroglycerin) can be rapidly and completely absorbed through the nasal mucosa into the blood circulation. The results indicated that propranolol, hydralazine, clofilium tosylate, ergotamine tartrate, disodium cromoglycate, progesterone, buprenorphine, naloxone, cocaine, hyoscine, atropine, and estradiol are all very rapidly and alsmost completely absorbed through the nasal mucosa (Table 3.9).

Table 3.9 Pharmacokinetic Data for Some Drugs Administered Intranasally

Drugs	Animal model	t_{max} [a]	Relative bioavailability[b] (%)	
			Nasal	Other[c]
Alsactide (109) (ACTH-17)	Rat	1 hr	12	
α^{1-18}-ACTH (110)	Human	<4 hr	12	
Buprenorphine (111)	Rat	2-5 min	95	9.7 (i.d.)
Buserelin (112)	Human	1-6 hr (LH), 2 hr (FSH)		
Calcitonin (113) (with sodium glycocholate)	Human	15 min		
[Asu^{1,7}]-eel calcitonin (114) (with polyacrylic acid)	Rat	30 min (pH 6.5) 1 hr (pH = 5.5 & 7.5)		
Cerulein (115)	Human		1	
Clofilium tosylate (116)	Rat	<10 min	69.6	1.3 (p.o.)
Cocaine	Human (117) Human (118) Human (119) Human (120)	15-60 min 60-120 min 30 min 57.6 (±5.8) min (solution) 35 (±13.2) min (crystalline)		

Drug	Species			
DDAVP (123)	Human (121)	60 min	10-20	
	Human (122)	36.9 (±7.4) min (64 mg)		
		41.2 (±5.5) min (96 mg)		
Cromoglycate disodium (124)	Human	20 min (plasma)	60 (plasma)	
	Rat	15–30 min (bile)	53 (bile)	
Dopamin (125)	Rhesus monkey	15 min		
Enkephalin analogs:				
1) Leucine enkephalin (126)	Rat		<10	
2) DADLE (in saline) (127)	Rat		59	
3) DADLE (1% sodium glycocholate in saline) (127)	Rat		94	
4) Metkephamid (127)	Rat	10 min	102	0.0 (p.o.)
Ergotamine tartrate (128)	Rat	20 min	62	12.7 (i.d.)
Ergotamine tartrate (with caffeine) (128)	Rat	20 min	65.4	5.1 (i.d.)
Gentamycin (129) (with sodium glycocholate)	Human	30 min (n = 4)		
		60 min (n = 3)		
GnRH (130)	Human	<30–90 min (LH)		
		<90–120 min (FSH)		

Table 3.9 (Continued)

Drugs	Animal model	t_{max} [a]	Relative bioavailability[b] (%)	
			Nasal	Other[c]
Glucagon (131) (with sodium glycocholate)	Human	10 min	50	
Growth hormone (132) (hpGRF-40)	Human	<30 min	1-2	
Hydralazine (133) at pH 3.0	Rat	30 min	127	
at pH 6.5		<10 min	83	
at pH 3.0 (+ **PL-9**, 0.5%)		<10 min	113	
Insulin (134)				
with promoter (135)	Rat		5 (no promoter)	
with saponin (1%) (136)	Rat		10	
with sodium glycocholate (1%)	Dog		30	
with BL-9 (1%)			25-33	
with sodium glycocholate (1%) (137)	Human	13.5 min	12.5	
with deoxycholate (138,139)	Human	10 min	10-20	
with hydrophobic bile salts (140)	Human	10 (±1) min	10-20	
with laureth-9 (141)	Human	<15 min	7-10	
freeze-dried powder with Carbopol 934 (142)	Dog	30 min	33	
LHRH (143)	Human	1 hr	1	
Lypressin (144)	Human		13.5	

Meclizine (145)	Rat	8.5 min	51	8
	Dog	11.9 min	89	22
Nafarelin acetate (146,147)	Rhesus monkey	<15 min 30 min	2 5	
Naxolone (111)	Rat	20 min	101	1.5 (i.d.)
Nitroglycerin (148,149)	Human	1-2 min		
Norethisterone	Rhesus monkey (150)	30 min		
	Rhesus monkey (151)	5 min		
Oxytocin	Human (152)	<10-20 min	<1-2	
	Human (153)		1	
	Human (154)			
	Human (155)	<10-15 min		
	Rabbit (156)		1-10	
	Human (157)		1	
Pentagastrin (158)	Human	<10 min	20-33	
Progesterone	Rhesus monkey (151)			
	Rat (159)	6 min	100	1.2 (i.d.)
	Rhesus monkey (160)	5.5 min	91	
	Rabbit (161)	5 min (spray) 20-30 min (device)	82.5 (spray) 72.4 (device)	7.9 (p.o.)

Table 3.9 (Continued)

Drugs	Animal model	t_{max}[a]	Relative bioavailability[b] (%)	
			Nasal	Other[c]
Propranolol	Rat (162)	5 min	100	15 (p.o.)
	Rat (163)	6.3 min	99.9	19 (p.o.)
	Dog (163)	5 min	102.6	6.8 (p.o.)
	Human (164)	5 min	109	
Secretin (165)	Rat		10	
Testosterone (166)	Rat	< 2 min	99 (25 μg)	1 (i.d.)
			90 (50 μg)	
Thyroxine-releasing hormone (TRH) (170)	Rat	15 min	20	

[a]t_{max}: The time required to reach the maximum plasma drug level following intranasal administration.
[b]Bioavailability as compared to intravenous administration
[c]Other routes of administration: Per Oral (p.o.) and intraduodenal (i.d.).

However, intranasal administration of peptide hormones was usually observed to achieve a very low systemic bioavailability as compared to that of intravenous administration. Enhancers, like bile salts, may be used to enhance the nasal absorption and systemic bioavailability for some peptides and proteins, such as insulin (Table. 3.9).

Thus, it can be concluded that intranasal administration is a useful nonparenteral route of administration for systemically effective drugs, which are either subjected to extensive degradation or poor absorption in the gastrointestinal tract and/or subjected to hepatic first-pass metabolism.

3.9 NASAL IRRITATION ASSESSMENT

The assessment of nasal irritation on the nasal mucosa is a difficult subject. There are great anatomical differences between the nasal organs of small laboratory animals and those of man, therefore different conditions for the spread and concentration of drugs administered are to be expected. Nevertheless, the nasal mucosa of experimental animals should be examined histologically to ensure that nasal absorption does not result from any damage to the absorption cells in the nasal mucosa (63). At times, no quantitatively histological damage is found, whereas in other situations an obviously subjective nasal irritation is observed (64).

A characteristic response during exposure of the upper respiratory tract to irritating airborne chemicals is a decrease in respiratory rate. This has been demonstrated for a variety of airborne chemical irritants in numerous species, such as cat, dog, mouse, rat, rabbit, guinea pig, and man (65). This reflex reaction has been exploited as a quantitative measure for evaluation of sensory irritation to airborne substances (66). It simply consists of measuring the percentage decrease in respiratory rate during exposure to various concentrations of a given gas, vapor, or aerosol. A dose-response relationship can be obtained by plotting the maximum percentage decrease from the control value in respiratory rate against the logarithm of the exposure concentrations. Chlorine and hydrogen chloride are well known for their irritating effects on the respiratory tract. To evaluate the degree of sensory irritation in mice, the measurement of the percentage decrease in respiratory rate was utilized in numerous studies (67-69). The response was reported as an upper respiratory tract phenomenon mediated via the trigeminal nerve endings located in the nasal mucosa, and was termed sensory irritation (67).

Although the information about the structure-activity of chemical irritants is limited, and there is no information on the nature of the receptor molecules with which they interact, it seems appropriate to define some possible

Table 3.10 Nasal Trigeminal Stimulation and Reflexes

Receptor →	Afferent Nerve →	Processor →	Efferent Nerves →	Effect on systems
Combination of specific chemicals with receptor molecule of free nerve endings of afferent trigeminal at surface of nasal epithelium	Increase impulse activity in the afferent trigeminal	Integration at CNS level: medulla	Change in activity of phrenic nerve Change in activity of efferent vagus nerve Change in activity of sympathetic splanchnic	Decrease in respiratory rate Decrease in heart rate Vasoconstriction and rise in blood pressure Others: reflex bronchconstriction, general reflex inhibition, bronchial spasm

Sources: Massion et al. (1962), Dawson (1962), Tucker (1962), Widdicombe (1964), Alarie (1966), Cauna et al. (1969), Ulrich et al. (1972).

mechanisms by which chemicals induce a change in the environment of the trigeminal nerve endings which yields a painful sensation of sensory irritation and initiating reflex reactions. The nasal trigeminal stimulation and reflex is illustrated in Table 3.10. Correlation between biological and chemical reactivity data suggests that compounds initiate the sensory irritation reaction by associating with the SH groups or a receptor molecule on the free nerve endings of the afferent trigeminal, which is located at the surface of the nasal mucosa (68).

In the late 1930s, sulfanilamide and its derivatives revolutionized the treatment of many serious bacterial infections. The spectacular results obtained from these drugs when they were administered internally prompted many clinicians to apply them for the local treatment of infections in the nose and paranasal sinuses. The effect of the highly alkaline nature of these solutions on nasal mucosa in the rabbit was studied. The results demonstrated that markedly alkaline preparations usually exert an irritating effect on the nasal tissue, impairing the ciliary function as well as damaging the olfactory lining (70).

That mucous membranes become resistant to the irritating effect of a drug was also reported (71). Sodium sulfathiazole in a 5% solution is an irritant to the nasal mucous membrane in the mouse. There is a marked inflammatory reaction in the first few days of its use. However, the inflammatory reaction subsides and almost no irritating effect is seen after 2 weeks, as noted by lack of epithelial change or purulent exudate. Olfactory membranes are also not permanently injured.

3.10 TOXICOLOGICAL EVALUATIONS

Toxicological evaluations on the nasal route of administration present a number of unique challenges (72). In addition to evaluating adverse local and systemic effects of a drug for intranasal administration, many other issues do arise for special considerations, such as administration of the appropriate dose to support the clinical use of a nasal formulation, the selection of concentration, and the volume of a test drug or formulation used in the animal models, which may differ greatly in nasal anatomy from humans, as well as the method of administration.

Both the drug and the final nasal dosage form for clinical use must be submitted to both acute and subchronic toxicology studies. The ingredients used in the nasal formulation are preferably those of GRAS materials (generally regarded as safe), so no major toxicity issues need to be concerned. If an excipient or an absorption enhancer is required in the formulation and its toxicity is unknown, an extensive program designed to define the absorption, distribution, metabolism, excretion, and toxicity/carcinogenicity of the agent may be in order.

Subchronic toxicity studies usually include a range of doses (or concentrations) and require testing in two different animal species. Other studies, including fertility, teratology, and carcinogenicity, should also be considered. In general, a 30-day toxicity test on the finished product is sufficient to support a single-dose clinical trial, whereas a 90-day toxicity test will be needed to substantiate the multiple-dose clinical trials. The nasal mucosa of the experimental animals should be examined histologically to ensure the integrity of the nasal membranes. The local effects, like irritation, cell damage, and mucociliary clearance, must also be evaluated. Gross examination of the nasal cavity of the subjects should be conducted by an ear, nose, and throat specialist during a clinical study.

REFERENCES

1. Su, K. S. E., and Campanale, K. M. Nasal drug delivery systems: Requirements, development and evaluates, in *Transnasal Systemic Medications* (Y. W. Chien, Ed.), Elsevier, Amsterdam (1985), pp. 139-159.
2. Hussain, A. A., Bawarshi-Nassar, R., and Huang, C. H. Physicochemical consideration in intranasal drug administrations, in *Transnasal Systemic Medications* (Y. W. Chien, Ed.), Elsevier, Amsterdam (1985), pp. 121-137.
3. Corbo, D. C., Huang, Y. C., and Chien, Y. W. Nasal delivery of progestational steroids in ovariectomized rabbits. II. Effect of penetrant hydrophilicity, *Int. J. Pharm.* (in press).
4. Hirai, S., Yashiki, T., Matsuzawa, T., and Mima, H. Absorption of drugs from the nasal mucosa of rat, *Int. J. Pharm., 7*:317 (198!).
5. Gordon, J. E. *Virus and Rickettsial Disease*, Harvard University Press, New Haven, Connecticut (1940).
6. Landsteiner, K., and Levaditi, C. Etude experimental le da la poliomyeliteaigue, *Ann. de Inst. Pasteur, 24*:833 (1910).
7. Klebs, A. C. The historical evolution of veriolation, *Bull. Johns Hopkins Hosp., 24*:69 (1913).
8. Peters, B. A. Intranasal immunisation against scarlet fever, *Lancet, 1*:1035 (1929).
9. Dserzgowsky, S. K. Uber die aktive Immunisierung des menschen gegen Diphtherie, *Immun.-Forsch.(II. Teil), 2*:602 (1910).
10. Zwillinger, H., Die lymphbahnen des oberen nasalschnittes und deren beziehungen zu den perimenigealen lymphraumen, *Arch. Laryngol. Rhinol.*, Bd *26*:S66 (1912).

11. Helenius, A., McCaslin, D. R., Fries, E., and Tanford, C. Properties of detergents, *Methods Enzymol., 56*:734 (1979).
12. Rubinstein, A. Intranasal administration of gentamicin in human subjects, *Antimicrob. Agents. Chemother., 23*:778 (1983).
13. Kaneo, Y. Absorption from the nasal mucous membrane: I. Nasal absorption of hydralazine in rats, *Acta. Pharm. Suec., 20*:379 (1983).
14. Pontiroli, A., Alberetto, M., and Pozza, G. Intranasal calcitonin and plasma calcium concentrations in normal subjects, *Br. Med. J., 290*: 1390 (1985).
15. Morimoto, K., Morisaka, K., and Kamada, A. Enhancement of nasal absorption of insulin and calcitonin using polyacrylic acid gel, *J. Pharm. Pharmacol., 37*:134 (1985).
16. Hussain, A. A., Hirai, S., and BAwarshi, R. Nasal absorption of natural contraceptive steroids in rats—Progesterone absorption, *J. Pharm. Sci., 70*:466 (1981).
17. Hussain, A. A., Kimura, R., and Huang, C. H. Nasal absorption of testosterone in rats, *J. Pharm. Sci., 73*:1300 (1984).
18. Tonndorf, J., Hyde, R. W., Chinn, H. I., and Lett, J. E. Absorption from the nasal mucous membrane: Systemic effect of hyoscine following intranasal administration, *Ann. Otol. Rhinol. Laryngol., 62*:630 (1953).
19. Hyde, R. W., Tonndorf, J., and Chinn, H. I. Absorption from the nasal mucous membrane, *Ann. Otol. Rhinol. Laryngol., 62*:957 (1953).
20. Yokosuka, T., Omori, Y., Hirata, Y., and Hirai, S. Nasal and sublingual administration of insulin in man, *J. Jpn. Diabet. Soc., 20*:146 (1977).
21. Hirai, S., Ikenaga, T., and Matsuzawa, T. Nasal absorption of insulin in dogs, *Diabetes, 27*:296 (1978).
22. Hirai, S., Yashiki, T., and Mima, H. Effect of surfactants on the nasal absorption of insulin in rats, *Int. J. Pharm., 9*:165 (1981).
23. Hirai, S., Yashiki, T., and Mima, H. Mechanisms for the enhancement of the nasal absorption of insulin by surfactants, *Int. J. Pharm., 9*:173 (1981).
24. Moses, A. C., Gordon, G. S., Carey, M. C., and Flier, J. S. Insulin administered intranasally as an insulin-bile salt aerosol: Effectiveness and reproducibility in normal and diabetic subjects, *Diabetes, 32*:1040 (1983).
25. Nagai, T., Nishimoto, Y., Nambu, N., Suzuki, Y., and Sekine, K. Powdered dosage form of insulin for nasal administration, *J. Controlled Release, 1*:15 (1984).
26. Salzman, R., Manson, J. E., Griffing, G. T., Kimmerle, R., Ruderman, N., McCall, A., Stoltz, E. I., Mullin, C., Small, D., Armstrong, J., and Melby, J. C. Intranasal aerosolized insulin: Mixed-meal studies and long-term use in type I diabetes. *N. Engl. J. Med., 312*:1078 (1985).

27. Gordon, G. S., Moses, A. C., Silver, R. D., Flier, J. S., and Carey, M. C. Nasal absorption of insulin: Enhancement by hydrophobic bile salts, *Proc. Natl. Acad. Sci. (U.S.A.)*, *82*:7419 (1985).
28. Mygind, N., and Vesterhauge, S. Aerosol distribution in the nose, *Rhinology*, *XI*:79 (1978).
29. Mygind, N. *Nasal Allergy*, 2nd ed., Blackwell, Oxford, England (1979), pp. 257-270.
30. Proetz, A. W. *Applied Physiology of the Nose*, Annals Publishing Company, St. Louis (1953).
31. Unno, T., Okude, Y., Yanai, O., and Onodera, S. Distribution of beclomethasone dipropionate aerosol particles in the nasal cavity, *Jpn. J. Otol. (Tokyo)*, *85*:277 (1982).
32. Hardy, J. G., Lee, S. W., and Wilson, C. G. Intranasal drug delivery by spray and drops, *J. Pharm. Pharmacol.*, *37*:294 (1985).
33. Hussain, A. A., Hirai, S., and Bawarshi, R. Nasal absorption of propranolol from different dosage forms by rats and dogs, *J. Pharm. Sci.*, *69*:1411 (1980).
34. Buri, P. P. Hydrogels destines a la muqueuse nasal controled physiologique, *Pharm. Acta Helv.*, *41*:88 (1966).
35. Buri, P. P., Gumma, A., and Mirimanoff, A. Nouvelles observations sur le controle physiologique d'un hydrogel destine a la muqueuse nasal, *Pharm. Acta Helv.*, *41*:480 (1966).
36. Corbo, D. C., Huang, Y. C., and Chien, Y. W. Nasal delivery of progestational steroids in ovariectomized rabbits. I. Progesterone-comparison of pharmacokinetics with intravenous and oral administration, *Int. J. Pharm. 46*:133 (1988).
37. Hounam, R. F., Black, A., and Walsh, M. The deposition of aerosol particles in the nasopharyngeal region of the human respiratory tract, *Aerosol Sci.*, *2*:47 (1971).
38. Proctor, D. F. The upper airways. 1. Nasal physiology and defense of the lungs, *Am. Rev. Respir. Dis.*, *115*:97 (1977).
39. Hatch, T. F. Distribution and deposition of the inhaled particles in respiratory tract, *Bact. Rev.*, *25*:237 (1961).
40. Proctor, D. F. Nasal physiology in intranasal drug administration, in *Transnasal Systemic Medications* (Y. W. Chien, Ed.), Elsevier, Amsterdam (1985), pp. 101-106.
41. Stuart, B. O. Deposition of inhaled aerosols, *Arch. Intern. Med.*, *131*:60 (1973).
42. Wolfsdorf, J., Swift, D. L., and Avery, M. E. Mist therapy reconsidered: An evaluation of the respiratory deposition of labelled water aerosols produced by jet and ultrasonic nebulizer, *Pediatrics*, *43*:799 (1969).
43. Dirnagel, K., TröpfchengröBen-analyse einem treibgas-zerstäuber zur behandlung von rhinopathien, *Arzneim. Forsch.*, *13*:497 (1963).

44. Yu, C. D., Jones, R. E., Wright, J., and Henesian, M. Characterization of the dose delivery and spray pattern of a metered-dose flunisolide nasal delivery spray, *Drug Devel. Ind. Pharm., 9*:473 (1983).
45. Task Group on Lung Dynamics, *Health Phys., 12*:173 (1966).
46. Hiller, F. C., Mazumder, M. K., Wilson, J. D., and Bone, R. C. Aerodynamic size distribution, hygroscopicity and deposition estimation of beclomethasone dipropionate aerosol, *J. Pharm. Pharmacol., 32*:605 (1980).
47. Orr, C., Hurd, F. K., and Corbett, W. J. Aerosol size and relative humidity, *J. Colloid Sci., 13*:472 (1958).
48. Davis, S. S., and Bubb, M. D. Physicochemical studies on aerosol solutions for drug delivery. III. The effect of relative humidity on the particle size of inhalation aerosols, *Int. J. Pharm., 1*:303 (1978).
49. Yu, C. D., Jones, R. E., and Henesian, M. Cascade impactor method for the droplet size characterization of a metered-dose nasal spray, *J. Pharm. Sci., 73*:344 (1984).
50. Sciarra, J. J., McGinley, P., and Izzo, L. Determination of particle size distribution of selected aerosol cosmetics. I. Hair sprays, *J. Soc. Cosmet. Chem., 20*:385 (1969).
51. Sciarra, J. J., and Adelman, D. Determination of particle size distribution of selected aerosol cosmetics. II. Cascade impactor use in fluorometric and weight-by-difference methods, *J. Soc. Cosmet. Chem., 22*: 867 (1971).
52. Swift, D. L. Aerosol deposition and clearance in the human upper airways, *Ann. Biomed. Eng., 9*:593 (1981).
53. Hallworth, G. M., and Malton, C. A. Recent in vivo methods for evaluating the deposition of aerosols in the respiratory tract, *Pharmacy Int. 00*:61 (1984).
54. Lendahl, H. D. On the removal of airborne droplets by human respiratory tract: The nasal passages, *Bull. Math. Biophys., 12*:161 (1950).
55. Scott, W. R., Taulbee, D. B., and Yu, C. P. Theoretical study of nasal deposition, *Bull. Math., Biol., 40*:581 (1978).
56. Pattle, R. E. Retention of gases and particles in the human nose, in *Inhaled Particles and Vapors* (C. N. Davies, Ed.), Pergamon, (1961), pp. 302-311.
57. Fry, F. A., and Black, A. Regional deposition and clearance of particles in the human nose, *J. Aerosol Sci., 4*:113 (1973).
58. Mygind, N. *Nasal Allergy*, 2nd ed., Blackwell, Oxford, England (1979), pp. 260-262.
59. Aoki, F. Y., and Crawley, J. C. W. Distribution and removal of human serum albumin-technetium[99m] instilled intranasally, *Br. J. Clin. Pharmacol., 3*:869 (1976).

60. Unno, T., Hokunan, K., Yanai, O., and Onodera, S. Deposition of sprayed particles in the nasal cavity, *Auris Nasus Larynx, 10*:109 (1983).

61. Colaizzi, J. L. Pharmacokinetics of intranasal drug administration, in *Transnasal Systemic Medications* (Y. W. Chien, Ed.), Elsevier, Amsterdam (1985), pp. 107–119.

62. Freestone, D. S., and Wingerg, A. L. The administration of drugs and vaccines by the intranasal route, *Br. J. Clin. Pharmacol., 3*:827 (1976).

63. Su, K. S. E., Campanale, K. M., and Gries, C. L. Nasal drug delivery system of a quarternary ammonium compound: Clofilium tosylate, *J. Pharm. Sci., 73*:1251 (1984).

64. Su, K. S. E., and Campanale, K. M. Unpublished data.

65. Barrow, C. S., Alarie, Y., Warrick, J. C., and Stock, M. F. Comparison of the sensory irritation response in mice to choline and hydrogen chloride, *Arch. Environ. Health, 32*:68 (1971).

66. Alarie, Y. Sensory irritation by airborne chemicals, *CRC Crit. Rev. Toxicol., 2*:299 (1973).

67. Alarie, Y. Irritating properties of airborne materials to the upper respiratory tract, *Arch. Environ. Health, 13*:433 (1966).

68. Alarie, Y. Sensory irritation of the upper airways by airborne chemicals, *Toxicol. Appl. Pharmacol., 24*:279 (1973).

69. Alarie, Y., and Keller, L. W. Sensory irritation by capsaicin, *Environ. Physiol. Biochem., 3*:169 (1973).

70. Fabricant, N. D. Significance of the pH of nasal secretions in situ, *Arch. Otolaryngol., 34*:150 (1941).

71. Hunnicut, L. G. Reaction of mucous membranes to five percent solution of sodium sulfathiazole, *Arch. Otolaryngol., 36*:837 (1942).

72. Dorato, M. A. Nasal delivery of peptides and proteins: Toxicologic considerations, presented at a *Symposium on Nasal Administration of Peptide and Protein Drugs*, Princeton, New Jersey, October 1987.

73. Kristensson, K., and Olsson, Y. Uptake of exogenous proteins in mouse olfactory cells, *Acta Neuropathol. (Berl.), 19*:145 (1971).

74. Svedberg, T., and Nichols, J. G. The molecular weight of egg albumin I in electrolyte-free condition, *J. Am. Chem. Soc., 48*:3081 (1926).

75. Yoffey, J. M., Sullivan, E. R., and Drinker, C. K. The lymphatic from the nose and pharynx: The absorption of certain proteins, *J. Exp. Med., 68*:941 (1938).

76. HochstraBer, M. K. Tierexperimentelle untersuchungen zur aufnahme von amino sauren nach applikation auf die nasenschleimhaut, *Z. Laryngol. Rhinol. Otol., 52*:144 (1973).

77. Weiss, P., and Holland, Y. Neuronal dynamics and axonal flow, II. The olfactory nerve as model test object, *Proc. Natl. Acad. Sci. (U.S.A.), 57*:258 (1967).

78. Schulz, R. Z., Warren, M. F., and Drinker, C. K. The passage of rabbit

virulent type III pneumococci from the respiratory tract of rabbits into the lymphatics and blood, *J. Exp. Med., 68*:251 (1938).

79. Bloomfield, A. L. The fate of bacteria introduced into the upper air passages. II. E. coli and staphylococcus albus, *Bull. Johns Hopkins Hosp., 31*:14 (1920).

80. Su, K. S. E., Campanale, K. M., and Gries, C. L. Nasal drug delivery system of a quaternary ammonium compound: Clofilium tosylate, *J. Pharm. Sci., 73*:1251 (1984).

81. Anand Kumar, T. C., David, G. F. X., Kumar, K., Umberkoman, B., and Krishnamoorthy, M. S. A new approach to fertility regulation by interfering with neuroendocrine pathways, in *Proceedings of International Symposium on "Neuroendocrine Regulation of Fertility"* (T. C. Anand Kumar, Ed.), Karger, Basel (1976), pp. 314-322.

82. Yoffey, J. M. The lymphatic pathway for absorption from the nasopharynx, *Lancet 1*:530 (1941).

83. Yoffey, J. M., and Drinker, C. K. The lymphatic pathway from the nose and pharynx: The absorption of dyes, *J. Exp. Med., 68*:629 (1938).

84. Clark, W. E., and Le, G. Anatomical investigation into the routes by which infections may pass from the nasal cavities into the brain, in *Great Britain Report Public Health and Medical Subjects*, Ministry of Health, London, No. 54 (1929).

85. Rake, G. Absorption through the nasal mucosa of mice, *Proc. Soc. Exp. Biol. Med., 34*:369 (1936).

86. Faber, W. M. The nasal mucosa and the subarachnoid space, *Am. J. Anat., 62*:121 (1937).

87. Ohman, L., Hahnenberger, R., and Johansson, E. D. B. 17β-estradiol levels in blood and cerebrospinal fluid after ocular and nasal administration in women and female rhesus monkeys (*Macaca mulatta*), *Contraception, 22*:349 (1980).

88. Anand Kumar, T. C., David, G. F. X., Umberkoman, B., and Saini, K. D. Uptake of radioactivity by body fluids and tissues in rhesus monkeys after intravenous injection or intransasal spray of tritium-labeled estradiol and progesterone, *Curr. Sci., 43*:435 (1974).

89. Anand Kumar, T. C., David, G. F. X., and Puri, V. Nasal spray contraceptive, in *Recent Advances in Reproduction and Regulation of Fertility*, (G. P. Talwar, Ed.), Elsevier/North Holland, New York (1979).

90. Gopinath, P. G., Gopinath, G., and Kumar, T. C. A. Target site of intranasally sprayed substances and their transport across the nasal mucosa: A new insight into the intranasal route of drug delivery, *Curr. Ther. Res., 23*:596 (1978).

91. Dzerniawska, A. Experimental investigations on the penetration of [198]Au from nasal mucous membrane into cerebrospinal fluid, *Acta Otolaryngol. (Stockh.), 70*:58 (1970).

92. Blumgart, H. L. A study of the mechanism of absorption of substances from the nasopharynx, *Arch. Int. Med., 33*:415 (1924).

93. Blumgart, H. L. Lead studies. VI. Absorption of lead by the upper respiratory passages, *J. Ind. Hyg., 5*:153 (1923).

94. Cuddihy, R. G., and Ozog, J. A. Nasal absorption of CsCl, $SrCl_2$, $BaCl_2$ and $CeCl_3$ in Syrian hamsters, *Health Phys. Pergamon Press, 25*:219 (1973).

95. Orosz, A., Foldes, I., Kosa, C. S., and Toth, G. Radioactive isotope studies of the connection between the lymph circulation of the nasal mucosa, the cranial cavity and cerebrospinal fluid, *Acta. Physiol. Acad. Sci. Hung., 11*:75 (1957).

96. McAuliffe, G. W., and Mueller, G. C. Aerosol penicillin administered in paranasal sinusitis with balanced suction and pressure, *Arch. Otolaryngol., 46*:67 (1947).

97. Johnson, R. T. The pathogenesis of herpes virus encephalitis, *J. Exp. Med., 119*:343 (1964).

98. Burnet, F. M., and Lush, D. Studies on experimental herpes infection in mice, using the chorio-allantoic technique, *J. Pathol. Bacteriol., 49*: 241 (1939),

99. Slavin, H. B., and Berry, G. P. Studies on herpetic infection in mice, *J. Exp. Med., 78*:315 (1943).

100. Friedemann, U. Permeability of the blood-brain barrier to neurotropic viruses, *Arch. Pathol., 35*:912 (1943).

101. Savin, A. B., and Olitsky, P. K. Influence of host factors on neuroinvasiveness of vesicular stomatitis virus, *J. Exp. Med., 66*:15 (1937).

102. Blumgart, H. L. A study of the mechanism of absorption of substances from the nasopharynx, *Arch. Intern. Med., 33*:415 (1924).

103. Flexner, S. The mode of infection in epidemic poliomyelitis, *J.A.M.A., 59*:1371 (1912).

104. Flexner, S., and Clark, P. F. A note on the mode of infection in epidemic poliomyelitis, *Proc. Soc. Exp. Biol. Med., 10*:1 (1912).

105. Clark, P. F., Fraser, F. R., and Amoss, H. L. The relation to the blood of the virus of epidemic poliomyelitis, *J. Exp. Med., 19*:223 (1917).

106. Yoffey, J. M., and Sullivan, E. R. The lymphatic pathway from the nose and pharynx, *J. Exp. Med., 69*:133 (1939).

107. Yoffey, J. M. Passage of fluid and other substances through the nasal mucosa, *J. Laryngol. Otolaryngol., 72*:377 (1958).

108. McCarrell, J. D. Lymphatic absorption from the nasopharynx, *Am. J. Physiol., 126*:20 (1931).

109. Baumann, G., Walser, A., Desaullels, P. A., Paesi, F. J. A., and Geller, L. Corticotropic action of an intranasally applied synthetic ACTH derivative, *Endocrinol. Metab., 42*:60 (1976).

110. Keenan, J., Thompson, J. K. B., Chamberlain, M. A., and Besser, G. M.,

Prolonged corticotrophic action of a synthetic substituted $\alpha^{1\text{-}18}$ ACTH, *Br. Med. J., 8*:742 (1971).

111. Hussain, A., Kimura, R., Huang, C. H., and Kashihara, T. Nasal absorption of naloxone and buprenorphine in rats, *Int. J. Pharm., 21*:233 (1984).
112. Wiegelman, W., Solbach, H. G., Kley, H. K., Nieschlag, E., and Kruskemper, H. L. A new LHRH analogue: d-Ser $(TBU)^6$-EA^{10} LHRH effects on gondotrophin and gonadal steroid secretion in men after intravenous and intranasal application, *Acta Endocrinol.* (Suppl.), *208*: 37 (1977).
113. Pontiroli, A., Albertto, M., and Possa, G. Intranasal calcitonin and plasma calcium concentrations in normal subjects, *Br. Med. J., 290*: 1390 (1985).
114. Morimoto, K., Morisaka, K., and Kamada, A. Enhancement of nasal absorption of insulin and calcitonin using polyacrylic acid gel, *J. Pharm. Pharmacol., 37*:134 (1985).
115. Agosti, A., and Bertaccini, G. Nasal absorption of caerulain, *Lancet 1*: 580 (1969).
116. Su, K. S. E., Campanale, K. M., and Gries, C. L. Nasal drug delivery system of a quaternary ammonium compound: Clofilium tosylate, *J. Pharm. Sci., 73*:1251 (1984).
117. Dyke, C. V., Barash, P. G., Jatlow, P., and Byck, R. Cocaine: Plasma concentration after intranasal application in man, *Science, 195*:859 (1977).
118. Byke, C. V., Jatlow, P., Ungerer, J., Barash, P. G., and Byck, R. Oral cocaine: Plasma concentrations and central effects, *Science, 200*:211 (1978).
119. Javaid, J. I., Fischman, M. W., Schuster, C. R., Dekirmenjian, H., and Davis, J. M. Cocaine plasma concentration: Relation to physiological and subjective effects in humans, *Science, 202*:227 (1978).
120. Wilkinson, P., Dyke, C. V., Jatlow, P., Barash, P., and Byck, R. Intranasal and oral cocaine kinetics, *Clin. Pharmacol. Ther., 27*:386 (1980).
121. Dyke, C. V., Ungerer, J., Jatlow, P., Barash, P., and Byck, R. Intranasal cocaine: Dose relationship of psychological effects and plasma levels, *Int. J. Psychiatry Med., 12*:1 (1982).
122. Javaid, J. I., Musa, M. N., Fischman, M., Schuster, C. R., and Davis, J. M. Kinetics of cocaine in humans after intravenous and intranasal administration, *Biopharm. Drug Dispos., 4*:9 (1983).
123. Anderson, K. E., and Arner, B. Effects of DDAVP, a synthetic analogue of vasopressin in patients with cranial diabetes insipidus, *Acta Med. Scand., 192*:21 (1982).
124. Fisher, A. N., Brown, K., Davis, S. S. Parr, G. D., and Smith, D. A. The nasal absorption of sodium cromoglycate in the albino rat, *J. Pharm. Pharmacol., 37*:38 (1985).

125. Anand Kumar, T. C., David, G. F. X., Kumar, K., Umberkoman, B., and Krishnamoorthy, M. S. A new approach with neuroendocrine pathways, in *Neuroendocrine Regulation of Fertility* (T. C. Anand Kumar, Ed.), Karger, Basal (1976), p. 314.
126. Hussain, A., Faraj, J., Aramaki, Y., and Truelove, J. E. Hydrolysis of leucine enkephalin in the nasal cavity of the rat—A possible factor in the low bioavailability of nasally administered peptides, *Biochem. Biophys. Res. Commun., 133*:923 (1985).
127. Su, K. S. E., Campanel, K. M., Mendelsohn, L. G., Kerchner, G. A., and Gries, C. L. Nasal delivery of polypeptides. I: Nasal absorption of enkephalins in rats, *J. Pharm. Sci., 74*:394 (1985).
128. Hussain, A., Kimura, R., Huang, C. H., and Mustafa, R. Nasal absorption of ergotamine tartrate in rats, *Int. J. Pharm., 21*:289 (1984).
129. Rubinstein, A. Intranasal administration of gentamicin in human subjects, *Antimicrob. Agents Chemother., 23*:778 (1983).
130. Potashnik, G., Ben-Adereth, N., Lunenfeld, B., and Rofe, C. Assessment of pituitary response to nasal application of synthetic gonadotropin-releasing hormone in men, *Fertil. Steril., 28*:650 (1977).
131. Pontiroli, A. E., Alberetto, M., and Pozza, G. Intranasal glucagon raises blood glucose concentrations in healthy volunteers, *Br. Med. J., 287*:462 (1983).
132. Evans, W. S., Borges, J. L. C., Kaiser, D. L., Vance, M. L., Seller, R. P., Macleod, R. M., Vale, W., Rivier, J., and Thorner, M. O. Intranasal administration of human pancreatic tumor GH-releasing factor-40 stimulates GH release in normal men, *J. Clin. Endocrinol. Metab., 57*:1081 (1983).
133. Kaneo, Y. Absorption from the nasal mucosa membrane. I. Nasal absorption of hydralazine in rats, *Acta Pharm. Suec., 20*:379 (1983).
134. Hirai, S., Yashiki, T., Matsuzawa, T., and Mima, H. Absorption of drugs from the nasal mucosa of rat, *Int. J. Pharm., 7*:317 (1981).
135. Hirai, S., Yashiki, T., and Mima, H. Effect of surfactants on the nasal absorption of insulin in rats, *Int. J. Pharm., 9*:165 (1981).
136. Hirai, S., Ikenaga, T., and Matsuzawa, T. Nasal absorption of insulin in dogs, *Diabetes, 27*:296 (1978).
137. Pontiroli, A. E., Alberetoo, M., Secchi, A., Dossi, G., Bosi, I., and Pozza, G. Insulin given intranasally induces hypoglycemia in normal and diabetic subjects, *Br. Med. J., 284*:303 (1983).
138. Moses, A. C., Gordon, G. S., Carey, M. C., and Flier, J. S. Insulin administered intranasally as an insulin-bile salt aerosol: Effectiveness and reproducibility in normal and diabetic subjects, *Diabetes, 32*:1040 (1983).
139. Flier, J. S., Moses, A. C., Gordon, G. S., Silver, R. S., and Carey, M. C. Intranasal adminstration of insulin: Efficacy of mechanism, in *Trans-*

nasal Systemic Medications (Y. W. Chien, Ed.), Elsevier, Amsterdam (1985), p. 217.

140. Gordon, G. S., Moses, A. C., Silver, R. D., Flier, J. S., and Carey, M. C. Nasal absorption of insulin: Enhancement by hydrophobic bile salts, *Proc. Natl. Acad. Sci. (U.S.A.)*, *82*:7419 (1985).

141. Salzman, R., Manson, J. E., Griffing, G. T., Kimmerele, R., Ruderman, N., McCall, A., Stoltz, E. I., Mullin, C., Small, D., Armstrong, J., and Melby, J. C. Intranasal aerosolized insulin: Mixed-meal studies and long-term use in type I diabetes, *N. Engl. J. Med.*, *312*:1078 (1985).

142. Nagai, T., Nishimoto, Y., Nambu, N., Suzuki, Y., and Sekine, K. Powder dosage form of insulin for nasal administration, *J. Controlled Release*, *1*:15 (1984).

143. Fink, G., Gennser, G., Liedholm, P., Thorell, J., and Mulder, J. Comparison of plasma levels of luteinizing hormone-releasing hormone in men after intravenous administration, *J. Endocrinol.*, *63*:351 (1974).

144. Moses, A. M. Synthetic lysine vasopressin nasal spray in the treatment of diabetes insipidus, *Clin. Pharmacol. Ther.*, *5*:422 (1964).

145. Chovan, J. P., Klett, R. P., and Rakieten, N., Comparison of meclizine levels in the plasma of rats and dogs after intranasal, intravenous and oral administration, *J. Pharm. Sci.*, *74*:1111 (1985).

146. Anik, S. T., McRae, G., Nerenberg, C., Worden, A., Foreman, J., Hwang, J. Y., Kushinsky, S., Jones, R. E., and Vickery, B. Nasal absorption of nafarelin acetate, the decapeptide [D-Nal(2)[6]] LHRH in rhesus monkeys I, *J. Pharm. Sci.*, *73*:684 (1984).

147. Vickery, B. H., Anik, S., Chaplin, M., and Henzl, M. Intranasal administration of nafarelin acetate: Contraception and therapeutic application, in *Transnasal Systemic Medications* (Y. W. Chien, Ed.), Elsevier, Amsterdam (1985), pp. 201–215.

148. Hill, A. B., Bowley, C. J., Nahrwold, M. L., Knight, P. R., Tait, A. R., Taylor, M. D., Kirsch, M. M., and Denlinger, J. K. Intranasal administration of nitroglycerin, *Anesthesiology*, *51*:S67 (1979).

149. Hill, A. B., Bowley, C. J., Nahrwold, M. L., Knight, P. R., Kirsch, M. M., and Denlinger, J. K. Intranasal adminstration of nitroglycerin, *Anesthesiology*, *54*:346 (1981).

150. Ohman, L., Hahnenberger, R., and Johansson, E. D. B. Topical administration of progestational steroids in the eye and nose—A rapid absorption to the blood, *Contraception*, *18*:171 (1978).

151. Anand Kumar, T. C., David, G. F. X., and Puri, V. Nasal spray contraceptives, in *Recent Advances in Reproduction and Regulation of Fertility* (G. P. Talwar, Ed.), Elsevier, Amsterdam (1979), p. 49.

152. Hendricks, C., and Gabel, R. A. Use of intranasal oxytocin in obstetrics. I. Laboratory evaluation, *Am. J. Obstet. Gynecol.*, *79*:780 (1960).

153. Hendricks, C. H., and Pose, S. V. Intranasal oxytocin in obstetrics, *J.A.M.A., 175*:384 (1961).
154. Stander, R. W., Thompson, J. F., and Gibbs, C. P. Evaluation of intranasal oxytocin in amniotic fluid pressure recordings, *Am. J. Obstet. Gynecol., 85*:193 (1963).
155. Devoe, K., Rigsby, W. C., and McDaniels, B. A. The effect of intranasal oxytocin on the pregnant uterus, *Am. J. Obstet. Gynecol., 97*:208 (1967).
156. Berde, B., and Cerletti, A. Uber die wirkung pharmakologischer oxytocindosen auf die milchdruse, *Acta Endocrinol. (Copenh.), 34*:543 (1960).
157. Sandholm, L. E. The effect of intravenous and intranasal oxytocin on intrammary pressure during early lactation, *Acta Obstet. Gynecol. Scand., 47*:145 (1968).
158. Wormsley, K. G. Pentagastrin snuff, *Lancet 1*:57 (1968).
159. Hussain, A. A., Hirai, S., and Bawarski, R. Nasal absorption of natural contraceptive steroids in rats—Progesterone absorption, *J. Pharm. Sci., 70*:466 (1981).
160. Anand Kumar, T. C., David, G. F. X., Sankaranarayanan, A., Puri, V., and Sundrani, K. R. Pharmacokinetics of progesterone after its administration to ovariectomized rhesus monkeys by injection, infusion or nasal spraying, *Proc. Natl. Acad. Sci. (U.S.A.), 79*:4185 (1982).
161. Corbo, D. C., Huang, Y. C., and Chien, Y. W. Nasal delivery of progestational steroids in ovariectomized rabbits. I. Progesterone—Comparison of pharmacokinetics with intravenous and oral administration, *Int. J. Pharm., 46*:133 (1988).
162. Hussain, A. A., Hirai, S., and Bawarshi, R. Nasal absorption of propranolol in rats, *J. Pharm. Sci., 68*:1196 (1979).
163. Hussain, A. A., Hirai, S., and Bawarshi, R. Nasal absorption of propranolol from different dosage forms by rats and dogs, *J. Pharm. Sci., 69*:1411 (1980).
164. Hussain, A. A., Foster, T., Hirai, S., Kashihara, T., Batenhorst, R., and Jones, M. Nasal absorption of propranolol in humans, *J. Pharm. Sci., 69*:1240 (1980).
165. Ohwaki, T., Ando, H., Watanabe, S., and Miyake, Y. Effect of dose, pH and osmolarity on nasal absorption of secretin in rats, *J. Pharm. Sci., 74*:550 (1985).
166. Hussain, A. A., Kimura, R., and Huang, C. H. Nasal absorption of testosterone in rats, *J. Pharm. Sci., 73*:1300 (1984).
167. Sandow, J., and Petri, W. Intranasal administration of peptides: Biological activity and therapeutic efficacy, in *Transnasal Systemic Medications* (Y. W. Chien, Ed.), Elsevier, Amsterdam (1985), pp. 183-199.

4
Intranasal Delivery of Peptide/Protein Drugs

Since amino acids are the building blocks in peptides, proteins, and the more complex biological products consisting of protein chains, the intranasal delivery of amino acids is discussed in this chapter together with peptides, proteins, and other biological products despite the fact that the amino acids are not macromolecules. In general, all except the small peptides are referred to as *polypeptides*. As the peptide size increases, a point is reached when general usage suggests that the term *protein* be used instead of polypeptide. The distinction between the terms protein and polypeptide is not clear-cut, but in general a peptide larger than 70 amino acid residues is referred to as a protein.

4.1 AMINO ACIDS

The nasal absorption of amino acids in the rabbit was found to be dependent upon the physicochemical characteristics of the individual amino acids (1). Amino acids were reportedly absorbed into the nasal mucosa and penetrated into the cells by an active transport process resembling that in the intestinal epithelium.

L-Tyrosine has been studied as a model amino acid to examine the effects of polarity and the absorption pathway by a carrier-mediated mechanism on the nasal absorption (2-4). L-Tyrosine has three polar functional groups, which can produce a significant effect on its nasal absorption. The extent of nasal absorption of L-tyrosine in rats was found to be about 13% at both pH 4 and 7.4 (4). However, the nasal absorption was found to be concentration dependent. If the mechanism of nasal absorption for amino acid follows the Michaelis-Menten process, then Equation (1) is valid:

$$\frac{1}{R_i} = \frac{K_m}{V_{max} S} + \frac{1}{V_{max}} \tag{1}$$

A plot of the reciprocal of the initial rate of disappearance $(R_i)^{-1}$ versus the reciprocal of the initial concentration of the substrate $(S)^{-1}$, like L-tyrosine, should yield a straight line (Figure 4.1). From the slope and intercept of this linear Lineweaver-Burk plot, K_m and V_{max} can be calculated, and the values were found to be 4.8×10^{-4} M and 3.39×10^{-4} M/hr, respectively, for L-tyrosine. The data indicated that L-tyrosine is absorbed from the nasal cavity in its zwitterion form and that its absorption is probably via a carrier-mediated process.

To determine the contribution of the hydroxyl group in the L-tyrosine molecule, O-acyl derivatives of L-tyrosine were prepared, and their nasal absorption has been studied (2,4). The results showed that the apparent rates of nasal absorption for the O-acyl esters of L-tyrosine are not significantly different from that of L-tyrosine, despite the fact that their partition coefficients (in octanol/water) are considerably different (Table 4.1). The observation may be attributed to the similarity in the ionic character of these compounds.

The significance of the ionic character was further examined using the carboxylic acid esters of L-tyrosine and N-acetyl-L-tyrosine. The results indicated that these ester derivatives exhibit both a higher partition coefficient and a greater absorption rate (4-10 times) than L-tyrosine, the parent amino acid. However, the acylation of L-tyrosine at the amino group neither changed the partition coefficient nor enhanced the rate of nasal absorption. These esters were found to be hydrolyzed enzymatically to regenerate L-tyrosine in the presence of pseudocholinesterase and human plasma. The data suggested that the nasal absorption of L-tyrosine may be facilitated by the formation of carboxylic acid esters as a result of the masking of the negative charge on the carboxylate moiety. This negative charge has contributed to the similar rate of nasal absorption among L-tyrosine, O-acetyl-L-tyrosine and N-acetyl-L-tyrosine, despite the significant variation in their partition coefficients.

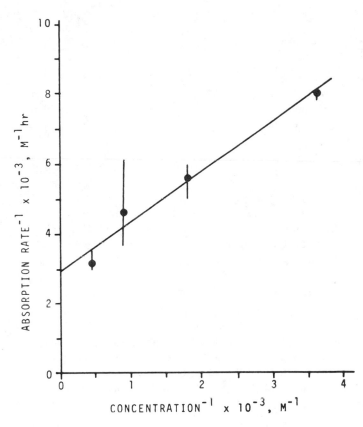

Figure 4.1 Linear dependency of in situ nasal absorption rate of L-tyrosine on a L-tyrosine concentration (at pH 7.4 and 37°C). Values are Mean ± SEM (n = 4-5). (From Ref. 2, used with permission.)

Table 4.1 Apparent Partition Coefficients and Observed Nasal Absorption Rate Constants of L-Tyrosine and Its O-Acyl Derivatives

Compound	Apparent partition coefficinet	K_{obs}, min^{-1} (mean ± SEM)
L-Tyrosine	0.0256	0.0023
O-Acetyl-L-tyrosine	0.0468	0.0026
O-Valeryl-L-tyrosine	1.17	0.0029

Source: From Ref. 2, used with permission.

4.2 PEPTIDES

The nasal absorption of peptides showed a lower bioavailability than that of amino acids. This low nasal bioavailability was shown to be unrelated to the size of the peptide, but rather was attributed to the following factors: high polarity, possible absorption via a specific carrier-mediated mechanism, possible hydrolysis in the nasal cavity, and/or the combination of the factors outlined above (2).

4.2.1 Dipeptides

The nasal absorption of a dipeptide, L-tyrosyl-L-tyrosine and its methyl ester, has also been studied to determine whether a similar esterification can also enhance the absorption of peptides as it did in the amino acids (2). The results demonstrated that L-tyrosyl-L-tyrosine undergoes considerable hydrolysis in the perfusate owing to the presence of peptidase in the nasal cavity, and the concentration of L-tyrosine formed is dependent upon the initial concentration of L-tyrosyl-L-tyrosine. The more lipophilic methyl derivative was also hydrolyzed rapidly to l-tyrosine and its methyl ester. Another two dipeptides, L-glycyl-L-tyrosine and L-glycyl-L-tyrosinamide, were also found to be cleaved enzymatically in the perfusate (2). In summary, all the studies conducted to date suggested a poor bioavailability for peptides as the result of hydrolysis by the peptidase in the nasal cavity during the absorption process.

4.2.2 Thyrotropin-Releasing Hormone

Thyrotropin-releasing hormone (TRH) is a tripeptide neurotransmitter which exists in the brain as well as in the peripheral neural tissue. It has been frequently used in the diagnosis of thyroid functions.

The nasal absorption of TRH has been studied in rats by instillation through a polyethylene-sheated cannula into one nostril (5). The results showed a rapid increase in the serum thyroid-stimulating hormone (TSH) concentration with its peak level being reached at 15 min. The nasal bioavailability of TRH was estimated to be about 20% (compared with i.v. administration). The results showed that intranasal administration of TRH yields a rapid stimulation of the TSH release with a maximum level achieved within 20-30 min (5). It was also reported that the use of TRH-nasal spray for clinical diagnosis of thyroid functions can reduce its side effects, such as the flushing and hypotensive reactions associated with the intravenous TRH test.

4.2.3 Enkephalins

Enkephalins are a group of naturally occuring pentapeptides isolated from extracts of the brain and pituitary glands possessing pharmacological properties similar to those of opioids. The feasibility of nasal absorption of the following enkephalin analogs has been evaluated.

4.2.3.1 DADLE

The nasal absorption of DADLE (Tyr—D—Ala—Gly—L—Phe—D—Leu—OH) has been investigated in rats (6). The results showed that nasal absorption has achieved a relative bioavailability of 59% as compared to subcutaneous administration; when 1% sodium glycocholate is incorporated into the formulation, the nasal bioavailability is enhanced to 94% (6) (Table 4.2). The plasma concentration profiles of DADLE in rats following intranasal and intravenous administration exhibited triphasic elimination kinetics.

4.2.3.2 Metkephamid

The intranasal delivery of metkephamid, a stable analog of enkephalins, was observed to produce a much higher plasma concentration than that of subcutaneous administration in rats (6) (Figure 4.2). The AUC (area under the plasma concentration versus time curve) of metkephamid from nasal absorp-

Table 4.2 Comparison of Blood Levels of Total Radioactivity Equivalents[a] of [^{3}H] DADLE in Rats After Various Routes of Administration[b]

Route of administration	n	AUC (μg · min/g ± SEM)	Relative bioavailability[c] (%)
Subcutaneous			
[^{3}H] DADLE in saline	3	590.4 (±41.4)	100
Intranasal			
[^{3}H] DADLE in saline	3	348.1 (±48.3)	59.0
[^{3}H] DADLE in saline plus 1% sodium glycocholate	4	555.9 (±85.1)	94.1

[a]Expressed as microgram equivalents in tritium in blood.
[b]2 mg/kg dose (the dose volume was maintained at 0.1 ml).
[c]$(AUC)_{in}/(AUC)_{sc} \times 100\%$.
Source: Modifed from Ref. 6, used with permission.

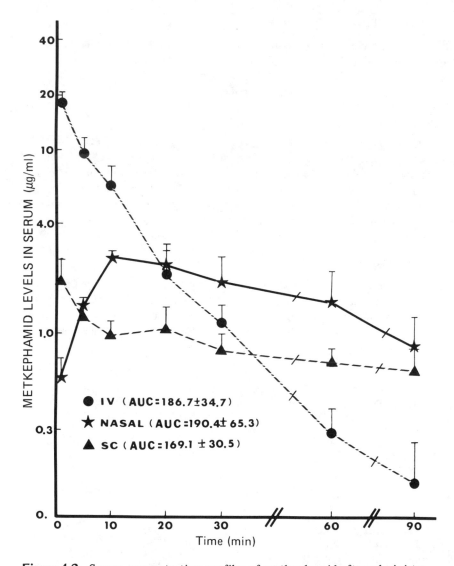

Figure 4.2 Serum concentration profiles of metkephamid after administration of a 25 mg/kg dose in rat ($n = 3-4$). Key: (●), intravenous administration; (▲), subcutaneous administration; (*), intranasal administration. No compound was detected after oral administration. (From Ref. 6, used with permission.)

tion was found to be approximately equivalent to that of the intravenous injection, whereas subcutaneous administration yielded a bioavailability of 91%. The influence of surfactant on the nasal absorption of metkephamid was found to be insignificant, which may be due to the fact that metkephamid is a more stable analog of enkephalins, and is therefore less susceptible to enzymatic degradation (7). A linear relationship between the AUCs and the doses was observed in the dosage range of 12.5-50.0 mg/kg (with a correlation coefficient of 0.95). The results suggested that the amount of metkephamid absorbed nasally is directly proportional to the dose administered. The plasma concentrations of metkephamid in rats following intravenous, intranasal, and subcutaneous administrations were observed to decline at biphasic kinetics. Histological examinations of the nasal mucosa after the experiments revealed only a slight irritation which is probably recoverable. These experiments have also demonstrated that metkephamid can be absorbed nasally with a rapid onset of absorption.

4.2.3.3 Leucine enkephalin

The nasal absorption of leucine enkephalin (Tyr–Gly–Gly–Phe–Leu) has been studied in rats (8). Using the in situ nasal perfusion technique, a solution of this enkephalin analog was recirculated through the nasal cavity of anesthetized rats. The diappearance of leucine enkephalin from the nasal perfusate was found to be a result of absorption and hydrolysis. The extent of absorption was calculated to be less than 10%. When administered at low concentrations, leucine enkephalin undergoes an extensive hydrolysis in the nasal mucosa. However, the extent of hydrolysis in the perfusate was considerably reduced by the addition of excess dipeptides, such as L-tyrosyl-L-tyrosine, at 20-fold molar concentration. The results demonstrated that the nasal bioavailability can be improved by the coadministration of a competing pharmacologically inactive peptide.

4.2.4 Octapeptides

Nasal absorption of an octapeptide, called SS-6(Cyclo[Pro–Phe–D–Trp–Lys–Thr–Phe]), with a molecular weight of around 800, was recently investigated in male Wistar rats (9). A nasal bioavailability of 73% was achieved.

4.2.5 Substance P

Substance P is an undecapeptide (Arg–Pro–Lys–Pro–Gln–Gln–Phe–Phe–Gly–Leu–Met–NH$_2$) with a molecular weight of 1347.66. It is present in the brain of all vertebrates, including the human, in the spinal ganglia, and in the intestines, especially the duodenum and jejunum. Substance P acts as a vasodilator, as a depressant, stimulates salivation, and produces increased capillary permeability.

The possibility of nasal absorption of substance P was recently investigated in rats (10). Results indicated that 18 of the 22 rats tested showed a rapid increase in the plasma levels of immunoreactive substance P (IR-SP), with peak concentrations reached within 2-5 min, and a return to baseline levels at 20 min after intranasal administration. It was concluded that nasal delivery achieves a more sustained systemic level than that by intravenous administration.

4.2.6 Calcitonin

Calcitonin is a calcium-regulating hormone secreted from the mammalian thyroid gland. It has a molecular weight of 3418, and contains 32 amino acid residues. Its activities include reduction of the plasma concentration of calcium.

The intranasal administration of calcitonin has been studied using nose drops (Cibacalcin/Ciba-Giegy) in six normal subjects (11). The results demonstrated that the intranasal administration of calcitonin has achieved a similar effect on the reduction of plasma calcium level as that of intravenous injection, even though the plasma calcitonin concentrations from intravenous injection are higher than those by intranasal administration. The data also illustrated that while a higher plasma calcitonin concentration is established by intranasal administration at a higher dose of calcitonin, the decrease in plasma calcium concentrations shows no difference between 500 and 1000 μg. The extent of side effects between the intravenous and intranasal administration or between the two nasal doses was not different.

The aqueous gel of polyacrylic acid (carbopol gel) has been reported to improve the absorption of calcitonin following intranasal and rectal administrations (12,13). The intranasal administration of [Asu^{1,7}]-eel calcitonin (10 U/kg) has been conducted in rats via a syringe. The results showed that delivery by polyacrylic acid gel at three different pHs (4.5, 5.5, and 7.5), the plasma calcitonin concentrations have all been shown to decrease rapidly, but the maximum hypocalcemic effect is obtained at 30 min for pH 6.5 and at 1 hr for pH 5.5 and 7.5. Furthermore, the intranasal administration of [Asu^{1,7}]-eel calcitonin (1 U/kg) in saline solution was found to produce no hypocalcemic effects. The dose-response relationship after the intranasal administration of [Asu^{1,7}]-eel calcitonin in the polyacrylic acid gel at pH 6.5

has also been investigated at a dose range of 1-10 U/kg. The result demonstrated a rapid decrease in the plasma calcium concentrations after doses of 5 and 10 U/kg, whereas at the 1 U/kg level only a small hypocalcemic effect was noted. The results suggest that polyacrylic acid gel may be used as the delivery system for the intranasal administration of peptides with enhanced absorption.

4.3 POLYPEPTIDES AND PROTEINS

4.3.1 Horseradish Peroxidase

The feasibility of nasal absorption of native horseradish peroxidase, a protein molecule with a molecular weight of around 34,000, was recently investigated in the mouse, rat, and squirrel monkey (14). Results indicated that by intranasal administration, horseradish peroxidase passes freely through the intercellular junctions of the olfactory epithelia and reaches the olfactory bulbs in the central nervous system (CNS) extracellularly within 45-90 min.

The transnasal bioavailability of horseradish peroxidase was also evaluated in comparison with an octapeptide (with a molecular weight of around 800) in male Wistar rats (9). Results suggested that a systemic bioavailability of only 0.6% has been achieved for horseradish peroxidase as compared to 73% for the octapeptide. The observations led the investigators to conclude that the nasal route is suitable for an efficient, rapid delivery of molecules with a molecular weight of less than 1000; and with the use of adjuvants, this limit can be extended to molecular weights of at least 6000 and possibly much higher.

4.3.2 Albumins

Egg albumin, a protein molecule with a molecular weight of 34,500, has reportedly been shown to be absorbed from the nasal mucosa and to enter the lymph stream just as readily as the dye T-1824 in monkeys, dogs, cats, and rabbits (15-17). With the exception of one experiment, egg albumin was always found in the lymph within a short interval following intranasal delivery. The horse serum instilled into the nose was never detected in either the lymph or the blood of cats, but it was found in the lymph of rabbits. However, horse serum was also found to inhibit the nasal absorption of T-1824 by protein binding. Intranasal instillation of protein tracers, such as albumin labeled with Evans blue and horseradish peroxidase, in the mouse was found to produce a rapid accumulation of tracers in the epithelial cells, including nerve cells in the mucosa (18). On the other hand, peroxidase was found in small vesicles in the bulbous apical endings of the dendrites, which extend beyond the free surface of the epithelium. Both tracers were also detected in the submucosa, fila olfactoria, olfactory glomeruli, and leptomeninges around the olfactory bulbs. Therefore, the sensory nerve cells in the olfactory epithelium of the mouse have the capacity to take up Evans blue-labeled albumin and peroxidase from the nasal cavities. The study also suggested that the communication between the subarachnoid space and olfactory mucosa in the mouse is bidirectional for macromolecular substances.

A solution of technetium-99m (^{99m}Tc)-labeled human serum albumin, which is also a tracer, was administered intranasally as a nasal spray or nose drops (19). The nasal spray was found to deposit the albumin mainly anteriorly in the nasal cavity, with little reaching the turbinates, whereas the nose drops dispersed the albumin solution throughout the length of the nasal cavity from the atrium to the nasopharynx. The results suggest that instillation of three drops provides a greater coverage of the walls in the nasal cavity. All the studies demonstrated tht the tracer is not well absorbed from the nasal cavity, but is observed to clear into the pharynx. The solution administered as nose drops was removed more rapidly than that administered by nasal spray.

4.3.3 Pancreatic Hormones

4.3.3.1 Insulin

Insulin is a protein hormone with a molecular weight of about 6000. It consists of two peptide chains, each with 21 and 30 amino acid residues, respectively. These two peptide chains are held together by the disulfide linkages between cysteines. Insulin is an endogenous hormone secreted by the beta cells in the glandular tissue of the pancreas. It is subjected to degradation by the proteolytic enzymes (i.e., leucine aminopeptidase) during its passage through the mucous membrane (20,21).

Treatment of diabetes with insulin currently requires that patients receive daily parenteral injections. However, the local discomfort and the perceived lifestyle disruption caused by the daily hypodermic injections of insulin deter many patients with type I diabetes from accepting an intensive insulin treatment regimen. In addition, many patients with type II diabetes refuse to accept insulin therapy entirely. For these reasons, numerous efforts have been made to find a nonparenteral route for insulin delivery, such as sublingual (22,23), enteral (24-28), rectal (29,30), vaginal (27), subcutaneous implantation (31), and inhalation (32,33). However, the limited and variable absorption of insulin through these routes has limited the development of a practical nonparenteral application.

Surface-active agents are known to affect membrane transport and thus drug absorption. The direct effect of surfactants on the permeability of biological membrane was observed to result in an increased passage of drugs through the intestinal membrane (34,35). Nonionic and anionic surfactants and bile salts have been reported to enhance the gastrointestinal absorption of water-soluble, micelle-free drugs, such as antibiotics (36), vitamin B_1 (37), vitamin B_{12} (38), phenol red (39,40), erythritol (41), electrolytes, and monosaccharides (42). Moreover, the presence of nonionic surfactants or bile acids was also found to enhance the rectal absorption of insulin (43,44). Bile salts have been known to promote the transmembrane movement of endogenous and exogenous lipids and small polar molecules (45). Furthermore, the bile salts' surface-active properties led them to be received as potential adjuvants for the transmucosal delivery of drugs (46). When surfactants or bile salts were incorporated into the nasal solution of insulin, they were observed to enhance significantly the biological activity of insulin, as shown by a prompt increase in the plasma concentration of immunoreactive insulin (IRI) and a reduction in the blood glucose level.

The first reported attempt to administer insulin by the nasal route can be traced back to 1922 (47). The intranasal administration of insulin was reported to yield a very weak, doubtful, or frankly negative effect, whereas intravenous and subcutaneous administration resulted in positive effects. In 1924 and 1925, the lowering of the blood sugar level in diabetes was observed to occur following the inhalation of insulin (48,49). In 1932, absorption of insulin through nasal mucous membrane was studied in human diabetics (50). Insulin solutions containing saponin were sprayed by an atomizer or applied using a small cotton pledget. The results showed a successful rate of 88.5%. This intranasal application achieved effects similar to those obtained by subcutaneous administration. However, this treatment produced some mild congestion in the nasal mucosa and some symptoms of rhinitis (51).

It has been reported that when insulin (100 IU/0.2 cc in ethylene glycol or trimethylene glycol) was applied, by either nose drops or nasal spray, a marked fall in blood glucose levels was produced in normal rabbits, dogs, and diabetic patients (52). However, the dose administered in this intranasal application was larger than that required for subcutaneous injection.

An investigation reported in 1958 indicated that the nasal absorption of insulin in both normal subjects and diabetic patients was achieved, and that 53% of the normoglycemic effect was obtained as compared to that of subcutaneous injection (53). Unfortunately, the effect was found to be rather unstable and variable.

The nasal absorption of insulin has also been compared with oral and intravenous administrations (54). The results demonstrated that the plasma glucose level in rats is decreased significantly following intranasal delivery, whereas the plasma glucose level is only scarcely decreased after oral administration. For the intranasal administration of insulin, about 10 times the intravenous dose was found necessary in order to obtain the same degree of pharmacological effect (Figure 4.3).

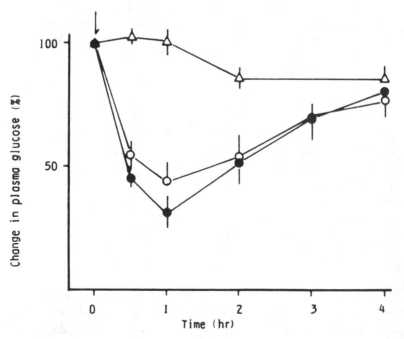

Figure 4.3   Reduction in plasma glucose levels following administration of insulin through various routes in rats. Each value is the mean ± SE for 5 animals. Key: (O), nasal 20 U/kg; (△), oral 100 U/kg; (●), intravenous 2 U/kg. (From Ref. 54, used with permission.)

The effect of several surfactants on the nasal absorption of insulin has been studied in 18 healthy adults (55). In this investigation, crystalline procine insulin (10, 30, and 50 IU) was dissolved in 0.1 ml of saline solution (pH 7.6) containing 1% sodium glycocholate. Without the surfactant, the intranasal administration of insulin yielded no measurable increase in the serum level of immunoreactive insulin (IRI). Following the intranasal application of insulin solution containing 1% sodium glycocholate, insulin was promptly absorbed with a significant increase in the plasma level of IRI, which was similar to that by intravenous injection, but not to that by subcutaneous administration. In addition, a decrease in both glucose level and C-peptide immunoreactivity (CPR) was observed. A dose-response relationship was noted between the peak serum levels of IRI and the administered dose of insulin. Substitution of sodium glycocholate with other surfactants, such as lysozyme chloride, HCO-60, Byco-E, the nasal absorption of insulin was found to be negligibly small. When 1% sodium ursodeoxycholate was added, the glucose level was not observed to decrease, in spite of the observation of an increase in the plasma IRI level.

The effect of surfactants, like saponin, sodium glycocholate, and polyoxyethylene-9-lauryl ether (BL-9), on the nasal absorption of insulin has also been studied in dogs (56). The results indicated that after the intranasal administration of insulin at pH 3.1 by nebulizer spray at a dose of 50 IU/dog, the plasma IRI level increases substantially from 32.8 to 296.7 μU/ml at 30 min, whereas the blood glucose level decreases from 90.8 to 20.4 mg/100 ml within 1-2 hr (Figure 4.4). However, the blood glucose level in the controls remained constant throughout the experimental period. The hypoglycemia induced by the intranasally delivered insulin was found to be dependent upon the pH of the preparations. The nasal absorption was enhanced significantly when it was dissolved in an acid medium rather than in a neutral medium. At pH 6.1, only a slight hypoglycemia occurred, whereas at pH 3.1, the decrement in the blood glucose level corresponded to a reduction of about 55% (Figure 4.5). The addition of 1% of saponin, sodium glycocholate, or BL-9 to insulin at pH 7.4 was found to enhance significantly the extent and the duration of hypoglycemia, with a reduction in blood glucose concentration down to 25% of the control level within 1-2 hr after administration. In contrast, in the absence of surfactant the nasal insulin preparation produced only a slight hypoglycemia at this pH, and its hypoglycemic effect also showed dependency on its solution pH. On the other hand, when 1% BL-9 was added the nasal absorption of insulin was remarkably enhanced, and its hypoglycemic effect became less dependent upon its solution pH.

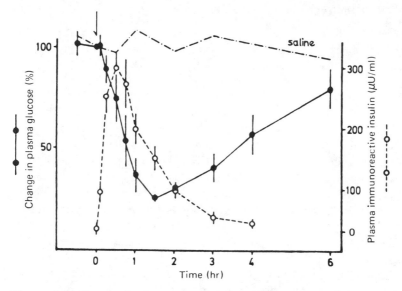

Figure 4.4 Changes in the plasma levels of glucose (●) and immunoreactive insulin (○) following intranasal administration of insulin (50 U/dog; pH = 3.1). The data are expressed as mean ± SE (*n* = 5). (From Ref. 56, used with permission.)

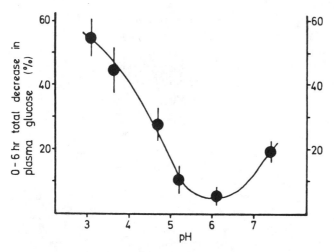

Figure 4.5 Effect of pH in nasal insulin solution on the reduction of plasma glucose levels in dogs (dose: 50 U/dog). The data are expressed as mean ± SE (*n* = 4). (From Ref. 56, used with permission.)

With the enhancing effect of 1% sodium glycocholate, the hypoglycemic action of nasally delivered insulin has been observed to be more effective at pH 7.4 than at 3.1. The nasal dose of insulin needed to achieve the equivalent hypoglycemia was estimated to be about three to four times of that for intravenous administration. This investigation suggested that alteration of the nasal mucosa in the presence of surfactants, such as saponin, sodium glycocholate, or BL-9, appears to increase the permeability of the nasal mucosa to insulin. It was also concluded that nasal spray for the intranasal delivery of insulin would be useful as a simple and painless dosage form or the long-term therapy of diabetes.

A variety of surfactants were screened in rats for their potential in enhancing the nasal absorption of insulin (57). The results showed a dose-dependent decrease in the blood glucose level at pH 8.1, but not at pH 5.5 and 7.4, at which no hypoglycemic effect was produced (Figure 4.6). On the other

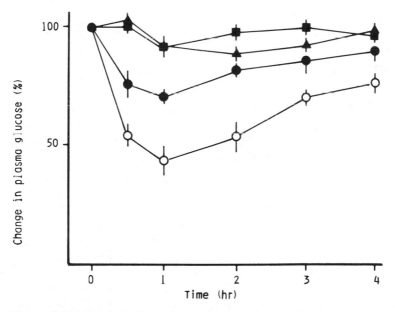

Figure 4.6 Effect of pH on the time course for the change in plasma glucose after intranasal adminstration of insulin in rats. Key: (○), pH 3.1 (20 U/kg); (●), pH 3.1 (10 U/kg); (■), pH 5.5 (10 U/kg); (▲), pH 7.4 (10 U/kg). The data are expressed as mean ± SE of four animals. (From Ref. 54, used with permission.)

hand, when 1% sodium glycocholate, saponin, or BL-9 was added to the insulin solution at pH 7.4, the extent and the duration of hypoglycemia was enhanced significantly with a peak effect observed at 2-3 hr after administration. The hypoglycemic effect gradually became greater as the surfactant concentration increased from 0 to 0.5% and then leveled off. The results also demonstrated that the blood glucose level is reduced by surfactants of nonionic ether, anionic, and amphoteric types as well as by bile salts, saponin, and surfactin. The nonionic ester-type surfactants were found to be less effective than the ether-type ones. Among the nonionic surfactants, addition of an ether type having a HLB value of 8-14 was found to produce the highest promoting effect on the nasal absorption of insulin, with the exception of polyoxyethylene butyl ethers and the ester-type surfactants. The reduction of the blood glucose levels was found to be linearly proportional to the logarithm of insulin doses. This linearity was found to be parallel between intranasal and parenteral administrations. The bioavailability of insulin by intranasal administration was 5%, as estimated from the hypoglycemic effect, at pH 3.1 when there was no promotor used. With the addition of a promotor, such as 1% sodium glycocholate or polyoxyethylene-9-lauryl ether, the nasal bioavailability of insulin was increased to about 30%. The results suggested that surfactants appear to facilitate the permeability of the nasal mucosa or to reduce the proteolytic enzyme activity in the nasal mucosa, and thereby promote the nasal bioavailability of insulin.

The mechanism of the promoting effect of surfactants on the nasal absorption of insulin has been studied in rats. The effects of surfactants on the morphology of the nasal mucosa have also been examined using the scanning electron microscope (SEM) (58). The addition of a surfactant significantly reduced the blood glucose levels, whereas the insulin solution without surfactant was noted to produce only a slight hypoglycemia. The reduction of blood glucose levels showed the maximum of 55.5% with the addition of polyoxyethylene-9-lauryl ether, and diminished gradually with the increase or the decrease in the number of ethylene oxide units. Both the hemolytic and protein-releasing effects of surfactants on the nasal mucous membrane were also observed to reach the maximum magnitude with polyoxyethylene-9-lauryl ether, and to decrease as the number of ethylene oxide units increased or decreased from 9. There appeared to be a linear correlation of the hemolytic activity and the protein-releasing effect with the reduction of the blood glucose level (0-4 hr). There existed a good correlation between the effect on the nasal mucous membrane and the absorption-promoting action of the nonionic surfactants, anionic surfactants, and saponin. On the other hand, bile salts (i.e., taurocholate, cholate, and glycocholate) showed lesser effects on both hemolytic activity and protein-releasing effect.

The addition of polyoxyethylene-9-lauryl ether in the nasal solution yielded a slight inhibition of the enzymatic degradation of insulin, whereas sodium glycocholate significantly inhibited the enzymatic hydrolysis. The activity of leucine aminopeptidase was observed to decrease as the concentration of surfactants was increased. A more marked effect on the enzyme was noted when sodium glycocholate rather than polyoxyethylene-9-lauryl ether was used. Bile salts were found to affect not only the permeability of the nasal mucosa, but also the activity of proteolytic enzyme. The studies also suggested that bile salts, like sodium glycocholate, are less irritating than nonionic ether-type surfactants, like polyoxyethylene-9-lauryl ether, on the nasal mucosa.

The efficacy and safety of the intranasal administration of insulin have been investigated in normal subjects as well as in insulin-dependent diabetic patients (59). In all the normal subjects, a fall in blood glucose levels was observed to occur at 12.3 (±1.5) min after intranasal administration, which lasted for 51.5 (±4.7) min with a reduction of 41.9% (±6.4%) in the basal blood glucose level. The serum concentrations of immunoreactive insulin (IRI) were observed to increase in all subjects with peak levels of 67.1 (±16.6) mU/L being achieved at 13.5 (±0.7) min. In three normal subjects, the potency ratio of hypoglycemia induced by intranasal and intravenous insulin administrations was found to be about 1:8. On the other hand, in the four insulin-dependent diabetic patients, insulin was administered once intranasally and once subcutaneously at a dose ratio of 9:1. During the 1-hr observation period, lower blood glucose levels were achieved after the nasal dose than after the subcutaneous dose. This investigation showed that in normal subjects, insulin administered intranasally is well absorbed to sufficient levels to induce hypoglycemia. Serum insulin concentrations lose sharply after intranasal administration, and showed a good correlation with the insulin doses administered, whereas the serum concentrations of C-peptide were either unaffected or decreased, indicating that pancreatic beta-cell function was inhibited, and that the hypoglycemia observed was due to the insulin administered intranasally.

The efficacy and reproducibility of the intranasal administration of insulin have been studied using sodium deoxycholate as an enhancer in normal and diabetic subjects (60,61). When insulin was administered alone in buffered saline solution (pH 7.4) at a dose of 0.5 IU/kg, neither an increase in plasma insulin concentrations nor a decrease in blood glucose levels was observed. When 1% sodium deoxycholate was incorporated in the insulin solu-

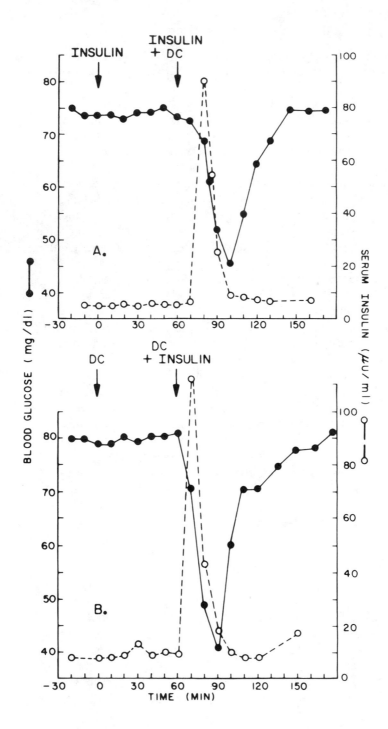

tion, the blood glucose levels were observed to fall promptly within 10-20 min (Figure 4.7). After intranasal administration of 0.5 IU/kg of insulin with 1% (w/v) of deoxycholate to 25 normal subjects, a prompt increase in the serum insulin concentrations was obtained with a peak level of 103 μIU/ml achieved at 10 min, which returned to baseline level within 40-60 min. On the other hand, blood glucose levels began to fall by 10 min, reached 54% ($\pm$14%) of the control value by 30 min, and returned to the baseline by 60-80 min (Figure 4.8). A linear dose-response relationship was established between the mean increment in the serum insulin levels and the nasal dose of insulin administered. In contrast, following the intravenous administration of the same dose, the peak serum insulin levels in the same subjects were attained within 2 min, and returned to baseline about 30-40 min. The nasal absorption of insulin from the nasal spray was calculated to be approximately 10-20% as efficient as the intravenous injection by comparing the area under the serum insulin concentration time curves (AUCs).

On the other hand, following the intranasal administration of insulin (0.5 IU/kg) with sodium deoxycholate in type I and type II diabetic patients, the blood glucose levels were observed to fall steeply for the first hour to a level which was approximately 30-40% below the pretreatment level. In addition, a prolonged hypoglycemic response to intranasal insulin was observed that persisted for as long as 4–6 hr (Figure 4.9 and 4.10).

In another study, when insulin was administered intranasally to diabetic patients within 15-30 min after the beginning of the mealtime, it was found to be extremely effective in reducing or ablating the meal-related hyperglycemia. Moreover, the risk of postprandial hypoglycemia associated with this medication appeared to be very low. The results suggest that when insulin is administered intranasally with 1% deoxycholate in an aerosol formulation, it traverses the nasal mucosa and rapidly reaches the systemic circulation with reproducible kinetics and good efficiency. The investigation also suggested that the intranasal administration of insulin together with a bile salt in aerosol

---

Figure 4.7   (A) Time course for the variation in serum insulin (○- -○) and blood glucose (●—●) concentrations in a normal volunteer following intranasal aerosol administration (arrow) of 0.5 U/kg insulin without and with 1% (w/v) deoxycholate (DC). (B) Time course for the variation in serum insulin (○--○) and blood glucose (●—●) concentrations in a normal volunteer following intranasal aerosol administration (arrow) of 1% deoxycholate (DC) without and with 0.5 U/kg insulin. (From Ref. 60, used with permission.)

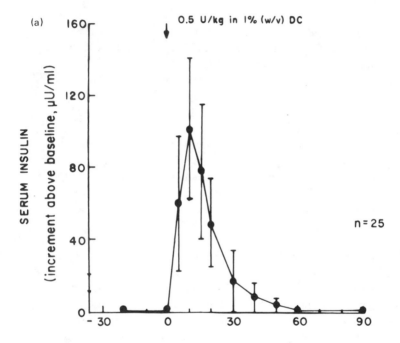

Figure 4.8 (a) Serum insulin concentration (mean ± 1 SD) profile for 25 normal subjects who received a nasal spray of 0.5 U/kg insulin in 1% (w/v) deoxycholate at time 0. (b) Blood glucose as percentage of the value at time 0 (mean ± 1 SD) versus time for 29 normal subjects who received 0.5 U/kg insulin in 1% (w/v) deoxycholate aerosol at time 0. (From Ref. 60, used with permission.)

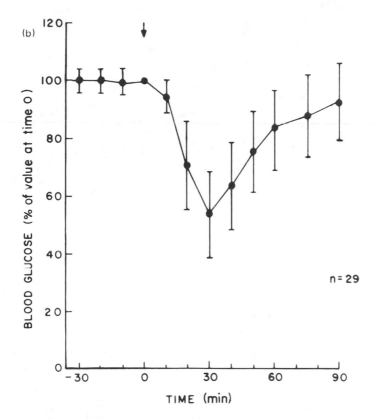

Figure 4.8 (Continued)

form may provide several advantages over other routes of administration, such as ease of administration, wide patient acceptability, and rapid onset of action.

The adjuvant potency of a series of bile salts with subtle differences in the number, position, and orientation of their nuclear hydroxyl groups and the alterations in side chain conjugation has been evaluated (59). Their potency in enhancing the nasal absorption of insulin was noted to correlate positively with the increase in the hydrophilicity of the bile salts' steroid nucleus on the basis of their HPLC retention factors (62). The potency of the unconjugated bile salts showed a rank order of: deoxycholate > chenodeoxycholate > cholate > ursodeoxycholate. The nasal absorption of insulin in the

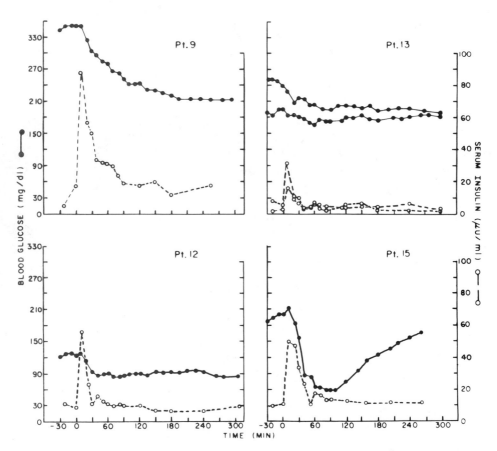

Figure 4.9 Time course for serum insulin (O--O) and blood glucose (●──●) concentrations for four subjects with Type I diabetes mellitus. At time zero, 0.5 U insulin/kg was administered with 1% (w/v) deoxycholate as a nasal spray. One patient (subject 13) was studied on two occasions. (From Ref. 60, used with permission.)

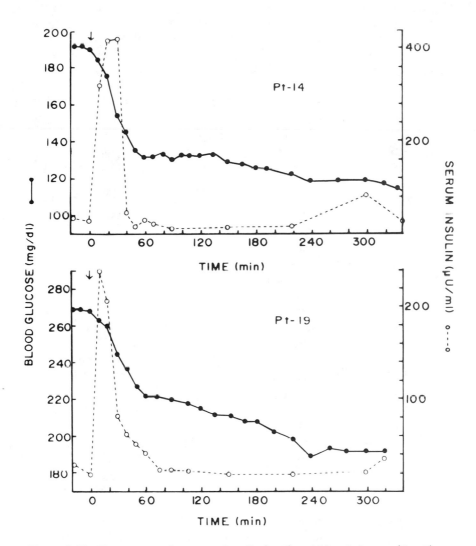

Figure 4.10 Time course for serum insulin (○--○) and blood glucose (●——●) concentrations for two patients with type II diabetes. The patients received 0.5 U insulin/kg body weight in 1% (w/v) deoxycholate as a nasal spray at time 0. (From Ref. 60, used with permission.)

presence of bile salts, all achieved peak serum insulin levels within 10 ($\pm$1) min following intranasal administration, with 10-20% of the administered insulin dose being absorbed into the circulation. The most hydrophilic of the bile salts, sodium ursodeoxycholate, did not produce an appreciable promotion of insulin absorption or lowering of the blood glucose level, whereas the most lipophilic bile salt, sodium deoxycholate, yielded a marked elevation in serum insulin concentrations and about 50% reduction in blood glucose levels. However, as the bile salts were conjugated with glycine or taurine, the overall lipophilicity of the molecules decreased, yet adjuvant activity was still retained. This suggests that the lipophilicity of the steroid nucleus is the major determinant of the adjuvant activity.

Nasal absorption of insulin appears to begin at the critical micellar concentration (CMC) of the bile salt and reaches the maximal level as micelle formation is well established (62). The CMC values for bile salts (sodium deoxycholate, sodium chenodeoxycholate, sodium ursodeoxycholate, and sodium cholate) are approximately 3, 3, 5, and 7 mM, respectively. Sodium deoxycholate, which has a CMC value of 3 mM, was found to be only slightly effective at 2.5 mM, 50% effective at 6 mM, and maximally effective at 12-24 mM. The increase of sodium deoxycholate concentration from 6 to 12 mM was observed to affect the magnitude of the serum insulin peak, but not the time to reach the peak level. The following mechanisms were hypothesized for the adjuvant effect of bile salts: (a) to produce a high juxtamembrane concentration of insulin monomers via solubilization in the mixed bile salt micelles, and (b) to form reverse micelles within the nasal membrane through which insulin monomers can diffuse through the polar channels from the nares into the blood stream.

The efficacy of the intranasal administration of aerosolized insulin containing polyoxyethylene-9-lauryl ether (BL-9) as the adjuvant has been recently studied in the patients with type I diabetes, in which eight patients were on fasting, 15 patients were on mixed meals, and eight patients were on long-term home use (63). In the fasting normal subjects, who were used as the controls, the intranasal administration of insulin at a dose of 0.1 IU/kg was observed to produce a minimal and transient effect on the levels of immunoreactive insulin (IRI) and blood glucose. At 0.5 IU/kg, the IRI level reached the maximal value within 15-30 min, and lasted for 60-90 min, whereas the blood glucose level was reduced to 50% of its pretreatment value at 45 min, and was returned to the pretreatment level at 90 min. At 1 IU/kg, the IRI peaked higher and later, and the peak level also lasted longer, producing the lowest blood glucose level at 45 min with no return to the pretreatment level for 2 hr. All the subjects who received 1 IU/kg of insulin had symptomatic hypoglycemia.

In the fasting subjects with type I diabetes, a more delayed and more prolonged response to nasal insulin was observed than in the normal controls. At a dose of 1 IU/kg, the mean blood glucose level was found to drop from 247 ($\pm$59) to 122 ($\pm$30) mg/dl within 2 hr and remained below the levels in the placebo group for at least 3-4 hr. Intravenously injected insulin at 0.1 IU/kg also produced a prolonged reduction in the blood glucose levels in the diabetic group. With 1% of BL-9, the potency of nasal insulin was approximately one-tenth to one-fifteenth of that obtained with intravenous insulin, as judged from the dose of insulin needed to produce the same magnitude of reduction in the blood glucose level. Intranasal administration of insulin with 1% of BL-9, immediately before a meal at doses of 1.0 and 1.5 IU/kg was noted to reduce the postprandial hyperglycemia significantly as compared with placebo. At 0.5 IU/kg, however, the postprandial glucose level was indistinguishable from that of the placebo group ($p > 0.05$). The effect of the variation in BL-9 concentration on the postprandial hyperglycemia has also been studied at a fixed nasal insulin dose (1 IU/kg). The result demonstrated that the glucose-lowering potency of nasal insulin depends not only on the insulin dose, but also on the surfactant concentration.

The irritation of various ingredients in the aerosol spray has also been assessed. The results revealed that the surfactant is responsible for the nasal irritation observed, such as nasal stinging, congestion, and rhinorrhea. The degree of nasal irritation varied widely among patients and was found to depend upon surfactant concentrations: Half the patients reported nasal discomfort with 1% BL-9, whereas most tolerated 0.25%, and all tolerated 0.1%.

The capability of sodium taurodihydrofusidate (STDHF) to enhance the transmucosal permeation of insulin was recently evaluted in sheep (64). At equivalent concentrations, STDHF was found to be five- to 10-fold less lytic than the bile salts, and at least 100-fold less lytic than nonionic surfactants, like laureth-9. At the concentrations greater than its critical micellar concentration, STDHF was noted to greatly enhance the nasal absorption of insulin, with the optimum absorption being attained at a molar ratio of 5:1 (STDHF/insulin). The nasal absorption of insulin was observed to be linearly dependent upon the applied insulin dose (0.25-1.0 U/kg), with a mean systemic bioavailability of 16.4%. It was also reported that without STDHF, the sodium salt of insulin cannot be absorbed to any appreciable extent; and, no difference in the nasal absorptivity of insulin was observed between the Zn and sodium salts in the presence or absence of STDHF. The results led the investigators to conclude that STDHF is an excellent enhancer for the transnasal absorption of insulin.

A 3-month study of the intranasal administration of aerosolized insulin before meals as a supplement to ultralente insulin illustrated that the aerosol is well tolerated for glycemic control, as compared to that observed in the conventional subcutaneous insulin administration. The results also demonstrated that insulin administered intranasally in the presence of BL-9 rapidly penetrates the nasal mucosa and reduces postprandial hyperglycemia. When administered before a meal, it is feasible as a long-term adjunct to subcutaneous insulin in the treatment of type I diabetes.

The aqueous gel of polyacrylic acid was reported to improve the rectal absorption of peptide hormones, such as insulin and calcitonin. The effect of polyacrylic acid gel on the nasal absorption of insulin has also been investigated in rats (65). The preparation (at pH 6.5) was administered into the nasal cavity through a syringe at a volume of 0.05 ml/kg. The maximum hypoglycemic effect was obtained at 0.5 and 1.0 hr for 0.1 and 1.0% of polyacrylic acid gel, respectively. On the other hand, intranasal administration of insulin in a 1% carboxymethylcellulose (CMC) solution produced no hypoglycemic effect at the same insulin dose (1 IU/kg). Further studies indicated that nasal absorption of insulin is not influenced by the pH of polyacrylic acid gel.

A powder dosage form of insulin has also been developed for intranasal administration (66). The effect of various pharmaceutical excipients (e.g., lactose, mycrocrystalline cellulose [MCC], hydroxypropylcellulose (HPC), and neutralized Carbopol 934 [Cp-Na]) on the bioavailability of insulin from such a powder dosage form was compared with liquid dosage forms in dogs. The powder preparations were sprayed into the nasal cavity by a special sprayer, whereas the liquid preparations were administered with an Eppendorf pipette. The powder preparations were found to bring about only a noticeable hypoglycemia, with the maximal reduction in blood glucose levels being reached within 1.0-1.5 hr after administration. The extent of reduction in blood glucose levels showed no pH dependency. On the other hand, the liquid preparations at pH 5.7 produced only a slight hypoglycemia, whereas the preparation at pH 3.4 reduced the blood glucose level by 61.4% (±5.6%). With the addition of MCC, the nasal absorption of insulin from the liquid dosage form was found to be rapid, and the blood glucose levels were reduced by 68% (±7.6%) after 1.5 hr. Correspondingly, the plasma concentration of immunoreactive insulin (IRI) was increased from 17.3 (±3.4) μIU/ml to a maximum of 455.3 (±180.1) μUI/ml after 30 min. The minimum glucose levels achieved from the formulation containing HPC and the formulation containing Carbopol 934 [Cp-Na] were 39.1% (±2.3%) and 42.0% (±8.3%), respectively. Lactose was the least effective among the four excipients investigated, and the minimum glucose level obtained was 46.6% (±6.4%) after 1 hr, which reversed rapidly 1 hr later. Furthermore, the addition of Cp-Na appeared to prolong the duration of the hypoglycemic effect of the powder dosage form, which seems to increase as increasing the concentration of Carbopol 934 [Cp-Na]. The powder dosage form of insulin with Cp-Na appeared to require a nasal dose of about three times the intravenous dose to produce the same extent of hypoglycemic effects.

4.3.3.2 Glucagon

Glucagon, the hyperglycemic glycogenolytic factor, is a polypeptide hormone secreted by the alpha cells in the pancreatic islets of Langerhans. It is known to stimulate the adenylate cyclase-cyclin adenosine monophosphate (AMP) system in the liver, which leads to the activation of phosphorylase in the conversion of glycogen to glucose. Glucagon plays an important role in the physiological regulation of blood sugar. Any defect in the control of glucagon secretion has been shown to be a factor in certain types of diabetes mellitus.

Hypoglycemic shock emergencies are common in the daily management of insulin-dependent diabetes, especially those with unstable diabetes. The subcutaneous or intramuscular administration of glucagon is known to be an effective treatment. A study was conducted to assess the efficiency of glucagon given intranasally in raising blood glucose levels in seven normal subjects (67). Nasal drops of porcine glucagon with sodium glycocholate was administered. In all the subjects, the intranasal administration of glucagon was observed to produce a sharp increase in plasma concentrations of immunoreactive glucagon (C_{max} = 1300 ng/dl at t_{max} of 10 min), and thereafter to produce an increase in blood glucose levels (Figure 4.11). In addition, the plasma concentrations of immunoreactive insulin were also significantly increased, indicating that glucagon given intranasally exerts its traditional metabolic effect. In the controls, however, blood glucose levels as well as plasma immunoreactive insulin and glucagon concentrations were observed to remain steady. After the intranasal administration of glucagon, the peak level of glucagon was found to be similar to that of intramuscular injection, whereas the fall in the plasma glucagon concentrations was observed to occur earlier with lower blood glucose levels being attained.

The results concluded that glucagon can be well-absorbed through the nasal mucosa to increase blood glucose levels. The efficacy of nasal glucagon seems to be slightly lower than that of intramuscular glucagon with a potency ratio of 1:2.

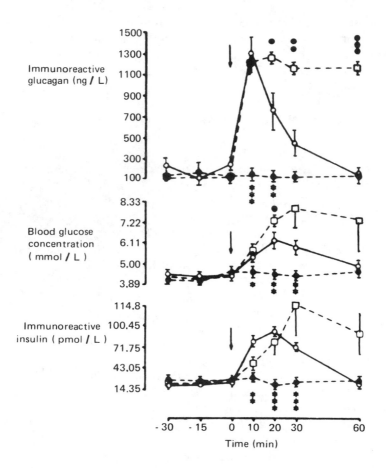

Figure 4.11 Effects of intranasally administered glucagon (1 mg, seven subjects, ○–○), of the diluent (four subjects, ●--●) and of intramuscular glucagon (two subjects, □---□) on plasma immunoreactive glucagon, blood glucose and plasma insulin concentration profiles. Means (± SEM) are indicated. Statistical differences: *p < 0.05; **p < 0.01; ***p < 0.001 (when comparing diluent and glucagon intranasally); ● p < 0.05; ●● p < 0.01; ●●● p < 0.001 (when comparing glucagon by intranasal and intramuscular route). (From Ref. 67, used with permission.)

4.3.4 Anterior Pituitary Hormones

4.3.4.1 Growth hormones

Growth hormone (GH) can affect the metabolism of proteins, carobhy-drates, fats, and electrolytes, which in turn influence the weight and height of the human body. It also exerts a prominent effect on the kidney's functions (68). When human pancreatic tumor GH-releasing factor 40 (hpGRF-40) is administered intravenously, it can selectively stimulate the secretion of GH in normal subjects (68) and in GH-deficient patients (69). The feasibility of intranasal administration of hpGRF-40 has been evaluated in normal sub-jects, and the results indicated that hpGRF-40 can be effectively absorbed nasally, which produces a significant stimulation and release of GH (70).

4.3.4.2 Adrenal corticotropic hormone (ACTH)

Natural ACTH

Adrenal corticotropic hormone (adrenocorticotropin, corticotropin) is a polypeptide which consists of 39 amino acid residues with a molecular weight of 4500. It is widely used in clinical practice for the diagnosis of various adrenal disorders and to differentiate primary and secondary insuf-ficiencies. In addition, it is also useful in the symptomatic treatment of a variety of conditions, like rheumatoid arthritis and asthma (71).

Clinically, ACTH is administered by either intramuscular or intravenous injection. The feasibility of intranasal administration of ACTH has been investigated in 20 normal volunteers by nasal insufflation (72). The lyo-philized ACTH powder was delivered to the nasal mucous membrane using a powder insufflator. The eosinopenic responses were found to be signifi-cant at the second hour, and reached the maximum level by the fourth hour.

Another study has also been performed in six normal subjects to investi-gate the effect of intranasal administration of ACTH on circulating eosino-phils (73). A solution of ACTH was dispensed intranasally using a hand nebulizer or the Vaponefrin nebulizer. No significant drop in the circulat-ing eosinophil levels was reported. However, a reduction of circulating eosinophil levels was achieved in 112 rheumatoid patients by daily intra-nasal administration of ACTH at a dose of 30-50 U, which induced the re-mission of rheumatoid arthritis (74). It was also reported that intranasal administration of ACTH at a daily dose of 40 IU can achieve sufficient nasal absorption to reduce the circulating eosinophil in normal subjects by more than 50%, and to produce a considerable increase in urinary 17-keto-steroids (75).

Tetracosactrin

Tetracosactrin (β^{1-24}-corticotropin) is a synthetic polypeptide with a molecular weight of 2900. It has been reported that this polypeptide can stimulate the synthesis and release of certain adrenal steroids in humans (71). The feasibility of nasal absorption of tetracosactrin has been studied in six healthy dexamethasone-suppressed subjects by nasal insufflation using a Marvic inhaler (76). A pronounced increase in the plasma level of fluorogenic corticosteroids was observed, suggesting that tetracosactrin is well absorbed nasally.

α^{1-18}-ACTH

A long-acting ACTH (D–Ser^1, Lys^{17,18}-α^{1-18}-ACTH) has been administered intranasally in a liquid suspension form via a nebulizing flask (77). The plasma corticosteroid level was observed to increase following the intranasal administration at a dose of 0.1-1.0 mg, and the duration of action appeared to be dose-dependent. The results suggested that intranasal administration is a viable means to circumvent the difficulties associated with the repeated administration of α^{1-18}-ACTH by injection. Further studies have been conducted to compare the potency and duration of adrenocorticotropic actions of α^{1-18}-ACTH following intranasal, intramuscular, subcutaneous, and sublingual administration in normal subjects (78). After intranasal administration, the α^{1-18}-ACTH was found to be well absorbed. The mean plasma concentration of corticosteroid rose rapidly, reaching a peak level of 37 ($\pm$3.7) μg/100 ml within 4 hr, and remained at the elevated level for about 24 hr.

The pharmacokinetic profiles were similar to the results achieved by intramuscular and subcutaneous injections. By sublingual administration, on the other hand, α^{1-18}-ACTH was not shown to produce any rise in the plasma level of corticosteroids, suggesting that α^{1-18}-ACTH can be rapidly and efficiently absorbed across the nasal membrane, but not through the buccal mucosa.

The intranasal administration of α^{1-18}-ACTH in an aerosol formulation has also been evaluated in 14 normal volunteers (79). α^{1-18}-ACTH was formulated as a suspension in oil and then administered nasally, using an automatic dose-controlled nebulizer. The results indicated that the plasma cortisol concentrations and the urinary levels of 17-ketogenic steroids and 17-ketosteroids rose substantially in all subjects. In conclusion, the intranasal administration of α^{1-18}-ACTH may provide a simple and effective way to stimulate the secretion of the endogenous corticosteroids.

Alsactide (HOE 433)

Alsactide is a potent ACTH derivative (β-Ala^1, Lys^{17}-ACTH$^{1-17}$ heptade-capeptide-4-amino-butylamide) with potency a five to eight times greater than natural ACTH and tetracosactrin. A nasal dose of 100 μg alsactide (Synchrodyn) was found to be equally effective as a subcutaneous dose of 9 μg in activating the release of corticosterone in dexamethasone-blocked rats. Based on its effect on the corticosterone release and adrenal ascorbic acid depletion, a nasal bioavailability of alsactide was estimated to be 12% as compared to the subcutaneous dose (79). In dose-response studies in humans, the nasal spray of 100 μg alsactide was observed to induce a significant prolongation in the duration of cortisol release for more than 4 hr, whereas the aldosterone secretion was not stimulated at this dose.

4.3.4.3 Gonadotropin-Releasing Hormones (GnRH)

Natural luteinizing hormone-releasing hormone

Luteinizing hormone-releasing hormone (LHRH) stimulates the gonadotrophs of the anterior pituitary to secrete both luteinizing hormone (LH) and follicle-stimulating hormone (FSH) (80,81).

Luteinizing hormone-releasing hormone, a decapeptide, is known to be secreted in a pulsatile fashion in order to trigger and to maintain the release of gonadotropins, like LH (Figure 4.12). The continous administration of LHRH has been reported to result in a down-regulation of the homologous pituitary receptors and interruption of the normal release patterns of gonadotropins (82,83).

The LHRH agonists are defined as a group of LHRH analogs which act initially to stimulate the release of gonadotropins, followed by the progressive desensitization of gonadotropin secretion and testicular/ovarian down-regulation, resulting in a suppression of the gonadal steroid secretion (84). Prolonged clinical treatment with high doses of agonists has been reported to achieve a reversible pituitary suppression and the inhibition of gonadal function—effects which were previously expected only after taking LHRH antagonist. Luteinizing hormone-releasing hormone and its analogs have a relatively short circulatory half-life and require a repeated daily administration in order to achieve a desired effect. Luteinizing hormone-releasing hormone agonists have distinct clinical advantages as potent therapuetic agents which can be self-administered by nasal spray.

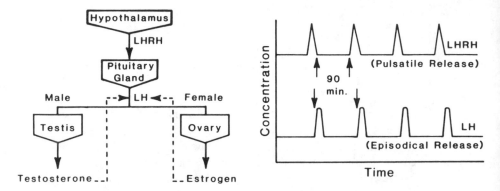

Figure 4.12 Diagram showing the relationship between LHRH and LH, between LH and testosterone (in male) and estrogen (in female), as well as the physiological rhythmic patterns for the release of LHRH and LH.

Synthetic LHRH

Some highly potent agonistic analogs of LHRH have been synthesized, and these synthetic agonists have the same biological properties as the natural LHRH (85-89). The synthetic LHRH analogs have been considered valuable in the diagnosis of the functionality of hypothalamic-pituitary gonadal axis as well as having therapeutic potentials in treating many diseases (80,90).

There are two principal groups of agonist analogs: The first group consists of LHRH decapeptide analogs with amino acid substitutions, and the second group comprises LHRH$^{1-9}$-nonapeptide-ethylamine agonists, Pro^9-ethylamide, which differ from LHRH in their C-terminal sequence.

For clinical applications, the following highly potent LHRH agonists have been of great importance in the development of nasal sprays and vaginal pressaries for self-administration. However, a bioavailability of as low as 1-5% has been reported for LHRH and its agonists (89,91-95).

D—Leu^6-ethylamine. D—Leu^6-des-Gly^{10}-LHRH-EA^{10} (HOE 471/Hoechst AG, West Germany) shows a potency which is slightly less than the buserelin (HOE 766). HOE 471 was shown to be slightly more effective by intravenous injection than by subcutaneous administration. With intranasal administration of HOE 471 at a dose of 50 μg, the release of gonadotropins was relatively small. This was found to be approximately equally effective as a subcutaneous dose of 5 μg, and lasted for about the same duration as an intravenous injection at a 5-μg dose; i.e., 7-9 hr (96). However, the net increase in the serum LH level produced by intranasal administration of 50 μ HOE 471 was observed to be equivalent to that achieved by 25 μg LHRH administered intravenously. Intranasal administration of HOE 471 to 18 healthy men by nasal spray or rhinyl tube was reported to produce a significant release of LH, which occurred within 15 min and was sustained for as long as 12 hr (97). Its clinical applications are outlined as follows:

1. Pregnancy-terminating effect. In animals, it was observed that LHRH agonists can block the action of gonadotropins on the gonads. This observation suggests that it might be possible to interfere with the action of human chorionic gonadotropins on the ovary and to prevent the rescue of the corpus luteum. This would interrupt the pregnancy before the endometrium becomes dependent upon placental-produced progesterone for its maintenance. A single intranasal administration of D–Leu^6-ethylamine was found not to be effective in terminating pregnancy in the rats even at a dose as high as 20 mg/kg (98). On the other hand, when LHRH was administered twice nasally on day 9, its effectiveness was markedly increased, and with the addition of a surfactant its effectiveness increased by 26 times.

2. Treatment of cryptorchidism. Using human chorionic gonadotropin to treat cryptorchidism is an established therapy. Alternatively, the treatment of cryptorchidism can also be accomplished by activating temporarily the endogenous secretion of gonadotropins using LHRH or agonists. Table 4.3 summarizes the effects of D–Leu^6-ethylamine, administered as a nasal spray, in the treatment of cryptorchidism (99-107). The results have led to the conclusion that intranasal administration of LHRH agonists, like D–Leu^6-ethylamine, is effective in the treatment of unilateral and bilateral cryptorchidism, and that this simple, painless, and convenient method of administration is especially suitable for children.

D–Ser(TBU)^6-LHRH–EA^{10} (buserelin). Buserelin (HOE-766/Hoechst AG, West Germany) is a nonapeptide LHRH agonist. It contains a tert-butyl-D-serine residue instead of a glycine at the 6th position, and a terminal amino group has been added to the ethyl group. The biological activities of this synthetic analog are qualitatively about the same as the natural LHRH (108116), but quantitatively it is 50-70 times more potent (117). Following parenteral (i.v., i.m., or s.c.) adminstration, this LHRH agonist produced a prolonged effect on the release of LH and FSH, which lasted for 8-10 hr. Although intranasal administration of buserelin produced only a smaller rise in the serum concentration of gonadotropins as compared to intravenous administration, the investigations conducted to date have indicated that this route of administration is a safer, rather rapid, and more convenient means

Table 4.3 Treatment of Cryptorchidism by Nasal Delivery of Gonadotropin-Releasing Hormones

Study[a]	Dosage	Delivery method	Treatment	Subjects	Results
A (99)	HOE 471 100 µg/nostril	Nasal spray	Maldescended testes	17 Boys	Testes descended in 94.1% of subjects. No adverse side effects observed.
B (100)	HOE 471 200 µg, 6x/day)	Nasal spray	Prepubertal boys with uni- or bilateral cryptorchidism	53 Boys	After 4 weeks therapy in 27 patients with 38 undescended tests, 14 testes improved position, 16 were in scrotum, and eight stayed at same position. In 26 placebo-treated patients, 10 out of 36 undescended testes improved position, one was in scrotum, and 25 remained at same position.
C (101)	HOE 471 200 µg, 6x/day, for 4 weeks	Nasal spray	Uni- or bilateral cryptorchidism	84 Boys	After 4-weeks therapy, complete descent in 38% of 61 testes, with improved position in 28% and no response in 19%. 15% of testes were never palpated. After placebo treatment, 25% of 51 testes improved position and 75% showed no response. The effect showed no dependency on the patients' age, but it was influenced by the initial testicular position. The success rate was inversely proportional to the percentage of testes initially not palpable.

D (102) HOE 471 200 µg, 6x/day, for 4-5 weeks	Nasal spray	Cryptorchidism	55 Prepubertal boys	Descent in 35.8% of 67 undescended testes by the end of the treatment period.
E (103) HOE 471 200 µg, 6x/day)	Nasal spray	Uni- or bilateral cryptorchidism	25 Boys	Of the 11 treated patients with bilateral cryptorchidism, there was a complete descent of both testes in six patients. Of the 14 patients with unilateral cryptorchidism, treatment was completely successful in 10 patients, partially successful in two patients, and unsuccessful in two patietns. A transitory increase of the LH responsiveness to GnRH in only four patients, and a slight but significant decrease of FSH responsiveness in all patients. This intranasal GnRH application represents a harmless, convenient, and very effective treatment of maldescended testes.
F (104) HOE 471 200 µg, 6x/day, for 4 weeks	Nasal spray	Uni- or bilateral cryptorchidism	19 Prepuberal boys	Increase in basal and peak LH levels and marked decrease in peak FSH values in the i.v. LHRH test. Basal testosterone remained unchanged. Testicular descent occurred most readily in boys with a large pool of easily releasable FSH and without a significant rise in testosterone.

Table 4.3 (Continued)

Study[a]	Dosage	Delivery method	Treatment	Subjects	Results
G (105) LHRH	100 μg, 6x/day, for 7 days	Nasal spray	Unilateral cryptorchidism	22 Prepubertal children	Descent of the testes into the scrotum seen in 7 children. Basal avlues for LH and FSH and pituitary LH and FSH reserves were not altered or different from those in control group. However, no correlation was found between responses to treatment and bone age, basal plasma testosterone level, basal values of LH and FSH, or pituitary reserves of LH and FSH. No side effects reported.
H (106) LHRH	1.2 mg/day for 4 weeks	Nasal spray	Undescended testes	188 Boys	Complete descent in 52% of the cases, and improved position in 21%, and no success in 27%. No side effects observed.
I (107) GnRH	400 μg, 3x/day, for 4 weeks	Nasal spray	Cryptorchidism	60 Cryptorchid boys (39 unilateral, 21 bilateral)	Those who did not respond favorably to the GnRH treatment immediately received follow-up therapy with 1500 or 2000 IU/week of HCG for 3 weeks. After completion of this therapy, the success rate was 80% (65/81 testes descended).

[a]Numbers in parentheses are reference numbers.
Source: Modified from Chien, Y. W., and Chang, S. F., Intranasal drug delivery for systemic medications, *CRC Crit. Rev. Ther. Drug Carrier Systems, 4*:67-194 (1987).

for the administration of LHRH agonist, and that it is an attractive alternative for long-term therapy (Table 4.4) (91-94,97,118-120).

Intranasal administration of buerelin has been clinically evaluated in the treatment of the following diseases

1. Precocious puberty. Precocious puberty is a disease characterized by premature hypothalamic activity, and its treatment requires daily subcutaneous injections of relatively high doses of LHRH agonists (120). The combined subcutaneous and intranasal administration of buserelin was reported to produce a sustained clinical suppression of both clinical sex characteristics and linear growth acceleration (121).

2. Delayed puberty. The intranasal administration of buserelin for a period of 3-6 months in seven male patients with delayed puberty yielded no significant clinical effects (122). In another study in which buserelin was administered intranasally three times a week for 1 year, however, it produced a delay but significant increase in the testosterone level among eight out of 10 boys (123).

3. Induction of ovulation. In normal cyclic women in whom appropriate follicular maturation occurred previously, a single injection of LHRH has been shown to induce ovulation readily (90). By suppressing the pituitary function with an LHRH agonist, gonadotropin injections can more effectively induce ovulation in women with infertility (124). Five of the eight anovulatory patients treated with clomiphene and nasal buserelin were found to ovulate, and three of them became pregnant (125). The results suggested that intranasal administration of buserelin, following clomiphene medication, can be effectively used for the induction of ovulation in chronically anovulatory patients.

4. Inhibition of ovulation. The neural mechanisms of controlling gonadotropin release during fetal development are organized differently in the two sexes (90). Thus, in the adult female, under appropriate environmental and steroidal feedback conditions, the hypothalamus will trigger rhythmically the surges of LH secretion, which is responsible for periodical ovulation and sexual cycles (126). Subcutaneous administration of buserelin has been reported to block ovulation in women (127). Buserelin administered nasally has been found to be effective in preventing ovulation and the luteal increases of progesterone (128-130). This intranasal administration has been well accepted by the medical profession and has been proven to provide a safe and effective method of birth control without serious side effects.

5. Contraception. Application of LHRH agonists for contraception requires different dosage forms and schedules of administration. In female contraception, a practical approach is to control ovulation by daily admini-

Table 4.4 Biological Effects of Synthetic LHRH

Study[a]	Dosage	Delivery method	Route of administration	Subjects	Biological Effects
A (91)	LH/FSH-RH 100 µg at 7-10 day intervals	Parenteral injection	i.v. (n = 3) i.m. (n = 3) s.c. (n = 3)	3 Healthy males	After parenteral administration, the effectiveness in prompting LH and FSH release, the magnitude of the responses, and their time course were the same among these three routes of administration. Following intranasal application, it was less effective in promoting gonadotropin release.
	2 mg	Pasteur pipette	i.n. (n = 2)		
B (92)	LHRH 100 µg 5 mg	Injection Nasal drops	i.v. i.n.	5 Healthy males	Intranasal administration produced rises in serum gonadotropin concentration similar to those found after i.v. injection. Maximum effect on LH was seen at i.n. dose of 2.5 mg. FSH responses were much smaller, and did not display the dose dependency of the LH changes.
C (118)	LHRH 2 mg	Nasal drops	i.n.	5 Young healthy males	A clear increase in the LH levels was observed in all subjects within 30 min, lasting for up to 180 min. A definite release of FSH was also noted in 2 subjects, whereas the other 3 showed no true reaction in FSH levels.
D (93)	LHRH 100 µg at the start, 500 µg	i.v. & small graded plastic nasal	i.v. & i.n.	5 Healthy males	Intranasal administration yielded an increase in the plasma LH concentrations, which are dose-dependent with the peak

				Results
after 2 hrs, and 1000 µg after 4 hrs	catheter (Rhinyle/Ferring AB)			LH levels reached 1 hr after the administration. The i.v. route was found to be approximately 100 times more effective than the i.n. route.
E (119) LHRH (Hoechst) 0.2, 0.5, 1.0, or 2.0 mg	Nasal spray	i.n.	10 Healthy volunteers (5 males & 5 females)	In males, it led to an apparent increase in LH release in all subjects with a linear dose dependency observed. However, FSH release was not apparent. In females, both LH and FSH release could also be observed.
F (94) LHRH (Hoechst) 2 mg	Nasal drops	i.n.	4 Young men	Initial rise in serum LHRH was seen at 2.5 min and the peak reached at 15 min. There was a rapid response in serum LH with peak occurring between 30 and 45 min, whereas FSH levels did not change significantly. Approximately 1.25% of the dose was absorbed.
G (97) HOE 471 (Hoechst) 800 µg/day	Nasal spray or Rhinyle tube	i.n.	18 Healthy men	A significant release of LH occurred within 15 min and was sustained for as long as 12 hr. Both delivery devices were effective in activating the release of LH.
H (120) Buserelin 500 µg	Nasal drops	i.n.	6 Normal adult men	It led to a transient increase in serum levels of 17-OH-progesterone, 5-androstene-3β, 17β-estradiol, and testosterone on the day of treatment followed by a loss of diurnal cyclicity and decrease in serum levels of the same steroids in the following days.

aNumbers in parentheses are reference numbers.

Source: Modified from Chien, Y. W., and Chang, S. F., Intranasal drug delivery for systemic medications, CRC Crit. Rev. Ther. Drug Carrier Systems, 4:67-194 (1987).

Table 4.5 Contraception by Nasal Delivery of Synthetic LHRH

Study[a]	Dosage	Delivery method	Treatment	Subjects	Biological Effects
A (131)	Buserelin (for 3-6 months) 0.4 mg/day, n = 13 0.6 mg/day, n = 14	Nasal spray	Contraception	27 Women	Ovulation was inhibited during all but 2 of the 89 treatment months. 77.8% of the women had slight menstrual-like anovulatory bleeding. The remaining 22.2% had amenorrheic ovulatory menstrual cycles which were rapidly returned after discontinuation of treatment. Treatment was found to be well tolerated and capable of of inhibiting ovulation without producing any side effects. The majority of the women found the nasal spray very convenient and practical to use.
B (132)	Buserelin (for 13-55 weeks) 0.4 mg/day, n = 5 0.6 mg/day, n = 7	Nasal spray	Contraception	12 Women	Ovulation was inhibited during all but 2 of the 102 treatment cycles. No pregnancy and no dysfunctional uterine bleeding occurred. 50% of the women had slight menstrual-like bleeding, and others had amenorrhea during the 78 to 380 days of treatment, the dominating histological picture of the 17 endometrial biopsies showed inactive or weak proliferative glands with slightly atrophic stroma. After discontinuation of treatment, ovulatory menstrual cycles rapidly returned.

C (133) Buserelin (for 20 months) 0.4 mg/day, n = 28	Nasal spray	Contraception	24 Normally ovulating women and 4 women with pre-existing endocrine dysregulation	Ovulation was inhibited in 87.2% of the 156 treatment months. In 20 treatment months, progesterone levels temporarily increased, indicating luteinization of follicles or ovulation with defective corpus luteum function. Estradiol secretion showed a tendency to reduce as treatment progressed. Bleeding pattern ranged from menseslike bleeding, in in regular as well as irregular intervals, to amenorrhea. The morphological alterations indicated that unopposed estrogen stimulation of the endometrium is the main problem of long-term contraception.
D (134) Buserelin (for 3-12 months) 0.4 mg/day, n = 27 0.6 mg/day, n = 24	Nasal spray	Inhibition of ovulation	51 Female volunteers	No pregnancies occurred during the 283 treatment months. No severe bleeding disturbances or serious side effects was observed. No signs of hyperplastic changes were found in endometrial biopsies. Ovulation promptly returned after cessation of the prolonged treatment. Thus, long-term treatment with intranasal buserelin proved to be a safe, effective, acceptable, and rapidly reversible method for contraception.
E (135) Buserelin (for up to 24 weeks) 0.8 mg/day, n = 7 1.2 mg/day, n = 2	Nasal spray	Castration	9 Fertile women	Both doses produced sustained suppression of ovarian function, accompanied by hot flushes. In 5 women, chemical castration was established within 1-5 weeks, whereas in the other 4 volunteers, transient peaks of serum estradiol occurred in 6-19 weeks.

Table 4.5 (Continued)

Study[a]	Dosage	Delivery method	Treatment	Subjects	Biological Effects
					Thereafter low, persistent postmenopausal estradiol levels were observed. After cessation of the treatment, normal cyclical function occurred immediately. In summary, Buserelin can be used for chemical castration.
F (136)	Buserlin (for 4 months) 0.2 mg/day, $n = 4$ 0.4 mg/day, $n = 3$	Nasal spray	Contraception	7 Regularly menstruating women	Inhibition of normal ovulation occurred in all subjects. Four of the women reported 1–4 uterine bleedings during the 4-month study period, and the remaining 3 women developed amenorrhea. This tudy demonstrated that chronic LHRH agonist treatment effectively inhibits normal ovulation in the regularly mensturating woman.
G (137)	Buserelin (for 3–26 months) 0.2–0.6 mg/day	Nasal spray	Contraception	71 Normally ovulating women	Only the initial 3 treatment cycles in a total of 628 treatment months were found to be normal ovulatory. No pregnancy occurred. Endometrial biopsies ($n = 50$) did not show any evidence of hyperproliferation. After cessation of the prolonged treatment, normal ovulation and fertility rapidly returned.

[a]Numbers in parentheses are reference numbers.
Source: Modified from Chien, Y. W., and Chang, S. F., Intranasal drug delivery for systemic medications, *CRC Crit. Rev. Ther. Drug Carrier Systems,* 4:67–194 (1987).

stration of an agonist beginning with the follicular phase of the cycle (90). It is essential to administer the buserelin daily, since pituitary depletion requires several days to complete. Table 4.5 summarizes the effects of buserelin delivered by nasal spray for contraception in the human (131-137). These treatments were found to be well tolerated and capable of inhibiting ovulation without producing any side effects. Furthermore, when prolonged treatment with buserelin was stopped, normal ovulation and fertility were returned rapidly. This long-term treatment with nasal buserelin proved to be a safe, effective, acceptable, and rapidly reversible method for contraception.

6. Luteolysis. Luteolysis is defined as a reduction of plasma progesterone concentrations by shortening the luteal period. The induction of early luteolysis may require either excessive doses or daily administration of LHRH agonists during the luteal phase. Intranasal administration of buserelin in six women has been reported to result in a shortened luteal phase (2.7 days) and a reduced progesterone level (138). Another study found that intranasal administration of buserelin produces a significant luetolytic effect as measured by the shortening of the luteal phase and reduction of serum progesterone and estradiol levels (139). Both studies have indicated that intranasal administration of buserelin can induce luteolysis in normal women and control the time of the occurrence of menses.

7. Hypogonadotropic hypogonadism. In hypogonadotropic hypogonadism, the hypothalamic activity is temporarily or permanently deficient (90) and the pituitary gland is not immediately responsive to exogenous LHRH. By giving several consecutive injections of LHRH, however, the LH responses can be reestablished. Administration of buserelin by nasal spray to nine males with idiopathic hypogonadotropic hypogonadism yielded a remarkable rise of the testosterone level in only one of the patients, whereas the testosterone levels remained at prepubertal levels in the others (140). In another study, buserelin was administered as a nasal ointment to normal subjects with hypogonadism. The results showed that a nasal dose of 800 µg triggers a rise of LH levels which continue for 10 hr, and the extended FSH and testosterone responses are similar to those after intravenous injection (141). Intranasal administration of buserelin (200 µg/2 hr, eight times per day) by nasal spray to two men with hypogonadotropic hypogonadism was found to increase the testicular volume and the spermatozoa count (142). The studies conducted to date have suggested the possibility of using nasal buserelin for long-term therapy in the patients with hypogonadotropic hypogonadism.

8. Endometriosis. Currently, endometriosis is controlled by administration of steroidal compounds, like danazol. Danazol has been reported to

induce a gonadotropin-suppressive effect. Luteinizing hormone-releasing hormone agonists could be a valuable and more specific medical approach for the treatment of endometriosis. It has been demonstrated that intranasal administration of buserelin in humans with endometriosis has led to the suppression of ovarian steroid production and has resulted in the resolution of endometriotic tissue (143,144).

9. Secondary amenorrhea. Numerous attempts have been made to use either single or repeated daily injections of LHRH and agonists to stimulate the maturation of follicles in secondary amenorrhaoea (90). However, the clinical responses to this treatment have been unsatisfactory and often inconsistent. After a transient activation of the LH secretion, pituitary desensitization was noted to develop in all patients treated. Intranasal administration of buserelin has been reported to induce the release of LH, FSH, and estradiol in amenorrheic women (145-150). The high potency and prolonged duration of action have made buserelin a potential drug of choice in the treatment of amenorrhea.

10. Mammary carcinoma. Since the treatment with high doses of LHRH agonist can result in the suppression of estradiol secretion, it is expected that administration of a high LHRH agonist dose can have a beneficial effect in the treatment of hormone-dependent mammary carcinoma. In four premenopausal women with metastatic breast cancer, treatment with an infusion of buserelin at 3 mg/day for 3 days initially and subsequently with intranasal administration of buserelin at a maintenance dose of 200-400 μg/t.i.d. has yielded a remarkable improvement in two of the patients (151).

11. Uterine leiomyomas. Nine women with uterine leiomyomas have recently been treated with subcutaneous injections and then with intranasal insufflation of buserelin (a LHRH agonist) for a total treatment period of 6 months (152). After initial stimulation, the mean serum concentration of estradiol was observed to progressively decrease and stabilize at 36.8 (±4.9) pg/ml for the rest of the treatment period. The volume of uterine leiomyomas has been reduced by an average of 71%. Side effects and hot flashes were found to be less severe and better tolerated than in those patients treated with a sole subcutaneous dose.

12. Prostate carcinoma. Intranasal administration of buserelin to 18 patients with prostate carcinoma has been reported to produce a decrease in the plasma concentrations of testosterone, 17-OH-progesterone and dihydrotestosterone (153). The results indicated that the chronic intranasal administration of buserelin could be a safe and effective means of reducing the serum levels of androgens in patients with prostate cancer. In another

study in nine patients with advanced carcinoma of the prostate, treatment with initial subcutaneous administration of buserelin for 3 days following intranasal administration of buserelin for up to 24 weeks was found to produce a rise in LH and FSH levels during the first few days, which fell after 3 weeks (154). In patients who received a nasal buserelin dose of 0.6-1.2 mg/day, testosterone concentrations fell to a level of less than 1 ng/ml within 3 weeks. After 3-6 months of treatment with nasal buserelin, a moderate to significant regression in the prostatic cancer tissue resulted, which corresponded to that seen after surgical castration. Therefore, intranasal buserelin therapy could be a viable alternative to surgery in the treatment of advanced carcinoma of the prostate.

(6-D-[2-naphthyl] alanine)-LHRH. Nafarelin acetate, (6-D-[2-naphthyl] alanine)-LHRH or (D-Nal[2]^6)-LHRH (Syntex), has been reported to produce a biological activity of approximately 200 times the potency of LHRH (155,156). Subcutaneous administration of nafcrelin acetate to male dogs was noted to cause an immediate elevation of plasma levels of LH and testosterone (157). Daily intramuscular injections of naferelin acetate in female rhesus monkeys was observed to yield a dose-dependent inhibition of ovulation. A dose-dependent inhibition was also observed following the daily intranasal administration of nafarelin acetate from a metered-dose pump (95, 157). Nasal absorption of naferelin acetate in rhesus monkeys was found to be rapid and reproducible, with a peak level occurring within 15 min. A nasal bioavailability of about 2% was obtained as compared to the plasma levels from the subcutaneous dose. The result was noted to agree fairly well with the bioassay data of an effective dose for the inhibition of ovulation (250 mg or nasal vs. 5 mg for s.c.) (94). Intranasal administration of nafarelin acetate to the women was found to have a nasal bioavailability of 5% (157). Furthermore, intranasal administration of nafarelin acetate at a daily dose of 125-250 μg to 30 women was reported to produce inhibition of normal ovulation and corpus luteum function (158).

A group of 24 women with normal menstrual cycles have recently been treated with nafarelin acetate administered intranasally at daily doses of 125 or 250 μg for 6 months (159). There were significantly less presumed ovulatory cycles at the higher dose (two out of 60 cycles) than at the lower dose (10 out of 54 cycles) (p < 0.01). With the higher dose of nafarelin acetate there were significantly fewer bleeding episodes, less number of days of bleeding and longer cycles. With both doses, the acute responses of LH, FSH, and estradiol were significantly greater on day 1 than on either day 98 or 186. Side effects observed in this study included galactorrhea (two subjects) and vasomotor symptoms (seven subjects).

In order to determine the efficacy of nafarelin hormonal manipulation in the treatment of endometriosis, 213 patients with laparoscopically confirmed endometriosis were randomly assigned to receive for 6 months either nafarelin (400 or 800 μg per day) by nasal spray or oral danazol (800 mg per day) (160). Placebo nasal spray and placebo tablets were used as the controls in this double-blind study. The results demonstrated that more than 80% of the patients in each treatment group achieved a reduction in the extent of disease as assessed by laparoscopy. The mean laparoscopic scores decreased from 21.9 to 12.6 with 800 μg of nafarelin, from 20.4 to 11.7 with 400 μg of nafarelin, and from 18.4 to 10.5 with danazol (p = 0.0001). The percentage of women with severely painful symptoms of endometriosis decreased from about 40 to 5-10%, whereas the percentage of patients with no or minimal discomfort rose from 25 to 70%. Of the 149 patients who tried to become pregnant, 58 (39%) succeeded after the completion of treatment. It was thus concluded that nafarelin is an effective agent for treating endometriosis and has few side effects other than hypoestrogenism.

4.3.5 Posterior Pituitary Hormones

4.3.5.1 Oxytocin

Oxytocin is synthesized in neurons in the hypothalamus. It is known to stimulate the contraction of smooth muscle in the uterus and to induce the contraction of the myoepithelial cells around the breast and alveoli to squeeze milk into the large ducts and increase milk flow through the nipple. Therefore, oxytocin is the drug of choice for the induction and enhancement of labor. It has also been used to assist an ongoing abortion, utilized in the treatment of breast engorgement, or applied to increase milk flow to the infant.

Oxytocin has been administered intranasally as a powerful stimulant for uterine contractions during labor, using a nasal cotton pledget presoaked in a solution of posterior pituitary extracts (161). The results indicated that there is no marked change in the nasal mucous membrane following repeated applications of such a pituitary extracts-presoaked cotton pledget.

Intranasal administration of oxytocin in combination with castor oil and quinine has been used to induce labor in women whose pregnancy had progressed beyond the period of viability, with an efficiency of 98.7% (162). The nose drops of pituitary extracts were used to induce labor or to combat uterine inertia, which resulted in a definite increase in the frequency and the strength of uterine contractions within 5-10 min. These uterine contractions were noted to last for 30 min or longer (163).

Syntocinon (Sandoz) and Partocon (Ferring AB) are both synthetic oxy-tocin products, which have been used in different concentrations and meth-ods of administration to induce labor (163-185) or lactation (186-194) as well as to produce an increase in the secretion of insulin and glucagon (195). These are discussed as follows.

Induction and enhancement of labor

Table 4.6 summarizes the results of the studies of the effectiveness (164-174) and safety (165,167,169,173,176) of synthetic oxytocin delivered intranasal-ly on the induction and the enhancement of labor, on the uterine response (183,184), and on the feasibility of replacing the intravenous drip or intra-muscular injection with nasal spray (168,179,180) as well as the compara-tive efficiency of oxytocin delivery between intranasal and intravenous (181, 182) or between intranasal and transbuccal administration (173,183-185). The uterine activity was usually detected to increase within 5-9 min (164, 166,172,174,178), and the peak activity was normally attained within 10-20 min (164,174). The fraction of the applied dose that appeared to be absorbed was not more than 1-2% (169). Even with this low level of nasal absorption, however, synthetic oxytocin was found to produce a stimulation of the uterine contractility desirable for obstetric purposes. It has been concluded that the intranasal administration of synthetic oxytocin is an efficacious, safe, and convenient method for the induction and the enhance-ment of labor. The results demonstrated no statistical difference in the rates of success among nasal, transbuccal, and intravenous administrations (168,173,179-185), and that intranasal administration can be used to re-place intravenous or intramuscular administration (168,179,180).

There were only two studies which questioned the use of nasal synthetic oxytocin; i.e., the unpredicability of the amount absorbed makes the intra-nasal route relatively unsafe, whereas the intravenous administration of oxytocin was more precise and more readily controlled than the intranasal administration (182).

Stimulation of lactation

The smooth course of breast feeding is dependent upon an adequate func-tion of the milk let-down reflex (186). Stimulation of the nipple in lactating women activates the release of an oxytocin factor into the blood stream through the mediation of the central nervous system and the posterior lobe of the pituitary gland. This factor then acts on the myoepithelial elements surrounding the alveoli of the breast, causing them to contract and force milk to flow into the large mammary ducts, where it becomes readily avail-able for breast feeding.

Table 4.6 Induction and Enhancement of Labor by Nasal Delivery of Synthetic Oxytocin

Study[a]	Delivery method	Subjects	Purpose	Biological effects	Conclusions
A (164)	Nose drops	23 Women	Evaluate effect of Syntocinon (Sandoz)	Uterine activity usually detected to increase within 5–7 min, and the peak activity normally attained within 10–20 min.	Contractions stimulated by nasal oxytocin are indistinguishable in all characteristics from the spontaneously occurring contractions.
B (165)	Nasal spray Nose drops	Humans	Evaluate clinical applicability of oxytocin	Extent of increase in uterine activity and progress of actual labor are primarily dependent upon the "readiness to labor" of the uterus and at the time when the labor induction is started.	Nasal oxytocin has a high degree of safety without the risks of excessive uterine activities or excessive tonus.
C (166)	Nasal spray	266 Women	Study nasal oxytocin for induction of labor, enhancement of labor, and prelabor and sensitivity tests	Following the first nasal application, a rise in uterine activity was observed within 7 min. The fraction of applied dose absorbed was about 1–2%.	Nasal oxytocin is useful in enhancing uterine activity during the inertial periods in labor and in inducing labor when combined with an amniotomy as well as in the oxytocin-sensitivity test.
D (167)	Standard tuberculin syringe	100 Women	Study safety and effectiveness of nasal oxytocin	Effectiveness for the elective induction of labor with nasal oxytocin was 91.5% in 47 primiparas and 79.4% in 184 multi-	Nasal oxytocin appears to offer a satisfactory method for induction of labor and/or stimulation of uterine contractions.

	Form	Subjects	Purpose	Results	Conclusions
E (168)	Nasal spray	109 Women	Study clinical impression of nasal oxytocin	paras. Induction for medical reasons was successful in 85.6% of the 14 primiparas and in 94.4% of 36 multiparas. Uterine response was most satisfactory in cases of inert labor and when used as an adjuvant to artificial rupture of the membranes in the induction of labor.	Intranasal administration is as efficacious as the intramuscular injection, but is much safer.
F (169)	Aerosol-activated spray	Human	Evaluate efficacy and safety of nasal oxytocin using continuous recordings of amniotic fluid pressure	Level of uterine activity achieved with nasal oxytocin at 2 IU was approximated to the i.v. infusion of 2 ml/min for 10 min. Considerable variability and undesirable degrees of uterine activity were noted.	Approximately 1% of the nasal dose was actually absorbed, and this weak stimulus to uterine contractility was desirable in the obstetric condition which require only a minimal enhancement of uterine contractility.
G (171)	Nasal spray	39 Women	Evaluate induction and enhancement of labor by nasal oxytocin	Nasal oxytocin was found particularly useful in the induction of labor in women whose membranes have already been ruptured and also useful in cases with unruptured membranes.	Nasal oxytocin spray has the advantages of simplicity and ease of application; therefore it is useful in induction of labor and also in enhancement of uterine action in certain types of labor.

Table 4.6 (Continued)

Study[a]	Delivery method	Subjects	Purpose	Biological effects	Conclusions
G (175)	Nasal spray	102 Women	Determine safety of oxytocin nasal spray	Efficacy of nasal oxytocin in labor induction was confirmed, but lack of the required precision.	Intravenous infusion of oxytocin at a controlled rate is preferable to nasal oxytocin in complicated pregnancy.
I (177)	Nasal spray	15 Women	Determine sensitivity of uterus at or past term prior to induction of labor	A single dose of nasal spray was found to produce a uterine activity corresponded to that achieved with 0.01 and 0.02 IU by i.v. injection.	Sensitivity test using nasal oxytocin provides a safe and reasonably accurate guide to the prospects of a patient beginning her labor after surgical induction.
J (178)	Tuberculin syringe	15 Women	Evaluate uterine response to oxytocin administered intranasally	After intranasal application, the initial uterine response appeared in 5-7 min and the duration of response varied (16-60 min). Levels of uterine response were found comparable to infusion of 2 mU/min.	Unpredictability of the amount absorbed and the uterine response make intranasal application relatively unsafe, and is not routinely recommended for the management of pregnant patients.
K (179)	Nasal spray	Humans	Investigate feasibility of replacing i.v. drip of oxytocin by	After intranasal administration, contractions were soon observed and 2-4 applications were found to	Nasal oxytocin is useful in the induction of labor, primary and secondary inertia, even in the third stage of labor.

L (180)	Nasal spray	19 Women	Study number of patients in whom an oxytocin drip was made unnecessary	nasal spray for labor induction be sufficient to establish labor. Intravenous oxytocin infusion was made unnecessary in 68.4% of subjects by use of nasal spray.	Nasal delivery requires little supervision and carries no apparent risk to mother or baby.
M (181)	Polyethylene tube	96 Women	Compare effectiveness of oxytocin in induction and stimulating of labor by intranasal nasal drip administrations	Intranasal administration produces a rapid and reliable effect in inducing or stimulating labor with a successful rate of 88.5%, which is as good as i.v. drip (90.9%).	Intranasal application of oxytocin is a simple, practical, and convenient method for patients.
N (182)	Nasal spray	15 Women	Compare efficacy of oxytocin by intranasal and i.v. administration induction or stimulation of labor	Uterine activity resulting from the administration of one spray to each nostril was slightly greater than the response obtained by intravenous infusion of 0.7 mU/min for 15 min. Corresponding activity due to a second spray 41 min later was equal to the activity by infusion of 1.5 mU/min for 15 min.	Intravenous administration is more precise and more readily controlled than nasal spray.

Table 4.6 (Continued)

Study[a]	Delivery method	Subjects	Purpose	Biological effects	Conclusions
O (172)	Rhinyle	22 Women	Induce labor while measuring pressure through a saline-filled vinyl catheter induced transabdominally	Enhancement of uterine activity became visible within 5-6 min after first nasal dose. Duration of effect was about 20 min, after which level of activity remained higher.	Uterine activity was higher by intranasal administration than spontaneous activity.
P (173)	Nasal spray	300 Women	Evaluate effectiveness, safety, and convenience of oxytocin administered by i.v., i.n., and transbuccal routes	Rates of success for i.v. and transbuccal administrations were practically the same, whereas rate by nasal routes was somewhat lower. However, no substantial difference in degree of safety.	Transbuccal administration was considered to be most convenient to patients and medical staff.
Q (174)	Graded polyethylene tube	26 Women	Study effect and safety of nasal oxytocin on pregnant uterus using a continuous recording of amniotic fluid pressure	Nine minutes after nasal application, increase in intensity and frequency of uterine contractions occurred, and attained maximum effect in 10-15 min.	Intranasal administration can be safely used as a gentle stimulus to the antepartum uterus.
R (176)	Nose drops	1806 Women	Study the safety of oxytocin administered intranasally	In 1806 patients in which 75% for elective stimulation of labor and 25% for induction of labor, there	Nasal oxytocin is easy to administer and safe in the induction of labor.

	Preparation	No.	Objective	Results	Conclusions
				was a total success rate of 88%, with an overall cesarean rate of only 1.5% was obtained.	
S (183)	Nasal solution	175 Women	Compare effect on labor induction among intranasal, transbuccal, and i.v. administration	Percent of successful induction for nasal, i.v., infusion, and buccal administration was 79, 75, and 67%, respectively.	Intranasal, transbuccal and intravenous administrations of oxytocin are all useful tools for obstetricians
T (184)	Graded polyethylene tube	122 Women (110 primiparae) (112 multiparae)	Compare clinical effectiveness between nasal and buccal preparations in the induction of labor	Nasal oxytocin produced and immediate response and triggered off labor at a rate faster than buccal oxytocin, whereas buccal oxytocin initiated a higher proportion of labor in the later hour.	No statistical difference in the success rates between intranasal and buccal routes in induction of labor, either for primiparae or for multiparae.
U (185)	Transbuccal (Syntocinon) Nasal solution (Partocon)	468 Women	Compare effect of transnasal and transbuccal administration on the induction of labor	Nasal oxytocin led to delivery in 43% of the cases, transbuccal 54% (50 IU) and over 60% (100 IU). Differences were greatest in primiparae: 37% with intranasal administration and 60-61% with transbuccal therapy.	Administration of oxytocin by intranasal and transbuccal routes is simple and produces obvious difference in action.

[a]Numbers in parentheses are reference numbers.
Source: Modified from Chien, Y. W., and Chang, S. F., Intranasal drug delivery for systemic medications, CRC Crit. Rev. Ther. Drug Carrier Systems, 4:67-194 (1987).

Table 4.7 Stimulation of Lactation by Nasal Delivery of Synthetic Oxytocin

Study[a]	Delivery method	Subjects	Purpose	Results	Conclusions
A (186)	Oxytocin-soaked cotton applicator	19 Women	Test practicability and effectiveness of nasal oxytocin in triggering the let-down reflex	Intranasal application of oxytocin before the baby starts to nurse may help the mother overcome the inhibition of let-down reflex.	Use of nasal oxytocin appears to be an effective and practical method of overcoming the inhibition of let-down reflex.
B (187)	Syntocinon nasal spray	Human	Study milk let-down effect	Nasal spray exerts a good galactokinetic (milk let-down) effect. 3–4 IU of drug should be sufficient, if applied 5 min before breast feeding or pumping.	Use of nasal spray has advantages of avoiding repeated injection and permitting self-administration by the patients.
C (188)	Syntocinon nasal spray 40 IU/ml	Humans	Evaluate efficacy of Syntocinon in stimulating milk ejection from parturient and engorged breast	Good milk let-down phenomenon was produced in nursing and nonnursing mothers.	Intranasal administration of Syntocinon is of value in stimulating breast secretion, though it is perhaps not quite as efficient as the intramuscular route.
D (189)	Syntocinon nasal spray	351 Patients	Investigate effects of Syntocinon	Unilateral intranasal spraying before a feeding produced a milk ejection effect which is as effective as parenteral injection.	It helped to relieve painful tension due to engorgement of the breast.

E (190) Syntocinon	25 Women	Evaluate management of breast-feeding	Nasal spray was noted to produce an early establishment of breast-feeding and also improve a milk production.	Nasal oxytocin has a trace usefulness in the management of breast-feeding and lactation.
F (191) Oxytocin nasal spray	125 Women	Report clinical experience with intranasal administration of oxytocin	In 80% of patients, oxytocin nasal spray produced an increase in milk yield for up to a maximum of 26%. Under the influence of nasal oxytocin, an empty breast can still produce 30-80% of the previous milk output.	Nasal spray causes a moderate increase in the milk yeild in 86% of the subjects, a great rise in 13%, and no effect in 1%.
G (192) Syntocinon nasal spray	Rabbits	Study influence on lactating mammary glands	Intravenous administration of adrenaline transiently suppressed a long-lasting reaction to oxytocin.	It is necessary to give approximately 10-100 times as much by intranasal administration to elicit identical results in intensity and character with those produced by i.v. infusion.
H (193) Syntocinon nasal spray	Women	Compare with sublingual tablet on initiation, enhancement, and maintenance of early phase of lactation	Nasal spray produced very rapid, high-intensity, and short-lived milk ejection response. Major reactions were seen in 1.5-3.0 min, reached extremely high	Nasal spray gives only a short-acting, quickly dispelled actuation, whereas sublingual tablet produces a prolonged low-dosage stimulation of lactation.

Table 4.7 (Continued)

Study[a]	Delivery method	Subjects	Purpose	Results	Conclusions
				peaks of pressure, and lasted for not exceeding 2 min.	
I (194)	Partocon polyethylene tube	10 Lactating women	Compare response of intramammary pressure (IMP) to oxytocin given by i.v. infusion with that by intranasal administration	After intranasal administration, IMP showed increase within 1–1.5 min, which persisted for 10–20 min. Nasal dose required about 100 times greater than dose needed by i.v. infusion to produce comparable effect.	The IMP curve of nasal oxytocin resembles that of i.v. infusion or following suction stimulation of the contralateral nipple.

[a]Numbers in parentheses are reference numbers.
Source: Modified from Chien, Y. W., and Chang, S. F., Intranasal drug delivery for systemic medications, *CRC Crit. Rev. Ther. Drug Carrier Systems, 4:*67–194 (1987).

Table 4.7 summarizes the studies on the effect of the intranasal administration of synthetic oxytocin on milk let-down (186,187) and milk ejection (lactation) (188-192) as well as comparative effects between intranasal and transbuccal administration (187) and between intranasal administration and intravenous infusion (194). The results indicated that the intranasal administration of synthetic oxytocin exerts a good milk let-down effect and helps to relieve painful tension due to engorgement of the breast. Intranasal administration of synthetic oxytocin produced a very rapid, high-intensity, and short-lived milk-ejection response, whereas transbuccal administration of synthetic oxytocin yielded a prolonged, low-dosage stimulation of lactation. An about 100 times higher dose was found to be required for the nasal oxytocin than the dose needed by intravenous infusion to produce a comparable effect (194).

Secretion of insulin and glucagon

The effectiveness of synthetic oxytocin following intranasal administration in evoking the secretion of insulin and glucagon has been studied in dogs (195). A prompt and striking increase in all measurements of glucose, insulin, and glucagon in the plasma was observed, whereas similar instillation of saline yielded no effect. The effects of nasal oxytocin on the plasma concentrations of glucose, insulin, and glucagon were observed to be somewhat greater than those observed with the intravenous infusion.

4.3.5.2 Vasopressin

Natural vasopressin

Human vasopressin The form of vasopressin isolated from human and most mammalian animals is usually arginine vasopressin, which is also called antidiuretic hormone (ADH) because it promotes water retention and also enhances the secretion of sodium and chloride. Where there is a defect in the hypothalamicopituitary secretion of adenosine disphophate (ADH), diabetes insipidus develops with polyuria and polydipsia as the major symptoms.

$$\overline{\text{S}\text{S}}$$
NH$_2$—Cys—Tyr—Phe—GlN—AsN—Cys—Pro—(L)Arg—Gly

The long-term treatment of diabetes insipidus has been by the intramuscular injection of aqueous vasopressin (Pitressin/Parke-Davis), Pitressin tan-

Table 4.8 Treatment of Diabetes Insipidus with Nasal Delivery of Lypressin

Study[a]	Delivery method	Subjects	Results	Conclusions
A (201)	Nasal spray	Humans	Effective in patients with diabetes insipidus who experienced a generalized allergic reaction to natural vasopressin.	Antidiuretic effect identical to natural vasopressin and is therapeutically effective by intranasal administration.
B (202)	Nasal spray	Humans	Effective in patients with diabetes insipidus who experienced generalized allergic reaction to natural vasopressin.	Nasal Lypressin was well tolerated. It provided satisfactory clinical control of polyuria and raised specific gravity of urine.
C (203)	Nasal spray	9 Children with diabetes insipidus	Effectively controlled diabetes insipidus over a 6-month period.	By intramuscular or intranasal administration, it can effectively control diabetes insipidus in humans.
D (204)	Nasal spray	3 Female and 5 male patients with diabetes insipidus	Completely controlled diabetes insipidus of moderate severity and partially controlled severe cases.	Satisfactory control of diabetes insipidus can be obtained. This form of administration is prefered by many patients.
E (205)	Nasal spray	Same as above	In all cases, urinary volume became normal after spraying (3–7 times/24 hr) of Lypressin. In 7 of 8 patients, nasal spray could replace pitressin tanate-in-oil. Nasal regimen can be maintained from 1 month to more than a year.	Same as above

F (206) Nasal spray 35–125 U/day	13 Patients with diabetes insipidus	Effective in reducing the urine volume and increasing the concentration to a normal range. Duration of antidiuretic action was intermediate between subcutaneous dose of 1.0 and 3.5 U.	In hydrated normal subjects, it is 7.4 times as effective as the nasal spray preparation of vasopressin.
G (207) Nasal spray	19 Patients with diabetes insipidus	Rapidly cleared from plasma with a duration of effect of 3–5 hr. A slow appearance and peaking of plasma concentration were observed also, a concomitant fall in urine volume and elevation of urinary osmolality was observed.	Delivered by nasal spray, Lypressin is effective, rapidly absorbed, apparently nonsensitizing, and nonirritating. It could be used in the management of vasopressin-sensitive diabetes insipidus.
H (208) Nasal spray	20 Patients with vasopressin-deficient diabetes insipidus	Antidiuretic activity was fairly prompt with the onset of action within 1 hr and a duration of activity for 3–8 hr. Use of nasal spray, 2–8 times/day (50–625 U/day), produced satisfactory control of polydipsia, polyuria, and nocturia in all patients.	Lypressin nasal spray was recommended for clinical use, since it is easy to administer, has produced no significant water retention, and is free from any potential serious allergic reaction.
I (209) Nasal spray	3 Patients with diabetes insipidus	Patients were adequately controlled with spraying every 3 hr during the day.	Nasal Lypressin provided adequate control in some patients, but may not be adequate in others, particularly in nocturnal control of thirst and polyuria.

Table 4.8 (Continued)

Study[a]	Delivery method	Subjects	Results	Conclusions
J (210)	Nasal spray	6 Patients with diabetes insipidus	Average dose requirement was 10-20 IU/day. One patient experienced some local nasal irritation wth spray of 50 IU/day for 14 weeks.	66.7% of patients were well controlled, whereas others required a higher dose and their symptomatic control was still not satisfactory.
K (211)	Nasal spray	3 Patients with diabetes insipidus Hypophyseal sufficiency	Successfully controlled manifestations of diabetes insipidus with demonstrable neurohypophyseal insufficiency.	Lypressin nasal spray is expected to become the treatment of choice in diabetes insipidus with neurohypophyseal insufficiency.
L (212)	Nasal spray	5 Children with diabetes insipidus	Antidriuetic action was noted within 1 hr in all patients and the drug was cleared from plasma in 3-5 hr. Effective in the control of polydipsia and polyuria.	Lypressin nasal spray is an effective and nonirritating agent for the long-term treatment of diabetes insipidus in children.
M (213)	Nasal spray	3 Patients with diabetes insipidus who showed manifested allergic reactions to various antidiuretic hormone preparations.	Yielded good control of diabetes insipidus.	The use of Lypressin nasal spray was not attended by any allergic symptoms or other side effects.

[a]Numbers in parentheses are reference numbers.
Source: Modified from Chien, Y. W., and Chang, S. F., Intranasal drug delivery for systemic medications, *CRC Crit. Rev. Ther. Drug Carrier Systems,* 4:67-194 (1987).

nate in peanut oil, or the nasal insufflation of crude posterior pituitary powder (5-20 USP units, three times or more a day) (196,197). The intramuscular injection of Pitressin tannate in oil is painful and unpleasant. Posterior pituitary extracts containing vasopressin have been used in the treatment of cranial diabetes insipidus since 1913. Posterior pituitary snuff has the disadvantage of needing frequent administration, of uncertain action, and, in some patients, of producing nasal irritation (197), asthma (198), or pulmonary fibrosis (199). However, intranasal administration by spray of posterior pituitary extracts powder in the treatment of polyuria and polydipsia was found to be as effective as by parenteral administration.

Synthetic vasopressin

Lypressin (Lysine-8-vasopressin). The success of vasopressin synthesis has led to the commercialization of a nasal spray containing synthetic lysine-8-vasopressin (Lypressin/Sandoz). Such a preparation has proved effective in patients with diabetes insipidus. Lypressin nasal spray has a short duration of action, and the patients need repeated doses at 2- to 4-hr intervals. Table 4.8 summarizes the clinical results of intranasal administration of Lypressin (200-213).

$$
\begin{array}{c}
\overset{\displaystyle \lceil \!-\!\!S\!-\!\!-\!\!-\!\!-\!\!-\!\!-\!\!S\!-\!\rceil}{} \\
NH_2-Cys-Tyr-Phe-GlN-AsN-Cys-Pro-Lys-Gly
\end{array}
$$

4.3.5.3 PLV-2 (phenylalanyl-lysyl-vasopressin)

PLV-2, a posthypophyseal hormonelike substance, has been reported to be five times more effective than Lypressin on blood pressure and 10-40 times weaker than Lypressin in diuretic action (214). PLV-2 has been used as a nasal spray for topical and local vasoconstriction and has been found to be as effective as 4% cocaine in achieving nasal decongestion prior to nasotracheal intubation (214). PLV-2 has been proposed for application as a topical and local vasoconstrictor, with a greater degree of safety than epinephrine, for controlling hypertension.

4.3.5.4 DDAVP (1-desamino-8-D-arginine)vasopressin

DDAVP has a greater antidiuretic potency than either natural vasopressin or any other known synethetic vasopressin, and it also produces prolonged antidiuresis (215). On the other hand, the other activities of DDAVP (like pressor, galactogogic, vagal-like action on the gut) are simultaneously reduced

Table 4.9 Intranasal Administration of DDAVP for Diabetes Insipidus Therapy

Study[a]	Delivery method	Subjects	Results	Conclusions
A (215)	Nasal spray 0.2 ng/ml	Rats, dogs, humans	Had higher antidiuretic potency and lower pressor activity.	Has a prolonged antidiuresis activity and greater antidiuretic potency than either natural or synthetic vasopressin.
B (216)	Rhinyle 7.5 or 15 μg, once to twice daily	10 Patients with vasopressin-sensitive diabetes insipidus	By intranasal administration in doses of 15 μg, 1-3 times daily, normalized urine production, including those cases in which previous therapy failed. A nasal bioavailability of 10-20% was achieved.	Safe and effective in treatment of cranial diabetes insipidus. It is free from side effects, easy to administer, and has long duration of action.
C (217)	Calibrated plastic tube or Rhinyle, 10 μg/12 hr to 20 μg/8 hr	21 Patients with central diabetes insipidus	Within 1 hr of administration, there was a substantial decrease in thirst and in urine output as well as an increase in urine concentration. In each case there was relief of polydipsia and cessation of polyuria.	The preferred drug for the management of central diabetes insipidus.
D (219)	Disposable plastic tube	7 Children with 1 adult with vasopressin-sensitive diabetes insipidus	Average duration of action was 10-11 hr. Most frequent use dosage was 2.5-10.0 μg b.i.d. All subjects found it superior to other forms of therapy.	Provides good control of diuresis for patients with diabetes insipidus as a result of its potency and prolonged duration. Preferred by patients over vasopressin tannate-in-oil and Lypressin.

E (220) Rhinyle attached to an air-filled syringe, 2.5-10.0 μg	29 Patients with neurogenic diabetes insipidus	Provided excellent control of symptoms and urine volume. It was as good as vasopressin tannate-in-oil and was better than chlorpropamide and Lypressin nasal spray.	The preferred treatment for neurogenic diabetes because of its ease of administration, efficacy, long duration of action, and absence of pressor side effects.
F (221) Rhinyle	6 Patients with neurogenic diabetes insipidus	Had specific antidiuretic activity with prolonged duration of action and minimal side effects.	Should be the drug of choice for neurogenic diabetes insipidus in pediatric patients as a result of its ease and convenience of administration, long duration of action, purity, and absence of side effects.
G (218) Plastic tube 20 μg, b.i.d.	7 Patients with cranial diabetes insipidus and 2 with nephrogenic diabetes insipidus	Single nasal administration produced antidiuresis for up to 20 hr without side effects. Each patient was well controlled.	An ideal drug for the treatment of vasopressin-sensitive diabetes insipidus due to its slow metabolic clearance when absorbed through the nasal mucosa and its lack of side effects.
H (224) Rhinyle	Patients with diabetes insipidus (not complicated with other diseases)	After intranasal administration of 5-320 μg, changes occurred qualitatively similar to those induced by i.v. injection of 1-24 μg. Osmolality showed a dose-related increase during the second 12-hr period and the peak effect was gradually prolonged.	In the evaluation of DDAVP, the maximal antidiuretic ability and the prolongation of action have to be lyzed separately. Nasal absorption is 10-20% with low and usual therapuetic doses and 2.5-5.0% with high and excessive doses.

Table 4.9 (Continued)

Study[a]	Delivery method	Subjects	Results	Conclusions
I (222)	Metered-dose nasal spray	Patients with diabetes insipidus	Produced potent antidiuresis with rapid onset and sustained activity for 10-12 hr, followed by a gradual loss in control of diuresis over the next 12 hr.	Method simple and efficient and generally preferred by patients, and better than the Rhinyle.
J (223)	With clofibrate by plastic tube	Patients with diabetes insipidus	Without clofibrate, had practically no effect at a 10-μg dose. With clofibrate, induced a significant increase (71% [+6.4%]) in the 24-hr urine osmolality.	Duration of antidiuretic effect is prolonged as a result of a decrease in the metabolic degradation of DDAVP.
K (225)	Plastic tube	11 Patients with central diabetes insipidus	Slowly absorbed with peak levels reached within 1-5 hr. μg produced three- to 20-fold longer duration of response than 18.5 μg LVP. Duration of response varied from 8 to 20 hr. Eleven patients responded to treatment for up to 11 months and showed no side effects.	The best treatment available for central diabetes insipidus. Prolonged effectiveness is due to its slow absorption from nasal mucosa, prolonged plasma level, and enhanced effect on the renal medulla.

[a]Numbers in parentheses are reference numbers.
Source: Modified from Chien, Y. W., and Chang, S. F., Intranasal drug delivery for systemic medications, *CRC Crit. Rev. Ther. Drug Carrier Systems, 4*:67-194 (1987).

to a very low value. It has the advantages of greater antidiuretic potency with longer duration of action, less vasopressor activity, and no oxytocic activity. It also has unique and important advantages in the management of central diabetes insipidus. Table 4.9 summarizes the results of the intranasal administration of DDAVP (215-225).

$$\overline{S-S}$$
Cys–Tyr–Phe–GIN–AsN–Cys–Pro–(D)Arg–Gly

The effect of methylcellulose on the particle size distribution and dosing accuracy of the premetered spray pumping devices containing desmopressin (DDAVP) has been recently investigated (226). Also, the influence of methylcellulose on the in vivo deposition and clearance of nasal solutions, administered as drops or spray, has also been studied. The results indicated that nasal formulations containing 0-0.50% of methylcellulose produce a dose-dependent increase in average particle size (51-200 μm). However, no effect was observed on the dosing accuracy of the spraying pumps.

With the pump device, the spray droplets were deposited in the anterior region of the nasal cavity, mainly in the atrium, whereas the drops delivered by the Rhinyle plastic tube appeared to deposit solution more evenly over the nasal cavity, pharynx, and sinuses. However, the net effect of methylcellulose on the clearance of DDAVP was observed to follow a biphasic pattern which showed an increase in retention time for the 0.25% solution, followed by a decrease in retention time and an increase in clearance rate for the 0.50% solution. The nasal spray was found to deliver well-controlled doses to the nasal cavity. These findings suggested that viscosity, particle size, and nasal clearance are important parameters in the design of nasal delivery systems.

4.4 OTHER THERAPEUTICALLY IMPORTANT BIOLOGICAL PRODUCTS

4.4.1 Interferon

Interferon, a proteinaceous molecule, is present in all vertebrates, which is produced in the body in response to the presence of a virus or even certain bacteria. It is a species-specific and relative nontoxic biological substance with a broad spectrum of antiviral activities and a high therapeutic index (227). The investigation of interferon as an antiviral agent began immediately after its discovery in 1957 (228).

Table 4.10 Preventive and Therapeutic Uses of Interferon in Man

Source of interferon	Method of application	Prevention/therapy	Result[a]
Monkey	Intradermal	Vaccination	+
	Subcutaneous	Vaccinia gangrenosa	−
	Eye drops	Vaccinal keratitis	+
	Nose drops	Rhinovirus, coevirus, and parainfluenza	−
Human amnion	Eye drops	Herpes simplex keratitis	−
Human WBC	Intravenous	Leukemia, cytomegalovirus, and herpes virus infection	? +
	Nasal spray	Influenza A2	+
	Nasal spray	Influenza A2 epidemic	+
	Nasal spray	Rhinovirus	−
	Nasal spray	Influenza B	±
	Nasal spray	Rhinovirus 4	+
	Parenteral	Osteogenic sarcoma	+

[a]+, Beneficial effect; −, no effect; ±, equivocal effect; ?, unclear effect.
Source: Modified from Ref. 227, used with permission.

The mechanisms of action of interferons have been ascribed at the cellular level, which include the inhibition of cell division and tumor growth, the enhancement of phagocytosis of macrophages, the cytotoxicity of lymphocytes, the activity of natural killer cells, and the production of antibodies. Human interferons have been grouped into three major classes: (a) IFN-α (leukocyte), (b) IFN-β (fibroblast), and (c) IFN-γ (immune); all interferons are proteins made up of 146-166 amino acids. The first 17 amino acids are essential to the biological activities of human interferons. In addition, cysteine bonds, which play a central role in the spatial folding of proteins, are also critical to the antiviral activities of this proteinaceous molecule. The uses of interferons in man are summarized in Table 4.10.

During an influenza A2 epidemic, which involved 14,000 persons, interferon was applied intranasally for 3-7 days (229,230). Among the 3129 control subjects treated with placebo, 551 (17.6%) became ill; in contrast, among the 2994 subjects treated with interferon, only 231 (7.7%) were not protected.

However, the studies on the intranasal delivery of human leukocyte interferon for the prophylaxis of rhinovirus infections failed to show any protective effect when 180,000 U of interferon were given to each volunteer (231). Study on human leukocyte interferon to inhibit the infection by respiratory virus was also unsuccessful. In this study, 800,000 U of interferon was locally applied to the nasal epithelial barrier to minimize the systemic availability of interferon and to avoid the possibility of rapid disappearance of interferon from the circulation. Intranasal delivery of human leukocyte interferon on the day before the influenza challenge could only slightly delay the onset of influenza B infection. It did not prevent the occurrence of the illness nor reduce its severity. However, using a high daily dose (14,000,000 U) of interferon, with 1 day of prophylaxis and 3 days of treatment, a statistically significant decrease in the severity of symptoms and in the frequency of virus shedding was achieved. It was surprising that even with these high doses, the interferon titers in the nasal washing were low and never exceeded the level of 300 U/ml (232). These findings suggested the possible occurrence of either an extensive dilution, a rapid uptake, or the destruction of interferon in the nasal cavity and/or nasopharynx.

The human leukocyte interferon, which was applied intranasally at a dose of 10,000 U by a Pasteur pipette, could be recovered locally in nine out of 10 chimpanzees and all the human volunteers tested at a recovery rate ranging from 2 to 10% (233). The amount of interferon recovered at 5-60 min after the intranasal application was only 2-20% of the reference samples. The nasal epithelial cells in humans were found to respond equally to both leukocyte and fibroblast interferons with the development of a resistance to the replication of virus, which was time- and dose-dependent (234).

The antiviral activity of human leukocyte interferon has been investigated by delivering it in either nose drops or an interferon-saturated cotton pledget (235). The nasal drops were instilled once every 5 min for 1 hr using a Pasteur pipette, whereas the medicated cotton pledget was placed in the inferior turbinate for 1 hr. No significant reduction in the mean value of virus yield was found in the volunteers receiving 80,000 U of interferon by nose drops, whereas a significant reduction (p < 0.025) was achieved in the cells obtained 4 hr after application with the cotton pledget saturated with 20,000-80,000 U of interferon (Tables 4.11 and 4.12). The volunteers who took oral antihistamines prior to their receiving interferon by nose drops were also effectively treated. These investigations suggested that nasal epithelial cells can be made antiviral in vivo by the intranasal administration of human leukocyte interferon. Furthermore, a significant antiviral activity can be achieved, depending upon the method of delivery of interferon to the nasal mucosa and the extent of interferon contact with the nasal epithelial cells.

Table 4.11 Antiviral Activity of Human Leukocyte Interferon

Nasal dosage[a] (U/0.1 ml)[b]	VSV yield[c] (mean ± SEM)		Reduction in VSV yield ($\log_{10}$)
	Untreated cells	Treated cells	
50,000	6.05 ± 0.03 (3)	5.88 ± 0.02 (2)	0.17
80,000	5.24 ± 0.11 (8)	5.34 ± 0.09 (7)	+ 0.10
80,000 + Anti-H[d]	5.07 ± 0.16 (8)	4.53 ± 0.13 (7)	0.54[e]

[a]0.01 ml HuIFN was applied every 5 min for 1 hr by a calibrated Pasteur pipette. Nasal epithelial cells from the HuIFN-treated and untreated inferior turbinate were scraped 4 hr later.
[b]Expressed in HuIFN reference standard (69/19 U).
[c]Geometric mean virus yield of 24-, 48-, and 72-hr samples minus the 0-hr sample (± SEM). Numbers in parentheses indicate the number of test samples containing 3 X 10^5 cells per tube. Each experiment used pooled cells obtained from at least three volunteers.
[d]A 4-mg antihistamine (Anti-H) tablet was given each at 12- and 1-hr before application of HuIFN.
[e]$p < 0.025$ (by Student's t test).
Source: Modifed from Ref. 235, used with permission.

The prophylactic effect of human leukocyte interferon (HuIFN-α) against rhinoviral infection has been evaluated in human volunteers at lower doses (236). These subjects were given an antihistamine before the intranasal administration of either a single or multiple dose of HuIFN-α on a cotton pledget or by aerosol. Volunteers were then challenged with rhinovirus. The cotton pledgets (saturated with 5 X 10^5 U of HuIFN-α) were placed between the inferior and middle turbinates of each nasal cavity. For aerosol administration, a nebulizer, which sprays HuIFN-α at a mean particle diameter of 2 μm, was used with a total of 1 X 10^6 or 3 X 10^6 U of HuIFN-α delivered in 1 hr. The volunteers in the control group inhaled a placebo aerosol, which consists of 0.3 mg/ml of human serum albumin to make it comparable to the HuIFN-α preparation. A significant improvement in the mean symptom scores was observed only in the volunteers who received HuIFN-α by cotton pledget (Table 4.13).

Two approaches were proposed to increase the fraction of the HuIFN-α dose in contact with the epithelial surface: One is to administer a highly concentrated HuIFN-α formulation in an intermittent manner to the nasal mucosa, and the other is to administer a less concentrated preparation with prolonged contact with the nasal mucosa. A purified human leukocyte inter-

Table 4.12   Antiviral Activity of Human Leukocyte Interferon

Nasal doseage[a] (U/0.5 ml)[b]	Interval to nasal scraping (h)	VSV yield[c]		Reduction in VSV yield ($\log_{10}$)
		Untreated cells	Treated cells	
8,000	4	5.99 (1)	5.82 (1)	0.17
8,000 (+ Anti-H)[d]	4	6.23 (1)	6.18 (2)	0.05
20,000	4	6.65 (2)	6.11 ± 0.05 (6)	0.54[e]
50,000	4	5.55 ± 0.23 (7)	4.81 ± 0.13 (9)	0.74[e]
80,000	4	6.26 ± 0.16 (7)	4.97 ± 0.05 (10)	1.29[e]
80,000 (+ Anti-H)[d]	4	5.22 (2)	4.13 ± 0.17 (3)	1.09[e]
80,000	18	5.18 ± 0.03 (7)	4.70 ± 0.18 (5)	0.48[e]
80,000	24	5.91 (2)	5.55 (2)	0.36

[a]A cotton pledget (2 × 2 cm²) was saturated with HuIFN or placebo and placed on each inferior turbinate for 1 hr and then removed. Nasal epithelial cells from each inferior turbinate were scraped 4, 18, or 24 hr later.
[b]Expressed in HuIFN reference standard (69/19 U).
[c]Geometric mean virus yield of 24-, 48-, and 72-hr samples minus the 0-hr sample (± SEM). Numbers in parentheses indicate the number of test samples containing 3×10^5 cells per tube. Each experiment used pooled cells obtained from at least two volunteers.
[d]A 4-mg antihistamine (Anti-H) tablet was given each at 12- and 1-hr before application of HuIFN.
[e]$p < 0.025$ (by Student's t test).
Source: Modifed from Ref. 235, used with permission.

feron when administered as a nasal spray via the Pisdon spray gun, was found to reduce the incidence and the severity of colds in the volunteers as challenged with human rhinovirus 9 (237). Interferon activity was still detectable in the nasal washings for as long as 26 hr after the last dose.

Using nasal spray, the prophylactic effect of recombinant leukocyte A interferon (γIFN-αA) against the infection by rhinovirus type 13 was measured in 26 volunteers (238). Significant reduction was observed in terms of illness frequency, mean symptom scores, nasal secretion weights, and frequency, mean symptom scores, nasal secretion weights, and frequency of virus isolation. But, there was no significant difference in the rates of infection between γIFN-αA- and placebo-treated volunteers.

Table 4.13 Effect of Human Leukocyte Interferon on Clinical Response and Antiviral Activity in Rhinovirus Type 13-Challenged Healthy Adult Volunteers

Treatment[a]	Sick/Total[b]	Sick/Infected[c]	Mean Symptom Scores[d]		Mean Titer of rhinovirus[e]	No increase in (Titer/Total[f])
			Infected volunteers	Sick volunteers		
Aerosol spray						
Single-dose treatment						
PBS	7/16 (44%)	7/14 (50%)	4.2	8.4	−0.07 (±0.08)	13/16 (81%)
HuIFN (1-3 × 10⁶ U)[g]	4/15 (27)	4/13 (31)	2.6	8.2	0.04 (±0.10)	12/15 (80%)
Multiple-dose						
PBS	6/11 (55)	6/11 (55)	7.5	13.3	0.63 (±0.14)	9/11 (82%)
HuIFN (4 × 10⁶ U)[g]	3/10 (30)	3/9 (33)	5.1	12.0	0.45 (±0.15)	9/10 (90%)
Cotton pledget						
Single-dose treatment						
PBS	7/12 (58)	7/11 (64)	9.3[h]	13.9[h]	0.51 (±0.12)	10/12 (83%)
HuIFN (10⁶ U)[g]	4/13 (31)	4/10 (40)	4.8[h]	9.7[h]	0.21 (±0.10)	10/13 (77%)

[a]PBS = phosphate-buffered saline.

[b]Volunteers were considered to be sick if they had respiratory or systemic symptoms for at least 24 hr during days 1-8 after challenged with rhinovirus.

[c]Daily nasal wash specimens were obtained with veal infusion broth and assayed for rhinovirus in WI-38 fibroblasts (Flow Laboratories, Rockville, MD) on days 2-8 after challenged with rhinovirus. Volunteers with at least one positive isolate were considered to have been infected.

[d]Nasal obstruction and discharge, sore throat, cough, headache, and systemic disorders (chills, malaise, and muscle aches) were graded on a scale of increasing severity from 0 to 3+ on days 2-5 after challenged with rhinovirus. Data are the mean values of the sum of the symptom scores per patient.

[e]Positive nasal wash specimens were tested for titers of rhinovirus in WI-38 fibroblasts. Data are mean log values ± SEM for days 2-5 after challenged with rhinovirus.

[f]Data are number of volunteers with a fourfold or greater increase in serum neutralizing antibody titers to rhinovirus type 13 after challenge.

[g]Quantities of HuIFN are reported to 69/19 reference units (research standard B; Medical Research Council, Division of Biological Standards, London).

[h]$p < 0.05$ (by Student's t test).

Source: Modified from Ref. 236, used with permission.

The human tolerance and histopathological effects of long-term intranasal administration of interferon-α2 have been reported by Hayden et al. (239). Fifty-two volunteers were self-administered daily with HuIFN-α2 (8.4×10^6 IU), using a metered-pump sprayer, for 4 weeks. HuIFN-α2 was found to be associated with the signs of mucosal irritation (e.g., dry mucous membranes, crusts, and friability) and/or the symptoms of blood-tinged mucous in 23% of the recipients, and a moderate or marked acute epithelial inflammation with ulcertaion in 19% of the users. Additionally, pronounced submucosal lymphocytic and mononuclear cell infiltrates were found to develop in 58% of the volunteers. The results suggested that long-term or indefinite intranasal administration of HuIFN-α2 is not a feasible strategy for the prophylaxis of respiratory viral infections.

The prophylactic efficacy of interferons against rhinoviral and coronaviral infections, the tolerance, and the minimal dose of interferon which are both efficacious and tolerable are summarized in Table 4.14.

Interferon therapy can also be instituted by administering an inducer rather than interferon itself. The use of interferon inducers for antiviral activity in man is summarized in Table 4.15. Most inducers are complex macromolecules with some formidable toxic properties (227); for example, poly I:poly C (polyriboinosinic-polyribocytidylic acid) a double-stranded ribonucleic acid (RNA)-type synthetic interferon inducer (260-263). Intranasal application of aerosolized poly I:poly C to mice was found to provide protection against pneumonia and influenza viruses (261). The baboons treated with a combined intravenous and intranasal administration of poly I:poly C were reportedly protected against influenza A2/Hong Kong virus (262). The effect of poly I:poly C applied intranasally on upper respiratory virus was also evaluated in human subjects (263). The poly I:poly C was administered intranasally to volunteers for a 7-day period, beginning at 1 day prior to the innoculation of 10^2 TCD_{50} (median tissue culture dose) U of rhinovirus type 13 or 10^5 TCD_{50} U of type A2 influenza virus/Hong Kong/68. The results indicated that only a low-to-undetectable level of nasal interferon was detected, whereas the symptoms of viral infection were reduced with no detection of toxic effect as well as no detectable effect on the antibody production. This clinical observation was found rather encouraging, since a low level of interferon induced by the intranasal administration of poly I:poly C was detected and associated with the protection against the infection by respiratory tract virus.

A study has been undertaken to investigate the factors involved in the early onset of protection against the infectious bovine rhinotracheitis virus (IBR) following the intranasal administration of an avirulent strain of IBR

Table 4.14 Intranasal Administration of Interferons

Study[a]	Preparation	Delivery method	Subjects	Purpose	Results
A (240)	HuIFN-α	Nasal drops	86 Subjects	Prevent upper respiratory disease.	Rise in antibody tiers against the parainfluenza virus was less in the treatment group than in the control group. Fever higher than 39°C seen only in placebo recipients. Results indicated prophylactic administration of an HuIFN-α2 preparation can influence upper respiratory tract.
B (241)	HuIFN-α2	Nasal spray	Humans	Test if self-administration is effective and how prophylaxis against rhinovirus infection can be achieved by both interferon dose and dosing interval.	Substantial protective effect was demonstrated.
C (242)	Interferon	Nasal spray	Humans	Compare the efficiency between physician- and self-administered IFN by measuring residual interferon recovered from the nose.	Amounts recovered at 5 min after administration and decay profiles of recoverable antiviral and immunoreactive IFN were variable among volunteers, but similar for both administration methods. Confirmed that IFN persists in the nose for at least 24 hr and is not all recovered by nasal washings.

D (243) γIFN-αA	Nasal spray 3 or 15 $\times 10^5$ IU daily	109 Subjects	Test efficacy for contact prophylaxis against common cold in families.	Nasally applied γIFN-αA significantly reduces number of days of clinical signs of common cold at doses which were well tolerated. No side effects were observed.
E (244) IFN-α2	Nasal drops	55 Healthy adults	Assess the prophylactic efficacy against rhinovirus type 39 infection.	Efficacy of multiple-dose treatment for preventing infection, virus, shedding, and RV type 39-specific colds were 78, 78, and 100%, respectively. The corresponding rates for single daily treatment were 45, 64, and 75%, respectively. Both dosage regimens were associated with significant reductions in days of virus shedding and nasal mucus production. Suggested nasal IFN-α2 may prove to be a safe and effective method of preventing rhinovirus infection and illness.
F (245) γHIFN-α2	Nasal spray & nose drops	53 Healthy adults	Study therapeutic efficacy in experimental infection with rhinovirus type 39.	Did not prevent rhinovirus infection or colds. May not be therapeutically useful in treating naturally occurring rhinovirus colds.

Table 4.14 (Continued)

Study[a]	Preparation	Delivery method	Subjects	Purpose	Results
G (246)	HuIFN-α2 10^7 IU/day, for 22 days	Nasal spray	304 Adults	Determine prophylactic activity against natural rhinovirus colds.	8.5% of placebo recipients, but no HuIFN-α2 recipients had respiratory illness documented secondary to rhinovirus infection ($p = 0.0002$). Results were partially confounded by the nasal side effects of prolonged administration, but they showed that nasal HuIFN-α2 is efficacious in preventing rhinovirus colds when under natural conditions.
H (247)	γIFN-αA 0.7 or 2.4 M/day, for 4 days	Nasal spray	56 Adults	Find a dose that is both efficacious against rhinovirus challenge and is tolerable.	Frequency of illness was significantly lower in the 2.4-M group than in the 0.7-M and placebo groups. No significant local or systemic reactions were noted. In a 26-day tolerance study, 15% of 2.4-M group volunteers developed bloody mucus and nasal mucosal erosions, whereas no such local reactions were noted in 0.7-M or placebo group.

I (248)	IFN-α 50,000 IU/day	Nasal spray	73 Volunteers	Prevent natural acquired viral respiratory infection.	Rise in complement fixation antibody titers against influenza A virus was not significantly different between treatment and placebo groups. However, the number of subjects without elevated antibody titers and without symptoms in the interferon group was significantly higher than those in the placebo group. Prophylactic nasal spray seems to protect against upper respiratory viral infection.
J (249)	IFN-α	Nasal spray	68 Volunteers	Study tolerance of 1-month treatment.	None of the volunteers on the high interferon dose were thought to have a definite cold, but viruses were isolated from 4/6 of the volunteers on low interferon who had definite colds.
K (250)	IFN-α2 1 million IU, 2X/day	Nasal spray	413 Volunteers	Find lowest efficacious dose in field setting that would be tolerated over a 28-day period.	2×10^6 IU/day confers no identifiable clinical benefits on volunteers or families, despite an apparent reduction in rhinoviral shedding. The efficacious daily dose would be 2-10 $\times 10^6$ IU.

Table 4.14 (Continued)

Study[a]	Preparation	Delivery method	Subjects	Purpose	Results
L (251)	IFN-α2	Nasal spray	120 Adults	Test prophylactic efficacy against rhinovirus infection in family setting.	Well tolerated, and the rate of minor nasal bleeding (12%) did not increase with repeated courses. Compared with the control groups, the treatment group experienced 33% fewer days with nasal symptoms and 41% fewer episodes of "definite" respiratory illness. Suggested prevention of 6.8 definite respiratory illness per 100 courses of IFN-α2 used.
M (252)	IFN-α2 5 × 10⁶ IU/day	Nasal spray	448 Subjects	Determine whether intranasal IFN-α2 could prevent respiratory illness in healthy contacts of ill family members.	Postexposure prophylaxis with intranasal interferon may in some cases provide an effective strategy for controlling spread of natural colds, especially those caused by rhinovirus.
N (253)	IFN-α2b 1,500,000 IU, 2X/day	Nasal spray	550 Subjects	Evaluate efficacy of recombinant IFN-α by intranasal administration.	Rhinovirus infections were prevented (with protective efficacy of 76%). Parainfluenza infections were not prevented, but symptoms (i.e., blood-tinged

				mucus) in associated episodes of disease were significantly reduced. Medication was generally well tolerated.
O (254) γIFN-αA 0.3 or 1.5 $\times$ 10^6 IU/day	Nasal spray	587 Subjects (147 families)	Investigate prophylactic efficacy of low-dose γIFN-αA under field conditions.	Both doses failed to exert therapeutic effects on established common cold or to prevent spread of common cold within families. Prophylactic treatment with 1.5 $\times$ 10^6 IU did, however, shorten the duration of the cold and reduced the severity of any ensuing common cold. The local tolerance of the nasal γIFN-αA was excellent.
P (255) IFN-αA	Nasal spray	35 Subjects	Study prophylactic efficacy against experimental respiratory coronavirus infection.	Incidence of colds, severity of clinical symptoms and signs, and virus replication were all reduced.
Q (256) γIFN 2 $\times$ 10^6 IU/day	Nasal spray	66 Volunteers	Determine efficacy in preventing coronavirus colds.	The mean nasal symptom scores in the placebo and IFN groups were 9.2 and 5.4, respectively, and mean total symptom scores in the two groups were 23.2 and 9.4, respectively. Indicated that nasal γIFN effectively shortens duration and reduces severity of coronavirus cold symptoms.

Table 4.14 (Continued)

Study[a]	Preparation	Delivery method	Subjects	Purpose	Results
R (257)	γIFN-αA or γIFN-αA/D	Nasal aerosol	Cotton rats (*Sigmodon hispidus*)	Develop in vitro assay for determining protective effects of interferon in primary cotton rat tissue cells against vesicular stomatitis virus (VSV) replication.	Preliminary in vitro tests indicated both recombinant IFNs were effective in protecting primary cotton rat pulmonary cells against VSV replication. However, γIFN-αA/D was 20-fold more active than γIFN-αA.
S (258)	IFNs	Nasal spray	Humans	Study efficacy and tolerance of nasal interferons at the common cold unit.	Given 1 day before and for three days after virus challenge, IFNs can protect humans from infection with rhinoviruses, coronavirus, and influenza virus. Longer treatment

T (259) IFN-α2b 9×10^6 IU/day	Nasal spray	Humans	Determine whether γIFN-α2a also causes histological changes in nasal mucosa, how rapidly the changes develop after exposure, which specific types of cells are involved in the response, and whether changes could be detected in peripheral blood lymphocytes that correlate with changes in the nasal mucosa.	gives rise to nasal symptoms and signs, such as blood-stained nasal discharge. Combining IFNs with synthetic antiviral drugs can produce synergistic increases in antiviral activity. Increased degree of lymphocyte infiltration, as compared with preexposure samples, is 56% of IFN vs. 0% of placebo recipients on day 4 and 60% of IFN vs. 10% of placebo recipients at day 10.

[a]Numbers in parentheses are reference numbers.
Source: Modified from Chien, Y. W., and Chang, S. F., Intranasal drug delivery for systemic medications, *CRC Crit. Rev. Ther. Drug Carrier Systems, 4*:67-194 (1987).

Table 4.15 Antiviral Use of Interferon Inducers in Humans

Type of inducer	Method of application	Disease treated	Result[a]
Measles vaccine	Subcutaneous	Vaccinia	+
Sendai, NDV influenza A (PR8) influenza B (lu)	i.v. sequential	Acute myelogenous leukemia	+
Semliki Forest virus			
Sindbi virus			
Influenza A (swine)	Nasal spray	Influenza A2 epidemic	+
UV irradiated			
Pyran	i.v.	Advanced cancer	±
Poly I:poly C	i.v.	Herpes encephalitis	?
	i.n.	Rhinovirus type 13	
		Influenza A2	±
Propanediamine	i.n.	Rhinovirus type 21	±
	i.n.	Rhinovirus type 13	±
	i.n.	Rhinovirus type 21	+

[a]+, beneficial effect; ±, equivocal effect; ? unclear effect.
Source: Modifed from Ref. 227, used with permission.

(AV-IBR) (264). A high level of interferon was found to develop in the nasal secretions after the intranasal administration of AV-IBR. The time of first appearance of interferon was noted to coincide with the time at which resistance to the challenge of virulent IBR virus became evident.

The effect of a chemical interferon inducer, CP-20961 (N, N-dioctadecyl-N', N'-bis[2-hydroxylethyl] propanediamine), on the time course of viral shedding has been assessed. The nasal interferon level and activity caused by the infection with rhinovirus was measured in human subjects (265). In six of the 11 subjects challenged with $10^{0.5}$ TCD_{50} U of rhinovirus 21, nasal interferon was produced to a level which was sufficient to inhibit the replication of rhinovirus 21 in a tissue culture. In eight of the 14 subjects, who were similarly challenged after a 24-hr treatment with CP-20961 in a nasal spray emulsion, the nasal interferon was observed to be produced 24 hr earlier with a slightly higher level. If this alkyl-substituted propanediamine-type interferon inducer was applied intranasally alone, it was also found to induce interferon production in four out of eight subjects. Apparently, intranasal administration of this chemical interferon inducer can induce the production of nasal interferon and also enhance the fabrication of virus-induced interferon. However, the results suggested that there is no difference in the rates of infection or the incidences of illness between the drug- and placebo-treated groups, except that the severity of the symptoms is reduced.

Similar conclusions were also drawn from the intranasal administration of CP-20961, which was suspended in a glycerin-polysorbate 80 vehicle, in 29 volunteers infected with rhinovirus 13 (266). Using the same treatment protocol, another clinical trial was also initiated utilizing a modified interferon inducer preparation in which the size of the particles in the suspension was less than 2 μm (267). The data showed that the patients in the treatment group had achieved a significantly higher level of interferon. As a result, a decrease in virus shedding and a marked reduction in the symptoms of the illness were observed as compared to those in the control group.

4.4.2 Vaccines

4.4.2.1 Influenza virus vaccine

Influenza is a viral disease resulting from infection of the respiratory epithelium. To induce the production of antibody in the respiratory tract is thus important in the prevention of infection.

The use of the nasal route for vaccination against epidemic influenza offers several theoretical advantages as well as disadvantages (268). Intranasal administration of vaccine is considered to be easy, comfortable, and it is possible to produce a low incidence of side reactions. One of the most obvious objections to nasal vaccination is the possibility of establishing an infection which could then be transmitted from one individual to another. It was reported that only one among 11 human subjects showed some rise in antibody level following inoculation intranasally with the PR8 strain of the epidemic influenza virus. However, the other 10 subjects exhibited no significant signs or symptoms of infection. It was also observed in another study that 68-80% of the subjects did not show any significant changes in their antibody titer following the inhalation of an "attenuated" influenza virus preparation (269).

Inhalation of an active influenza virus has been reported to yield a modified form of the disease and result in a good antibody response (270). Using the antibody response determined serologically as the indicator for comparing the effectiveness between the intranasal and subcutaneous administration, it was concluded that the inhalation of an active or inactive virus is not as effective as the subcutaneous injection of vaccine (271).

The antigenic effect of inactivated virus has been conducted in 80 children by giving intranasally a single or multiple sprays and comparing the results with those of subcutaneous vaccination (272). The results indicated that a single intranasal inhalation of the inactivated influenza virus preparation produces a rather good antibody response, whereas the use of five daily sprays yields only a slightly higher level of antibody. Furthermore, the effect of two dose levels on the sera taken 5 months after the intranasal vaccination has been studied and the data suggested that the higher dose results in a more persistent evaluation in the antibody titer. Subcutaneous vaccination was also found to produce a higher and more persistent level of antibody responses even with a smaller dose, whereas only a minimal reaction was obtained following the intranasal inhalation of the inactivated virus. On the other hand, the live, attentuated influenza vaccine administered intranasally yielded better protection than the intramsucular administration (273).

A study has been undertaken to evaluate the effectiveness of a vaccine-containing aerosol by determining the rates of infection by influenza (274). The aerosolized vaccine of inactivated influenza virus was administered intranasally to 386 volunteers. The same vaccine was also given subcutaneously to 269 volunteers, while another 1490 volunteers (who received a saline solution or no inoculation) were used as the controls. The group receiving the aerosolized vaccine was found to have 79% fewer illnesses as compared to 27% of the subcutaneously immunized volunteers (Tables 4.16 and 4.17). In addition to its superior ability to protect the volunteers from the infection by naturally occurring influenza, the aerosolized vaccine was also noted to produce a significantly lower incidence of side effects and a substantial reduction in the duration of illness in those few who became ill.

4.4.2.2 Parainfluenza virus vaccine

Parainfluenza viruses are a major cause of lower respiratory infections in children, which can be life threatening. A study has been performed in 56 volunteers to compare the antibody levels in the serum and in the respiratory secretions following the intranasal aerosol spray or subcutaneous injection of an inactivated parainfluenza type 2 vaccine (275). The results indicated that the levels of neutralizing antibody in the nasal secretions and sputum rose at a rate which was greater in the group of men receiving the vaccine by nasal aerosol than in the group vaccinated by subcutaneous injection. Both intranasal and subcutaneous groups yielded a significant

Table 4.16 Influenza Infection and Severity

Subjects	No. Illness (%)	Illness (%)				
		1+	2+	3+	4+	Total (%)
Prisoner volunteers						
Vaccine by						
nasal aerosol	97.5 (312)[a]	0.0 (0)	0.3 (1)	0.3 (1)	1.9 (6)	2.5 (8)
s.c. injection	88.6 (78)	1.1 (1)	3.4 (3)	4.5 (4)	2.3 (2)	11.4 (10)
saline solution	90.9 (59)	1.5 (1)	1.5 (1)	1.5 (1)	4.6 (3)	9.1 (6)
Nonvolunteers						
Vaccine by						
s.c. injection	92.2 (153)	0.0 (0)	1.8 (3)	3.0 (5)	3.0 (5)	7.8 (13)
Nonimmunized	88.0 (~1,230)	0.4 (6)	1.7 (24)	4.3 (60)	5.6 (78)	12.0 (168)

[a]Numbers in parentheses are the number of volunteers.
Source: Modified from Ref. 274, used with permission.

Table 4.17 Duration of Illness by Influenza Infection

Subjects	No. subjects				Mean duration of illness (Days)
	1-2 days	3-4 days	5-6 days	>6 days	
Prisoner volunteers Vaccine by					
nasal aerosol	5	2	1	0	2.2
s.c. injection	2	1	2	5	5.8
saline solution	1	2	1	2	5.2
Nonvolunteers Vaccine by					
s.c. injection	5	5	2	1	3.5
Nonimmunized	10	84	36	38	4.8

Source: Modifed from Ref. 274, used with permission.

rise in the serum level of antibody as measured by both neutralizing and hemagglutination inhibitory tests. A greater rise was observed in the subcutaneous group, which however was not statistically different from the intranasal group.

4.4.2.3 Measles vaccine

Measles is a serious public health problem worldwide. The subcutaneous or intramuscular route has been generally employed for the inoculation of live measles vaccine. Via these routes of inoculation, measles virus is known to induce uniformly an effective immunity in susceptible children.

A study has been performed to compare the effectiveness of attenuated measles vaccine by subcutaneous injection, conjunctival instillation, and intranasal administration (276). The attenuated measles virus was administered intranasally in two groups of seronegative children by swabbing the anterior nares. The results indicated that immunization by the nasal route has a success rate of 36% as compared to a success rate of 100% by subcutaneous injection. Whereas a shortened incubation period was observed with subcutaneous injection, the intranasal vaccination resulted in an incubation period which is comparable to those associated with the natural infection.

Intranasal inoculation of the first generation of chorioallantoic passage measles virus in children was reported to yield mild measleslike symptoms, so-called "vaccination measles" in about one-quarter of the subjects as suggested by the antibody titer (277). After inoculation with the virus of the second or later generations, a rise in the antibody titer was observed in some subjects but without occurrence of vaccination measles. These subjects became immune against the natural infection. On the other hand, the monkeys vaccinated with the second generation of chorioallantoic passage measles virus by inhalation and injection were observed to yield a remarkable rise in the antibody titer witout any clinical manifestation.

The clinical and immunological reactions elicited in 71 children exposed to the measles vaccine propagated in a canine renal cell culture have been studied (278). The results indicated that intranasal administration of the attenuated measles virus in an aerosol formulation yields a milder response and a lower incidence of high fever than intramuscular injection or conjunctival instillation. It was concluded that humans can be rendered immune to measles by vaccination with a live attenuated measles virus. A group of 121 susceptible children were also successfully immunized with the live attenuated measles virus vaccine (279). However, vaccination by intranasal aerosol has been reported to have the disadvantages of a high reaction rate and unpredictable take-rate. Administration of pooled human gamma globulin following the parenteral inoculation of attenuated measles virus vaccine, was noted to produce a marked modification of clinically overt reaction.

The Toyoshima strain of measles virus can be serially cultivated over many generations in the amniotic cavity of a developing chick embryo (280). When a definite dose (>10 $TCID_{50}$/person) of this long-term egg-amniotic-passaged virus was given by nasal spray to children, vaccination measles appeared in nearly all the children, with a satisfactory antibody response at approximately 8-9 days after the vaccination.

The clinical and antibody responses following the inhalation of live attenuated measles virus have been studied in 51 home-dwelling seronegative children (281). The seroconversion rate obtained was found to be 79% in the 19 children vaccinated by inhalation as compared to 100% in the 32 children vaccinated by subcutaneous injection. However, the difference in the mean CF antibody titer at 1 month after the vaccination was not statistically significant between these two methods of vaccination. While the onset of fever and rash was much delayed and widely scattered in the inhalation group, the duration of fever and rash was not significantly different between these two groups of children. The mean value of maximal temperature was noticed to be somewhat higher by subcutaneous injection than by inhalation.

The combined use of killed and live measles vaccines seems to afford the best method for mass immunization against measles. Thus, an attempt was made to develop a practical method in which the live measles vaccine was given by inhalation using a newly devised nebulizer and a Nissho-type compressor, whereas the killed measles vaccines A, B, or C were injected subcutaneously (282). When live measles vaccine was inoculated following the injection of killed measles vaccine (A, B, or C), the children receiving vaccine A had in general the severest clinical symptoms, followed by those receiving vaccines B and C. It is interesting to note that inoculation with killed vaccine did not have any notable adverse effects. The combined use of live and killed measles vaccines also caused less clinical reaction than the inocualtion of live measles vaccine alone, though it did cause a fever of more than 39°C in some children. In practice, it was suggested that following two injections of killed measles vaccine, live measles vaccine should be administered by inhalation, by which most children will be expected to develop a sufficient level of immunity without developing the clinical symptoms.

Russian investigators reported that they achieved effective immunization of 1- to 8-year-old children by exposing them to an aerosol of attenuated measles vaccine in a large tent or chamber (283). In 1983, a study was carried out to determine whether the inhalation of an aerosolized measles vaccine, using a plastic nebulizer attached to a DeVilbiss Pulmo-Aide (561 series), might provide a practical approach to the elimination of measles in countries where measles is a serious problem during the first year of life (284). Inhalation of aerosolized, undiluted measles vaccine was 100% immunogenic in 4- to 6-month-old and older children with and without maternal antibodies. Prevaccination with the residual placentally transmitted plaque-neutralizing antibody has been reported to prevent an immune response to the subcutaneous injection of measles vaccine, but not to the inhalation of aerosolized vaccine. No immediate clinical reactions were noted in the 160 children who inhaled the aerosolized vaccine. Also, no significant subsequent reactions were reported among the 96 children who were successfully immunized.

4.4.2.4 Poliovaccine

Poliovirus antibody activity has been found in immunoglobulin A (IgA) in nasal and duodenal secretions. Oral administration of live, attenuated poliovaccine was also reportedly characterized by the regular appearance of IgAγ poliovirus antibodies in nasal and duodenal secretions, in addition to the antibody response in the circulation. On the other hand, parenteral

Table 4.18 Protection by Nasal Vaccination with Inactivated Rhinovirus Vaccine Against Challenge with Type 13 Rhinovirus[a]

Group	No. men challenged	Prechallenge serum neutral Antibody	No. men with indicated response[b]								Virus recovery
			Study 1		Study 2		Study 3		Total		
			Sick	Not sick	Sick	Not sick	Sick	Not sick	Sick	Not sick	
Nasal vaccination with rhinovirus (inactivated)	12	<1:4–1:28[c] (30.1)[d]	3	4	1	1	0	3	4[e]	8	8
Unvaccinated	13	<1:4[c]	5	0	5	1	1	1	11	2	13

[a]Challenge dose = $10^{1.7}$–$10^{2.5}$ TCD$_{50}$.
[b]Upper Respiratory tract illness.
[c]Range.
[d]Reciprocal of geometric mean.
[e]Significantly different from unvaccinated group (p < 0.05 Fisher exact test, two tails).
Source: Modified from Ref. 286, used with permission.

administration of inactivated vaccine produced no antibody activity in either nasal or duodenal secretions.

The secretory antibody response in nasal secretions following the intranasal inoculation of large doses of inactivated poliovaccine has also been investigated (285). From 60 to 100 days after the primary inoculation, four patients were reinoculated with a single nasal dose of inactivated vaccine (P-KVT), whereas another four were also administered orally with monovalent type I live poliovaccine (P-LVM$_1$) orally at various intervals. Six of the eight patients manifested antibody responses of varying degrees, whereas seven of them showed no significant rise in IgG levels. Secretory IgAγ antibody was detected in the nasal secretions as early as 5 days after the first nasal dose and disappeared by 77-100 days. A similar response to the second intranasal inoculation of inactivated vaccine was also noted at 3-4 months later.

4.4.2.5   Rhinovirus type 13 vaccine

The antigenicity and protective action of the inactivated rhinovirus type 13 vaccine have been studied in adult male volunteers (286). After intranasal vaccination, 14 of the 17 volunteers developed a fourfold or greater rise in nasal and/or serum antibody. Significant protection was obtained when the men were challenged with $10^{1.7}$-$10^{2.5}$ TCD$_{50}$ of type 13 virus with only four of the 12 vaccinees developing illness, whereas 11 of the 13 seronegative controls became ill (Table 4.18).

4.4.2.6   Respiratory syncytial virus vaccine

Respiratory syncytial (RS) virus is the most common viral agent implicated in bronchiolitis and pneumonia in infants and young children. The lack of success and the hazards associated with the inactivated RS virus vaccines have directed a research effort toward the development of a live, attenuated vaccine that could be administered intranasally. Respiratory syncytial virus ts-1, which is a temperature-sensitive mutant of RS virus, is a live, attenuated experimental vaccine. When administered intranasally at low dose by nose drops to 25 infants (287), eight of them were successfully infected with RS virus ts-1, with no transmission of the viurs to the nine control subjects receiving the placebo. However, the incidence of illness observed in the vaccinees during the trials was found to be comparable to that in the control subjects. Reinfection occurred in both vaccinees and control subjects in the subsequent epidemics by natural RS virus; however, there was no evidence of potentiation of natural illness by the live, attenuated RS virus vaccine.

REFERENCES

1. Hochstrasser, M. K. Tierexperimentelle untersuchungen zur aufnahme von aminosäuren nach applikation auf die nasenschleinhaut, *Z. Laryngol. Rhinol. Otol., 52*:144 (1973).

2. Hussain, A. A., Bawarshi-Nassar, R., and Huang, C. H. Physicochemical considerations in intranasal drug administrations, in *Transnasal Systemic Medications* (Y. W. Chien, Ed.), Elsevier, Amsterdam (1985), pp. 121-137.

3. Huang, C. H., Kimura, R., Nassar, R. B., and Hussain, A. A. Mechanism of nasal absorption of drugs. I. Physicochemical parameters influencing the rate of in situ nasal absorption of drugs in rats, *J. Pharm. Sci., 74*:608 (1985).

4. Huang, C. H., Kimura, R., Nassar, R. B., and Hussain, A. A. Mechanism of nasal absorption of drugs. II. Absorption of L-tyrosine and the effect of structural modification on its absorption, *J. Pharm. Sci., 74*:1298 (1985).

5. Sandow, J., and Petri, W. Intranasal administration of peptides: Biological activity and therapeutic efficacy, in *Transnasal Systemic Medications* (Y. W. Chien, Ed.), Elsevier, Amsterdam (1985), pp. 183-199.

6. Su, K. S. E., Campanale, K. M., Mendelsohn, L. G., Kerchner, G. A., and Gries, C. L. Nasal delivery of polypeptides. I. Nasal absorption of enkephalins in rats, *J. Pharm. Sci., 74*:394 (1985).

7. Gesellchen, P. D., Parli, C. J., and Fredcrickson, R. C. A. "Peptides: Synthesis—structure—function," in *Proceedings of the Seventh American Peptide Symposium* (D. H. Rich, and E. Gross, Eds.), Pierce Chemical Co., Rockford, Illinois, pp. 637-640.

8. Hussain, A., Faraj, J., Aramaki, Y., and Truelove, J. E. Hydrolysis of leucine enkephalin in the nasal cavity of the rat—A possible factor in the low bioavailability of nasally administered peptides, *Biochem. Biophys. Res. Commun., 133*:923 (1985).

9. Balin, B. J., Broadwell, R. D., Salcman, M., and El-Kalliny, M. Avenues for entry of peripherally administered protein to the central nervous system in mouse, rat and squirrel monkey, *J. Comp. Neurol. 251*:260 (1986).

10. Karasek, E., Rathsack, R., Fechner, K., and Gräfenberg, M. Nasal absorption of substance P in rats, *Pharmazie, 41*:289 (1986).

11. Pontiroli, A., Alberetto, M., and Pozza, G. Intranasal calcitonin and plasma calcium concentrations in normal subjects, *Br. Med. J., 290*: 1390 (1985).

12. Morimoto, K., Morisaka, K., and Kamada, A. Enhancement of nasal absorption of insulin and calcitonin using polyacrylic acid gel, *J. Pharm. Pharmacol., 37*:134 (1985).

13. Morimoto, K., Akatsuchi, H., Aikawa, R., Morishita, M., and Morisaka, K. Enhanced rectal absorption of [Asu^{1,7}]-eel calcitonin in rats using polyacrylic acid aqueous gel base, *J. Pharm. Sci., 73*:1366 (1984).

14. McMartin, C., Hutchinson, L. E. F., Hyde, R., and Peters, G. E. Analysis of structural requirements for the absorption of drugs and macromolecules from the nasal cavity, *J. Pharm. Sci., 76*:535 (1987).

15. Scedberg, T., and Nichols, J. G. The molecular weight of egg albumin. I. In electrolyte-free condition, *J. Am. Chem. Soc., 48*:3081 (1926).

16. Yoffey, J. M., Sullivan, E. R., and Drinker, C. K. The lymphatic pathway from the nose and pharynx: The absorption of certain proteins, *J. Exp. Med., 68*:941 (1938).

17. Yoffey, J. M. The lymphatic pathway for absorption from the nasopharynx, *Lancet, 1*:530 (1941).

18. Kristensson, K., and Olsson, Y. Uptake of exogenous proteins in mouse olfactory cells, *Acta Neuropathol. (Berl.), 19*:145 (1971).

19. Hardy, J. G., Lee, S. W., and Wilson, C. G. Intranasal drug delivery by sprays and drops, *J. Pharm. Pharmacol., 37*:294 (1985).

20. Klostermeyer, H., and Humbel, R. E. The chemistry and biochemistry of insulin, *Angew. Chem. Intern. Ed., 5*:807 (1966).

21. Smith, E. L., Hill, R. L., and Borman, A. Activity of insulin degraded by leucine aminopeptidase, *Biochim. Biophys. Acta, 29*:207 (1958).

22. Earle, M. P. Experimental use of oral insulin, *Isr. J. Med. Sci., 8*:899 (1971).

23. Walton, R. P., and Lacey, C. F. Absorption of drugs through the oral mucosa, *J. Pharm. Exp. Ther., 54*:61 (1938).

24. Harrison, G. A. Insulin in alcoholic solution by mouth, *Br. Med. J., 2*: 1204 (1923).

25. Engel, R. H., Riggi, S. J., and Fahrenbach, M. J. Intestinal absorption as water-in-oil-in-water emulsion, *Nature, 219*:856 (1968).

26. Crane, C. W., Path, M. C., and Luntz, G. R. W. Absorption of insulin from the human small intestine, *Diabetes, 17*:625 (1968).

27. Fisher, N. F. The absorption of insulin from the intestine, vagina and scrotal sac, *Am. J. Physiol., 67*:65 (1923).

28. Shichiri, M., Kawamori, R., Goriya, Y. I., Kikuchi, M., Yamasaki, Y., Shigeta, Y., and Abe, H. Increased intestinal absorption of insulin in a micellar solution: Water-in-oil-in-water insulin micelles, *Acta Diabetol. Lat., 15*:175 (1978).

29. Ichikawa, K., Ohata, I., Mitomi, M., Kawamura, S., Maeno, H., and Kawata, H. Rectal absorption of insulin suppositoried in rabbits, *J. Pharm. Pharmacol., 32*:314 (1980).

30. Yamaski, Y., Schichiri, M., and Kawamori, R. The effectiveness of rectal administration of insulin in normal and diabetic subjects, *Diabetes Care, 4*:454 (1981).

31. Davis, B. K. Control of diabetes with polyacrylamide implants containing insulin, *Experientia, 28*:348 (1972).
32. Lee, S. W., and Sciarra, J. J. Development of an aerosol dosage form containing insulin, *J. Pharm. Sci., 65*:567 (1976).
33. Wigley, F. M., Londono, J. H., and Wood, S. H. Insulin across respiratory mucosa by aerosol delivery, *Diabetes, 20*:552 (1971).
34. Gibaldi, M. Role of surface-active agents in drug absorption, *Fed. Proc., 29*:1343 (1970).
35. Gibaldi, M., and Feldman, S. Mechanisms of surfactant effects on drug absorption, *J. Pharm. Sci., 59*:579 (1970).
36. Kruetler, C. J., and Davis, W. W. Normal and promoted GI absorption of water-soluble substances. III. Absorption of antibiotics from stomach and intestine of the rat, *J. Pharm. Sci., 60*:1835 (1971).
37. Utsurm, I., Kohno, K., and Takeuchi, Y. Surfactant effects on drug absorption. III. Effects of sodium glycocholate and its mixtures with synthetic surfactants on absorption of thiamine disulfide compounds in rats, *J. Pharm. Sci., 63*:676 (1974).
38. Davis, W. W., and Kreutler, C. J. Normal and promoted GI absorption of water-soluble substances. II. Absorption of vitamin B_{12} from ligated stomach and intact intestine of the rat, *J. Pharm. Sci., 60*:1651 (1971).
39. Khalafallah, N., Gouda, M. W., and Khalil, S. Effect of surfactants on absorption through membranes. IV. Effect of dioctyl sodium sulfosuccinate on the absorption of a poorly absorbable drug, phenolsulfonphthalcin in humans, *J. Pharm. Sci., 64*:991 (1975).
40. Gouda, M. W., Khalatallah, N., and Khalil, S. A. Effect of surfactant on absorption through membrane. V. Concentration-depedent effect of a bile salt (sodium deoxycholate) on absorption of a poorly absorbable drug, phenolsulfonphthalein, in humans, *J. Pharm. Sci., 66*:727 (1977).
41. Birkett, D., and Silen, W. Alteration of the physical pathways through the gastric mucosa by sodium taurocholate, *Gastroenterology, 67*:1131 (1974).
42. Harries, J. T., and Sladen, G. E. The effects of different bile salts on the absorption of fluid, electrolytes and monosaccharides in the small intestine of the rat in vivo, *Gut, 13*:596 (1972).
43. Ichikawa, K., Ohata, I., Mitomi, M., Kawamura, S., Maeno, H., and Kawata, H. Rectal absorption of insulin suppositories in rabbits, *J. Pharm. Pharmacol., 32*:314 (1980).
44. Nishioka, Y., and Kawamura, T. Effect of surface-active agent on insulin absorption upon rectal administration of insulin suppository to rabbits, *Yakuzaigaku, 37*:119 (1977).
45. Carey, M. C. In *The Liver Biology and Pathobiology* (I. M. Aries, H. Popper, D. Schacter, and D. Shafritz, Eds.), Raven Press, New York (1982), pp. 429-465.

46. Carey, M. C. In *Bile Acids in Gastroenterology* (E. Roda, and L. Barbara, Eds.), MTP Press, Boston (1983), pp. 19-56.

47. Woodyatt, R. T. The clinical use of insulin, *J. Metab. Res.*, *2*:793 (1922).

48. Heubner, W., DeJough, S. E., and Laquer, E. Ueber inhalation von insulin, *Klin. Wochnschr.*, *3*:2342 (1924).

49. Gänsslen, M. Ueber inhalation voninsulin, *Klin. Wochnschr.*, *4*:71 (1925).

50. Collens, W. S., and Goldzieher, M. A. Absorption of insulin by nasal mucous membrane, *Proc. Soc. Exp. Biol. Med.*, *29*:756 (1932).

51. Major, R. H. The intranasal application of insulin, *J. Lab. Clin. Med.*, *21*: 278 (1935).

52. Major, R. H. The intranasal application of insulin: Experimental and clinical experiences, *Am. J. Med. Sci.*, *192*:257 (1936).

53. Hankiss, J., and Hadhazy, C. S. Resorption von insulin und asthmolysin von der nasenschkeimhas, *Acta Med. Acad. Sci. Hung.*, *12*:107 (1958).

54. Hirai, S., Yashiki, T., Matsuzawa, T., and Mima, H. Absorption of drugs from the nasal mucosa of rat, *Int. J. Pharm.*, *7*:317 (1981).

55. Yokosuka, T., Omori, Y., Hirata, Y., and Hirai, S. Nasal and sublingual administration of insulin in man, *J. Jpn. Diabet. Soc.*, *20*:146 (1977).

56. Hirai, S., Ikenaga, T., and Matsuzawa, T. Nasal absorption of insulin in dogs, *Diabetes*, *27*:296 (1978).

57. Hirai, S., Yashiki, T., and MIma, H. Effect of surfactants on the nasal absorption of insulin in rats, *Int. J. Pharm.*, *9*:165 (1981).

58. Hirai, S., Yashiki, T., and Mima, H. Mechanism for the enhancement of the nasal absorption of insulin by surfactants, *Int. J. Pharm.*, *9*:173 (1981).

59. Pontiroli, A. E., Alberetto, M., Secchi, A., Dossi, G., Bosi, I., and Pozza, G. Insulin given intranasally induces hypoglycaemia in normal and diabetic subjects, *Br. Med. J.*, *284*:303 (1982).

60. Moses, A. C., Gordon, G. S., Carey, M. C., and Flier, J. S. Insulin administered intranasally as an insulin-bile salt aerosol: Effectiveness and reproducibility in normal and diabetic subjects, *Diabetes, 32*:1040 (1983).

61. Flier, J. S., Moses, A. C., Gordon, G. S., Silver, R. S., and Carey, M. C. Intranasal administration of insulin: Efficacy and mechanism, in *Transdermal System Medications* (Y. W. Chien, Ed.), Elsevier, Amsterdam (1985), pp. 217-226.

62. Gordon, G. S., Moses, A. C., Silver, R. D., Flier, J. S., and Carey, M. C. Nasal absorption of insulin: Enhancement by hydrophobic bile salts, *Proc. Natl. Acad. Sci. (U.S.A.)*, *82*:7419 (1985).

63. Saltzman, R., Manson, J. E., Griffing, G. T., Kimmerle, R., Ruderman, N., McCall, A., Stoltz, E. I., Mullin, C., Small, D., Armstrong, J., and Melby, J. C. Intransasal aerosolizied insulin: Mixed-meal studies and long-term use in type I diabetes, *N. Engl. J. Med.*, *312*:1078 (1985).

64. Longenecker, J. P., Moses, A. C., Flier, J. S., Silver, R. D., Carey, M. C., and Dubovi, E. J. Effects of sodium taurodihydrofusidate on nasal absorption of insulin in sheep, *J. Pharm. Sci., 76*:351 (1987).

65. Morimoto, K., Morisaka, K., and Kamada, A. Enhancement of nasal absorption of insulin and calcitonin using polyacrylic acid gel, *J. Pharm. Pharmacol., 37*:134 (1985).

66. Nagai, T., Nishimoto, Y., Nambu, N., Suzuki, Y., and Sekine, K. Powder dosage form of insulin for nasal administration, *J. Controlled Release, 1*: 15 (1984).

67. Pontiroli, A. E., Alberetto, M., and Pozza, G. Intranasal glucagon raises blood glucose concentrations in healthy volunteers, *Br. Med. J., 287*: 462 (1983).

68. Thorner, M. O., Spiess, J., Vance, M. L., Rogol, A. D., Kaiser, D. L., Webster, J. D., Rivier, J., Borges, J. L., Bloom, S. R., Cronin, M. J., Evans, W. S., Macleod, R. M., and Vale, W. Human pancreatic growth hormone-releasing factor selectively stimulates growth hormone secretion in man, *Lancet, 1*:24 (1983).

69. Borges, J. L. C., Gelato, M. C., Rogol, A. D., Vance, M. L., Macleod, R. M., Loriaux, D. L., Rivier, J., Blizzard, R. M., Furlanetto, R., Evans, W. S., Kaiser, D. L., Merriam, G. R., Speiss, J., Vale, W., and Thorner, M. O. Effects of human pancreatic growth hormone-releasing factor on growth hormone and somatomedin C levels in patients with idiopathic growth hormone deficiency, *Lancet, 2*:119 (1983).

70. Evans, W. S., Borges, J. L. C., Kaiser, D. L., Vance, M. L., Seller, R. P., Macleod, R. M., Vale, W., Rivier, J., and Thorner, M. O. Intranasal administration of human pancreatic tumor GH-releasing factor-40 stimulates GH release in normal men, *J. Clin. Endocrinol. Metab., 57*:1081 (1983).

71. Landon, J., James, V. H. T., Cryer, R. J., Wynn, V., and Frankland, A. W. Adrenocorticotropic effects of a synthetic polypeptide–β^{1-24}-corticotropin in man, *J. Clin. Endocrinol. Metab., 24*:1206 (1964).

72. Smith, R. W., Dickson, L. C., Bryan, J. B., and Lowrie, W. D. Nasal administration of ACTH: Observations of effectiveness measured by blood eosinopenic response, *J. Clin. Endocrinol., 12*:958 (1952).

73. Glefand, M. L., and Shearn, M. A. Absence of eosinopenic response to ACTH administration by the aerosol route in normal subjects, *P.S.E.B.M., 80*:134 (1952).

74. Paulson, F., and Nordstrom. Pharmacologic and clinical results with ACTH in 112 cases, *Swed. Med. J., 49*:2998 (1952).

75. McKendry, J. B. R., Schwartz, H., and Hall, M. Intranasal corticotropin—Its physiological and clinical effects, *Can. Med. Assoc. J., 70*:244 (1954).

76. Keenan, J., and Chamberlain, M. A. Nasal mucosal absorption of tetra-

cosactrin as indicated by rise in plasma fluorogenic corticosteroids, *Br. Med. J., 4*:407 (1969).

77. Felber, J. P., Aubert, M. L., and Deguillaume, R. Administration by nasal spray of an 18 amino acid synthetic polypeptide with corticotropic action, *Experientia, 25*:1195 (1969).

78. Keenan, J., Thompson, J. B., Chamberlain, M. A., and Besser, G. M. Prolonged corticotropic action of a synthetic substituted [1-18]ACTH, *Br. Med. J., 3*:742 (1971).

79. Baumann, G., Walser, A., Desaulles, P. A., Paesi, F. J. A., and Geller, L. Corticotropic action of an intranasally applied synthetic ACTH derivative, *J. Clin. Endocrinol. Metab., 42*:60 (1976).

80. Zatuchni, G. I., Shelton, J. D., and Sciarra, J. J. *LHRH Peptides as Female and Male Contraceptives*, Harper & Row, Philadelphia (1976).

81. Schally, A. V., Arimura, A., Kastin, A. J., Matsuo, H., Baba, Y., Redding, T. W., Nair, R. M. G., and Debeljuk, J. Gonadotropin-releasing hormone: One polypeptide regulated secretion of luteinizing and follicle-stimulating hormones, *Science, 173*:1036 (1971).

82. Bergquist, C., Nillius, S. J., Skarin, G., and Wide, L. Inhibitory effects on gonadotropin secretion and gonadal function in men during chronic treatment with a potent stimulatory luteinizing hormone-releasing hormone analog, *Acta Endocrinol. (Copenh.), 91*:601 (1979).

83. Dekonig, J., Van Dieten, J. A. M. J., and Van rees, G. P. Refractoriness of the pituitary gland after continuous exposure to luteinizing hormone-releasing hormone, *J. Endocrinol., 79*:311 (1979).

84. Sandow, J. Inhibition of pituitary and testicular function by LHRH analogues, in *Progress Towards a Male Contraceptive* (S. L. Jeffcoate, and M. Sandler, Eds.), Wiley, London (1982), pp. 19-39.

85. Kastin, A. J., Shally, A. V., Gual, C., and Arimura, A. Release of LH and FSH after administration of synthetic LH-releasing hormone, *J. Clin. Endocrinol. Metab., 34*:753 (1972).

86. Yen, S. S. C., Rebar, R., Vandenberg, G., Naftolin, F., Ehara, Y., Engblom, S., Ryan, K. J., and Benirschke, K. Synthetic luteinizing hormone–releasing factor: A potent stimulator of gonadotropic release in men, *J. Clin. Endocrinol. Metab., 34*:1108 (1972).

87. Besser, G. M., McNeilly, A. S., Anderson, D. C., Marshall, J. C., Harsoulis, P., Hall, R., Ormston, B. J., Alexander, L., and Collins, W. P. Hormonal responses to synthetic luteinizing hormone and follicle stimulating hormone-releasing hormone in men, *Br. Med. J., 3*:267 (1972).

88. Gonzalex-Barcena, D., Kastin, A. J., Schalch, D. S., Bermuder, J. A., Lee, D., Arimur, A., Ruelas, J., Zepeda, I., and Schally, A. V. Synthetic LH-releasing hormone (LH-RH) administered to normal men by different routes, *J. Clin. Endocrinol. Metab., 37*:481 (1973).

89. Schally, A. V., Kastin, A. J., and Coy, D. H. LH-releasing hormone

and its analogues: Recent basic and clinical investigations, *Int. J. Fertil., 21*:1 (1976).

90. Sandow, J. Clinical applications of LHRH and its analogues, *Clin. Endocrinol., 18*:571 (1983).

91. Mortimor, C. H., Besser, G. M., Hook, J., and McNeilly, A. S. Intravenous, intramuscular, subcutaneous and intranasal administration of LH/FSH-RH: The duration of effect and occurrence of asynchronous pulsatile release of LH and FSH, *Clin. Endocrinol., 3*:19 (1974).

92. London, D. R., Butt, W. R., Lynch, S. S., Marshall, J. C., Owusu, S., Robinson, W. R., and Stephenson, J. M. Hormonal responses to intranasal luteinizing hormone-releasing hormone, *J. Clin. Endocrinol. Metab., 37*:829 (1973).

93. Fink, G., Gennser, G., Liedholm, P., Thorell, J., and Mulder, J. Comparison of plasma levels of luteinizing hormone-releasing hormone in men after intravenous or intranasal administration, *J. Endocrinol., 63*:351 (1974).

94. Bourguignon, J. P., Burger, H. G., and Franchimont, P. Radioimmunoassay of serum luteinizing hormone-releasing hormone (LH-RH) after intranasal administration and evaluation of the pituitary gonadotropic response, *Clin. Endocrinol., 3*:437 (1974).

95. Anik, S. T., McRae, G., Nerenberg, C., Worden, A., Foreman, J., Hwang, J. Y., Kushinsky, S., Jones, R. E., and Vickery, B. Nasal absorption of nafarelin acetate, the decapeptide [D-Nal(2)^6)] LHRH in rhesus monkeys I, *J. Pharm. Sci., 73*:684 (1984).

96. Happ, J., Hartmann, U., Weber, T., Cordes, U., and Beyer, J. Gonadotropin and testosterone secretion in normal human males after stimulation with gonadotropin-releasing hormone (GnRH) or potent GnRH analogs using different modes of application, *Fertil. Steril., 30*:666 (1978).

97. Gonzalez-Barcena, D., Kastin, A. J., Schalch, D. S., Coy, D. H., and Schally, A. Prolonged elevation of luteinizing hormone (LH) after intranasal administration of an analogue of LH-releasing hormone, *Fertil. Steril., 27*:1246 (1976).

98. Yamazaki, I. Differences in the pregnancy-terminating effectiveness of an LH-RH analogue by subcutaneous, vaginal, rectal and nasal routes in rats, *Endocrinol. Jpn., 29*:415 (1982).

99. Happ, J., Kollmann, F., Krawehl, C., Neubauer, M., and Beyer, J. Intranasal GnRH therapy of maldescended testes, *Horm. Metab. Res., 7*:440 (1975).

100. Illig, R., Exner, G. U., Torresani, T., Kellerer, K., Borkenstein, M., Gleispach, H., Kollman, F., Happ, J., Lunglmayr, G., and Spona, J. Treatment of cryptorchidism by intranasal application of synthetic LH-releasing hormone (LHRH): Results of a collaborative double blind study, *Acta Endocrinol. (Suppl.), 212*:27 (1977).

101. Illig, R., Kollmann, F., Borkenstein, M., Kuber, W., Exner, G. U., Kellerer, K., Lunglmary, L., and Prader, A. Treatment of cryptorchidism by intranasal synthetic luteinizing hormone-releasing hormone, *Lancet, 2*:518 (1977).

102. Illig, R., Bucher, H., and Prader, A. Success, relapse and failure after intranasal LHRH treatment of cryptorchidism in 55 prepubertal boys, *Eur. J. Pediatr., 133*:147 (1980).

103. Happ, J., Kollmann, F., Krawehl, C., Neubauer, M., Krause, U., Demisch, K., Sandow, J., Rechenberg, W. V., and Beyer, J. Treatment of cryptorchidism with pernasal gonadotropin-releasing hormone therapy, *Fertil. Steril., 29*:546 (1978).

104. Pirazzoli, D., Zappullam, F., Bernardi, F., Villa, M. P., Aleksandrowicz, D., Scandola, A., Stancari, P., Cicognani, A., and Cacciari, E. Luteinizing hormone-releasing hormone nasal spray as therapy for undescended testicle, *Arch. Dis. Child., 53*:235 (1978).

105. Illig, R., Torresani, T., Bucher, H., Zachmann, M., and Prader, A. Effect of intranasal LHRH therapy on plasma LH, FSH and testosterone, and relation to clinical results in prepubertal boys with cryptorchidism, *Clin. Endocrinol., 12*:91 (1980).

106. Zabransky, S. LHRH nasal spray (kryptocar), ein neuer aspekt in der hormonellen behandlung des hodenhochstandes, *Klin. Padiatr., 193*:382 (1981).

107. Hadziselimovic, F., Girard, J., Herzog, B., and Stalder, G. Hormonal treatment of cryptorchidism, *Horm. Res., 16*:188 (1982).

108. Wiegelmann, W., Solbach, H. G., Kley, H. K., Nieschlag, E., Rudorff, K. H., and Kruskemper, H. L. Effect of a new LH-RH analogue [D-Ser(TBU)^6-EA^{10}-LHRH] on gonadotrophin and gonadal steroid secretion in men, *Hor. Res., 7*:1 (1976).

109. Dericks-Tan, J. S. E., Hammer, E., and Taubert, H. D. The effect of [D-Ser(TBU)^6-EA^{10}-LHRH] upon gonadotrophin release in normally cyclic women, *J. Clin. Endocrinol. Metab., 45*:597 (1977).

110. Sandow, J., Rechenberg, W. V., Jerrabek, G., and Stoll, W. Pituitary gonadotropin inhibition by a highly active analog of luteinizing hormone-releasing hormone, *Fertil. Steril., 30*:205 (1978).

111. Bergquist, C., Nillius, S. J., and Wide, L. Reduced gonadotropin secretion in postmenopausal women during treatment with a stimulating LHRH analogue, *J. Clin. Endocrinol. Metab., 49*:472 (1979).

112. Wiegelmann, W., Solbach, H. G., Kley, H. K., and Kruskemper, H. L. LH and FSH response to long-term application of LH-RH analogue in normal males, *Horm. Metab. Res., 9*:521 (1977).

113. Wiegelmann, W., Solbach, H. G., Kley, H. K., Nieschlag, E., and Kruskemper, H. L. A new LHRH analogue: D-Ser(TBU^6-EA^{10}) LHRH effects on gonadographin and gonadal steroid secretion in

men after intravenous and intranasal application, *Acta Endocrinol.* (*Suppl.*), *208*:37 (1977).

114. Baumann, R., Kuhl, H., Taubert, H.-D., and Sandow, J. Ovulation inhibition by daily i.m. administration of a highly active LH-RH analog [D-Ser(TBU)^6-LH-RH-(109)-nonapeptide-ethylamide] , *Contraception, 21*: 191 (1980).

115. Nillius, S. J., Bergquist, C., and Wide, L. Inhibition of ovulation in women by chronic treatment with a stimulatory LRH analogue—A new approach to birth control? *Contraception, 17*:537 (1978).

116. Kerr-Wilson, R. H. J., Mackenzie, L., and Fraser, H. M. Effects of chronic LHRH agonist treatment on the endometrium and ovaries of the stumptailed Macaque, *Contraception, 24*:647 (1981).

117. Koch, H. Buserelin: Contraception through nasal spray, *Pharmacy Int., 72*:99 (1981).

118. Solbach, H. G., and Wiegelman, W. Intranasal application of luteinizing hormone-releasing hormone, *Lancet, 1*:1259 (1973).

119. Dahlen, H. G., Keller, E., and Schneider, H. P. G. Linear dose dependent LH release following intranasally sprayed LHRH, *Horm. Metab. Res., 6*:510 (1974).

120. Belanger, A., Labrie, F., Lemay, A., Caron, S., and Raynaud, J. P. Inhibitory effects of a single intranasal administration of [D-Ser(TBU)^6 des-Gly-NH$_2$^{10}] LHRH ethylamide, a potent LHRH agonist, on serum steroid levels in normal adult men, *J. Steroid. Biochem., 13*: 123 (1980).

121. Luder, A. S., Holland, F. J., Costigan, D. C., Jenner, M. R., Wielgosz, G., and Fazekas, A. T. A. Intranasal and subcutaneous treatment of central precocious puberty in both sexes with a long-acting analog of luteinizing hormone-releasing hormone, *J. Clin. Endocrinol. Metab., 58*:966 (1984).

122. Happ, J., Schmitz, V., Cordes, U., Krause, U., Atzpodien, W., and Beyer, J. Treatment of delayed puberty by intranasal application of gonadotropin-releasing hormone (GnRH), *Int. J. Fertil., 25*:247 (1980).

123. Mies, R. Effects of the LH-RH analogue [D-Ser(TBU)^6-EA^{10}-LHRH] in delayed puberty, *Acta Endocrinol.* (*Suppl.*), *234*:77 (1980).

124. Fleming, R., Adam, A. H., Barlow, D. H., Black, W. P., MacNaughton, M. C., and Coutts, J. R. T. A new systemic treatment for infertile women with abnormal hormone profiles, *Br. J. Obstet. Gynaecol., 89*:80 (1982).

125. Phansey, S. A., Barnes, M. A., Williamson, H. O., Sagel, J., and Nair, R. M. G. Combined use of clomiphene and intranasal luteinizing hormone-releasing hormone for induction of ovulation in chronically anovulatory women, *Fertil. Steril., 34*:448 (1980).

126. Harris, G. W., and Naftolin, F. The hypothalamus and control of ovulation, *Br. Med. Bull., 26*:3 (1970).

127. Nillius, S. J., Bergquist, C., and Wide, L. Inhibition of ovulation in women by chronic treatment with a stimulatory LRH analogue—A new approach to birth control? *Contraception, 17*:537 (1978).

128. Bergquist, C., Nillius, S. J., and Wide, L. Inhibition of ovulation in women by intranasal treatment with a luteinizing hormone-releasing hormone agonst, *Contraception, 19*:497 (1979).

129. Bergquist, C., Nillius, S. J., and Wide, L. Failure of positive feedback of oestradiol during chronic intranasal luteinizing hormone-releasing hormone agonist treatment, *Clin. Endocrinol., 16*:147 (1982).

130. Bergquist, C., Nillius, S. J., and Wide, L. Intranasal LHRH agonist treatment for inhibition of ovulation in women: Clinical aspects, *Clin. Endocrinol., 17*:91 (1982).

131. Bergquist, C., Nillius, S. J., and Wide, L. Intranasal gonadotropin-releasing hormone agonist as a contraceptive agent, *Lancet, 2*:215 (1979).

132. Bergquist, C., Nillius, S. J., Wide, L., and Lindgren, A. Endometrial patterns in women on chronic luteinizing hormone-releasing hormone agonist treatment for contraception, *Fertil. Steril., 36*:339 (1981).

133. Schmidt-Gollwitzer, M., Hardt, W., Schmidt-Gollwitzer, K., Von Der Ohe, M., and Nevinny-Stickel. Influence of the LH-RH analogue buserelin on cyclic ovarian function and on endometrium—A new approach to fertility control? *Contraception, 23*:187 (1981).

134. Bergquist, C., Nillius, S. J., and Wide, L. Long-term intranasal luteinizing hormone-releasing hormone agonist treatment for contraception in women, *Fertil. Steril., 38*:190 (1982).

135. Hardt, W., and Schmidt-Gollwitzer. Sustained gonadal suppression in fertile women with the LHRH agonist buserelin, *Clin. Endocrinol., 19*: 613 (1983).

136. Bergquist, C., and Lindgren, P. G. Ultrasonic measurement of ovarian follicles during chronic LHRH agonist treatment for contraception, *Contraception, 28*:125 (1983).

137. Nillius, S. J., Bergquist, C., Gudmundsson, J., and Wide, L. Superagonists of LHRH for contraception in women, *J. Steroid Biochem., 20*:1373 (1984).

138. Lemay, A., Labrie, F., Belanger, A., and Raynaud, J. P. Luteolytic effect of intranasal administration of [D-Ser(TBU)^6-des-Gly-NH$_2$ ^{10}]-luteinizing hormone-releasing hormone ethylamide in normal women, *Fertil. Steril., 32*:646 (1979).

139. Lemay, A., Faure, N., and Labrie, F. Sensitivity of pituitary and corpus luteum responses to single intranasal administration of [D-Ser(TBU)^6-des-Gly-NH$_2$ ^{10}]-luteinizing hormone-releasing hormone ethylamide (buserelin) in normal women, *Fertil. Steril., 37*:193 (1982).

140. Happ, J., Neubauer, M., Egri, A., Demisch, K., Schoffling, K., and Beyer, J. GnRH therapy in males with hypogonadotrophic hypogonadism, *Horm. Metab., 7*:526 (1975).

141. Wiegelmann, W., Solbach, H. G., Kley, H. K., Nieschlag, E., and Kruskemper, H. L. A new LH-RH analogue: [D-Ser(TBU)^{6}LH-RH-1-9 EA^{10}] effects on gonadotrophin and gonadal steroid secretion in men after intravenous and intranasal application, *Acta Endocrinol. (Suppl.)*, *208*:37 (1977).

142. Klingmüller, D., Meschi, M., and Schweikert, H. U. Successful intranasal administration of LH-RH in men with hypogonadotropic hypogonadism, *J. Steroid Biochem.*, *20*:1395 (1984).

143. Lemay, A., and Ouesnel, G. Potential new treatment of endometriosis: Reversible inhibition of pituitary-ovarian function by chronic intranasal administration of a luteinizing hormone-releasing hormone (LH-RH) agonist, *Fertil. Steril.*, *38*:376 (1982).

144. Shaw, R. W. Fraser, H. M., and Boyle, H. Intranasal treatment with luteinizing hormone-releasing hormone agonist in women with endometriosis, *Br. Med. J.*, *287*:1667 (1983).

145. Katz, M., Pimstone, B. L., Carr, P. J., and Hendricks, S. Plasma gonadotropin and gonadotropin-releasing hormone levels after intranasal administration of gonadotropin-releasing hormone, *J. Clin. Endocrinol.*, *43*:215 (1976).

146. Potashnik, G., Homberg, R., Eshkol, A., Insler, V., and Lunenfeld, B. Hormonal and clinical responses in amenorrheic patients treated with gonadotropins and a nasal form of synthetic gonadotropin-releasing hormone, *Fertil. Steril.*, *29*:148 (1978).

147. Potashnik, G., Homburg, R., Eshkol, A., Insler, V., and Lunenfeld, B. Hormonal responses to nasal application of synthetic gonadotropin-releasing hormone in amenorrheic patients pretreated with gonadotrophins, *Int. J. Fertil.*, *25*:234 (1980).

148. Katzorke, T., Propping, D., Ohe, M. V. D., and Tauber, P. F. Clinical evaluation of the effects of a new long-acting super-active luteinizing hormone-releasing hormone (LH-RH) analog, [D-Ser(TBU)^6-des-Gly-10-ethylamide-LH-RH], in women with secondary amenorrhea, *Fertil. Steril.*, *33*:35 (1980).

149. Etzrodt, A., and Friedrich, E. Treatment of functional amenorrhea and anovulation with [D-Ser(TBU)^{6}LH-RH 1-9 EA] (HOE766), *Acta Endocrinol. (Suppl.) (Copenh.)*, *234*:73 (1980).

150. Jeppson, S., Kullander, S. Rannevik, G., and Thorell, J. Intranasal administration of synthetic gonadotropin-releasing hormone, *Br. Med. J.*, *4*:231 (1973).

151. Klijn, J. G. M., and DeJong, F. H. Treatment with a luteinizing hormone-releasing hormone analogue (buserelin) in premenopausal patients with metastatic breast cancer, *Lancet*, *2*:1213 (1982).

152. Maheux, R., Lemay, A., and Merat, P. Use of intranasal luteinizing hormone-releasing hormone agonist in uterine leiomyomas, *Fertil. Steril.*, *47*:229 (1987).

153. Faure, N., Labrie, F., Lemay, A., Belanger, A., Gourdau, Y., Laroche, B., and Robert, G. Inhibition of serum androgen levels by chronic intranasal and subcutaneous administration of a potent luteinizing hormone-releasing hormone (LH-RH) agonist in adult men, *Fertil Steril., 37*:416 (1982).

154. Borgmann, V., Hardt, W., Schmidt-Gollwitzer, M., Andenauer, H., and Nagel, R. Sustained suppression of testosterone production by the luteinizing hormone-releasing hormone agonist Buserelin in patients with advanced prostate carcinoma, a new therapeutic approach, *Lancet, 2*:1097 (1982).

155. Vickery, B. H. Physiology and antifertility effects of LHRH and agonist analogs in male animals, in *LHRH Peptides as Female and Male Contraceptives* (G. I. Zatuchni, J. D. Shelton, and J. J. Sciarra, Eds.), Harper & Row, Philadelphia (1982), pp. 275-290.

156. Nestor, J. J., Ho, T. L., Simpson, R. A., Horner, B. L., Jones, G. H., McRae, G. I., and Vickery, B. H. Synthesis and biological activity of some very hydrophobic superagonist analogues of luteinizing hormone-releasing hormone, *J. Med. Chem., 25*:795 (1982).

157. Vickery, B. H., Anik, S., Chaplin, M., and Henzl, M. Intranasal administration of nafarelin acetate concentration and therapeutic applications, in *Transnasal Systemic Medications* (Y. W. Chien, Ed.), Elsevier, Amsterdam (1985), pp. 201-215.

158. Nillius, S. J., Bergquist, C., Gudmendsson, J., and Wide, L. Superagonists of LHRH for contraception in women, *J. Steroid Biochem., 20*:1373 (1984).

159. Brenner, P. F., Shoupe, D., and Mishell, D. R. Ovulation inhibition with nafarelin acetate nasal administration for six months, *Contraception, 32*:531 (1985).

160. Henzl, M. R., Carson, S. L., Moghissi, K., Buttram, V. C., Bergquist, C., and Jacobson, J. Administration of nasal nafarelin as compared with oral danazol for endometriosis: A multicenter double-blind comparative clinical trial, *N. Engl. J. Med., 318*:485 (1988).

161. Hofbuaer, J., and Hoerner, J. K. The nasal application of pituitary extracts for the induction of labor, *Am. J. Obstet. Gynecol., 14*:137 (1927).

162. Morton, D. G. Induction of labor by means of artificial rupture of membranes, castor oil and quinine, and nasal pituitrin, *Am. J. Obstet. Gynecol., 26*:323 (1933).

163. Bartholomew, R. A. Diagnostic and therapeutic uses of pituitary extracts in obstetrics, *J. Med. Assoc. Ga., 34*:110 (1945).

164. Hendricks, C., and Gabel, R. A. Use of intranasal oxytocin in obstetrics. I. Laboratory evaluation, *Am. J. Obstet. Gynecol., 79*:780 (1960).

165. Hendricks, C. Use of intranasal oxytocin in obstetrics. II. A clinical appraisal, *Am. J. Obstet. Gynecol., 79*:789 (1960).
166. Hendricks, C. H., and Pose, S. V. Intranasal oxytocin in obstetrics, *J.A.M.A., 175*:384 (1961).
167. Clement, J. E., Harwell, V. C., and McCain, J. R. Use of intranasal oxytocin for induction and/or stimulation of labor, *Am. J. Obstet. Gynecol., 83*:778 (1962).
168. Hinde, F. C. The value of intranasal oxytocin spray in obstetrics, *Med. J. Aust., 1*:268 (1963).
169. Stander, R. W., Thompson, J. F., and Gibbs, C. P. Evaluation of intranasal oxytocin by amniotic fluid pressure recordings, *Am. J. Obstet. Gynecol., 85*:193 (1963).
170. Turner, E. D. Clinical impressions of intranasal oxytocin in obstetrics, *N. Z. Med. J., 63*:29 (1964).
171. Jones, C. Clinical experience with intranasal oxytocin spray, *Med. J. Aust., 2*:1099 (1966).
172. Gent, I. V., Eskes, T., and Seelen, J. C. Changes in intrauterine pressure due to intranasal administration of oxytocin (Partocon), *Acta Obstet. Gynecol. Scand., 46*:340 (1967).
173. Müller, K., and Osler, M. Induction of labor: A comparison of intravenous, intranasal and transbuccal oxytocin, *Acta Obstet. Gynecol. Scand., 46*:59 (1967).
174. Devoe, K., Rigsby, W. C., and McDaniels. The effect of intranasal oxytocin on the pregnant uterus, *Am. J. Obstet. Gynecol., 97*:208 (1967).
175. Bradfield, A. Reservations on the safety of oxytocin nasal spray in obstetrics, *Aust. N.Z. J. Obstet. Gynaecol., 5*:138 (1965).
176. Hoover, R. T. Intranasal oxytocin, in eighteen hundred patients: A study on its safety as used in a community hospital, *Am. J. Obstet. Gynecol., 110*:788 (1971).
177. Baumgarten, K., and Hofhansl, W. A modified oxytocin sensitivity test, *Geburtshilfe Franenheilkd., 21*:10 (1961).
178. Talledo, E., Adams, S. F., and Zuspan, F. P. Response of pregnant human uterus to oxytocin given intranasally, *J.A.M.A., 189*:348 (1964).
179. Baumgarten, K., and Hofhansl, W. Induction of labor by means of oxytocin spray, *Zentralbl. Gynakol., 83*:154 (1961).
180. Stichbury, P. C. Intranasal synthetic oxytocin in the induction of labour, *N. Z. Med. J., 61*:160 (1962).
181. Borglin, N. E. Intranasal administration of oxytocin for induction and stimulation of labour, *Acta Obstet. Gynecol. Scand., 41*:238 (1962).
182. Cohen, J., Danezis, J., and Burnhill, M. S. Response of the gravid uterus at term to intranasal oxytocin as determined by intra-amniotic fluid pressure recording, *Am. J. Obstet. Gynecol., 83*:774 (1962).

183. Laine, J. Experience of the use of intranasal, buccal and intravenous oxytocin as methods of inducing labor, *Acta Obstet. Gynecol. Scand.*, *49*:149 (1970).

184. Bergsjö, P., and Jenssen, H. Nasal and buccal oxytocin for the induction of labor: A clinical trial, *J. Obstet. Gynecol., Cwlth.*, *76*:131 (1969).

185. Sjöstedt, S. Induction of labour: A comparison of intranasal and transbuccal administration of oxytocin, *Acta Obstet. Gynecol. Scand.*, (*Suppl. 7*), *48*:1 (1969).

186. Newton, M., and Elgi, G. E. The effect of intranasal administration of oxytocin on the let-down of milk in lactating women, *Acta Obstet. Gynecol. Scand.*, *76*:103 (1958).

187. Wenner, R. Galaktokinetische wirkung von synthetischem oxytocin bei nasaler anwendung, *Schweiz. Med. Wochenschr.*, *89*:441 (1959).

188. Stewart, R. H., and Nelson, R. N. Synthetic oxytocin. I. Evaluation of its results in milk letdown, *Obstet. Gynecol.*, *13*:204 (1959).

189. Hollenbach, C. Lactagogue action of oxytocin (oxytocin als lakagoges hormon), *Zentralbl. Gynakol.*, *81*:1980 (1959).

190. Huntingord, P. J. Intranasal use of synthetic oxytocin in the treatment of breast feeding, *Br. Med. J.*, *1*:709 (1961).

191. Heckmann, U. Clinical experiences with intranasal oxytocin spray, Zentralbl. Gynakol., 83:2042 (1961).

192. Berde, B., and Cerletti, A. Uber die wirkung pharmakologischev oxytocindosen auf die milchdruse, *Acta Endocrinol.*, *34*:543 (1960).

193. Friedman, E. A., and Sachtleben, M. R. Oxytocin in lactation: Clinical applications, *Am. J. Obstet. Gynecol.*, *82*:846 (1961).

194. Sandholm, L. E. The effect of intravenous and intranasal oxytocin on intrammary pressure during early lactation, *Acta Obstet. Gynecol. Scand.*, *47*:145 (1968).

195. Altszuler, N., and Hampshire, J. Intranasal instillation of oxytocin increases insulin and glucagon secretion, *Proc. Soc. Exp. Biol. Med.*, *168*:123 (1981).

196. Fraser, R., and Scott, D. J. Nasal spray of synthetic vasopressin for the treatment of diabetes insipidus, *Lancet, 1*:1159 (1963).

197. Pepys, J., Jenkins, P. A., Lachman, P. J., and Mahon, W. E. An iatrogenic auto-antibody: Immunological responses to "pituitary snuff" in patients with diabetes insipidus, *J. Endocrinol.*, *33*:viii (1965).

198. Mahon, W. E., Scott, D. J., Ansell, G., Mason, G. L., and Fraser, R. Hypersensitivity to pituitary snuff with miliary shadowing in the lungs, *Thorax, 22*:13 (1967).

199. Blumgart, H. L. The antidiuretic effect of pituitary extract applied intranasally in a case of diabetes insipidus, *Arch. Intern. Med.*, *29*:508 (1982).

200. Berde, B., and Cerletti, A. Über antidiuretische wirking von synthetischem lysin-vasopressin, *Helv. Physiol. Acta, 19*:135 (1961).

201. Guhl, V. U. Die antidiuretische und pressorische von arginin[8]-vaso-
pressin, lysin[8]-vasopressin und phenylalanin[2]-lysin vasopressin,
Schweiz. Med. Wochenschr., 91:798 (1961).

202. Spiegelman, A. R. Treatment of diabetes insipidus with synthetic vasopressin, *J.A.M.A., 184*:657 (1963).

203. Barltrop, D. Diabetes insipidus treated with synthetic lysine vasopressin, *Lancet, 1*:276 (1963).

204. Sjöberg, H., and Luft, R. Nasal spray of synthetic vasopressin for the
treatment of diabetes insipidus, *Lancet, 1*:1159 (1963).

205. Fabricant, N. D. Nasal spray treatment of diabetes insipidus, *Eye Ear
Nose Throat Monthly, 42*:64 (1967).

206. 'Moses, A. M. Synthetic lysine vasopressin nasal spray in the treatment
of diabetes insipidus, *Clin. Pharmacol. Ther., 5*:422 (1964).

207. Dashe, A. M., Kleeman, C. R., Czaczkes, J. W., Rubinoff, H., and
Spears, I. Synthetic vasopressin nasal spray in the treatment of diabetes
insipidus, *J.A.M.A., 190*:1069 (1964).

208. Dingman, J. F., and Hauger-Klevene, J. H. Treatment of diabetes insipidus: Synthetic lysine vasopressin nasal solution, *J. Clin. Endocrinol.,
24*:550 (1964).

209. Chirman, S. B., and Kinsell, L. W. Diabetes insipidus: Treatment with
8-lysine vasopressin in a nasal spray, *Calif. Med., 101*:1 (1964).

210. Martin, F. I. R., and Mathew, T. H. The treatment of diabetes insipidus
with synthetic lysine-vasopressin by inhalation, *Med. J. Aust., 2*:984
(1964).

211. Fogel, R. L. Treatment of diabetes insipidus with lysine vasopressin
spray, *J. Med. Soc. N. J., 63*:203 (1966).

212. Hung, W. Treatment of diabetes insipidus in children with synthetic
lysine-8-vasopressin nasal spray, *Med. Ann. Dis. Col., 36*:400 (1967).

213. Mimica, N., Wegienka, L. C., and Forsham, P. H. Lypressin nasal
spray: Usefulness in patients who manifest allergies to other antidiuretic hormone preparation, *J.A.M.A., 203*:802 (1968).

214. Green, H. D., and Blumberg, J. B. The use of a synthetic analogue of
post-hypophysial vasopressin (PVL-2) for local hemostasis, *Surgery,
58*:524 (1965).

215. Vavra, I., Machova, A., Holecek, V., Cort, J. H., Zaoral, and Sorm, F.
Effect of a synthetic analogue of vasopressin in animals and in patients
with diabetes insipidus, *Lancet, 1*:948 (1968).

216. Anderson, K. E., and Arner, B. Effects of DDAVP, a synthetic analogue of vasopressin, in patients with cranial diabetes insipidus, *Acta
Med. Scand., 192*:21 (1972).

217. Ziai, F., Walter, R., and Rosenthal, I. M. Treatment of central diabetes insipidus in adults and children with desmopressin, *Arch. Intern. Med.*, *138*:1382 (1978).

218. Edwards, C. R. W., Kitau, M. J., Chard, T., and Besser, G. M. Vasopressin analogue DDAVP in diabetes insipidus: Clinical and laboratory studies, *Br. Med. J.*, *3*:375 (1973).

219. Lee, W. N., Lippe, B. M., Franchi, S. H., and Kaplan, S. A. Vasopressin analog DDAVP in the treatment of diabetes insipidus, *Am. J. Dis. Child.*, *130*:166 (1976).

220. Cobb, W. E., Spare, S., and Reichlin, S. Neurogenic diabetes insipidus: Management with DDAVP (1-desamino-8-arginine vasopressin), *J. Intern. Med.*, *88*:183 (1978).

221. Brown, D. R., and Uden, D. L. The use of 1-desamino-8-D-arginine vasopressin (DDAVP) in the management of neurogenic diabetes insipidus, *Minn. Med.*, *62*:427 (1979).

222. Grossman, A., Fabbri, A., Goldberg, P. L., and Nesser, G. M. Two new modes of desmopressin (DDAVP) administration, *Br. Med. J.*, *280*: 1215 (1980).

223. Rado, J. P., and Marosi, J. Prolongation of duration of action of 1-desamino-8-D-arginine vasopressin (DDAVP) by ineffective doses of clofibrate in diabetes insipidus, *Horm. Metab.*, *7*:527 (1975).

224. Rado, J. P., Marosi, J., Szende, L., Borbely, L., Tako, J., and Fischer, J. The antidiuretic action of 1-desamino-8-arginine vasopressin (DDAVP) in man, *Int. J. Clin. Pharmacol.*, *13*:196 (1976).

225. Robinson, A. G., Seif, S. M., Ciarochi, F. F., Zenser, T. V., and Davis, B. B. DDAVP (1-desamino-8-D-arginine vasopressin)—Kinetics of prolonged antidiuresis in central diabetes insipidus, *Clin. Res.*, *24*:277A (1976).

226. Harris, A. S., Svensson, E., Wagner, Z. G., Lethagen, S., and Nilsson, I. M. Effect of viscosity on particle size, deposition and clearance of nasal delivery systems containing desmopressin, *J. Pharm. Sci.*, *77*: 405 (1988).

227. Ho, M., and Armstrong, J. A. Interferon, *Ann. Rev. Microbiol.*, *29*:131 (1975).

228. Isaacs, A., and Lindemann, J. Virus interference. I. The interferon, *Proc. R. Soc. Lond. (Biol.)*, *147*:258 (1957).

229. Soloviev, V. D. In *The Interferons* (G. Rita, Ed.), Academic Press, New York (1968), p. 233.

230. Soloviev, V. D. The results of controlled observations on the prophylaxis of influenza with interferon, *Bull. W.H.O.*, *41*:683 (1969).

231. Scientific committee on interferon; Progress towards trials of human interferon in man, *Ann. N.Y. Acad. Sci.*, *173*:770 (1970).

232. Merigan, T. C., Reed, S. E., Hall, T. S., and Tyrrell, D. A. J. Inhibition

of respiratory virus infection by locally applied interferon, *Lancet, 1*: 563 (1973).

233. Johnson, P. E., Greenberg, S. B., Harmon, M. W., Alford, B. R., and Couch, R. B. Recovery of applied human leukocyte interferon from the nasal mucosa of chimpanzees and humans, *J. Clin. Microbiol., 4*: 106 (1976).

234. Harmon, M. W., Greenberg, S. B., Johnson, P. E., and Couch, R. B. Human nasal epithelial cell culture system: Evaluation of response to human interferons, *Infect. Immun., 16*:480 (1977).

235. Greenberg, S. B., Harmon, M. W., Johnson, P. E., and Couch, R. B. Antiviral activity of intranasally applied human leukocyte interferon, *Antimicrob. Agents Chemother., 14*:596 (1978).

236. Greenberg, S. B., Harmon, M. W., Couch, R. B., Johnson, P. E., Wilson, S. Z., Dasco, C. C., Bloom, K., and Ouarles, J. Prophylactic effect of low doses of human leukocyte interferon against infection with rhino-virus, *J. Infect. Dis., 145*:542 (1982).

237. Scott, G. M., Phillpotts, R. J., Wallace, J., Secher, D. S., Cantrell, K., and Tyrrell, D. A. J. Purified interferon as protection against rhinovi-rus infection, *Br. Med. J., 284*:1822 (1982).

238. Samo, T. C., Greenberg, S. B., Couch, R. B., Ouarles, J., Johnson, P. E., Hook, S., and Harmon, M. W. Efficacy, and tolerance of intra-nasally applied recombinant leukocyte A interferon in normal volun-teers, *J. Infect. Dis., 148*:535 (1983).

239. Hayden, F. G., Mills, S. E., and Johns, M. E. Human tolerance and histologic effects of long-term administration of intranasal interferon-α2, *J. Infect. Dis., 148*:914 (1983).

240. Imanishi, J., Karaki, T., Matsuo, A., Oishi, K., Pak, C. B., Kishida, T., Toda, S., and Nagata, H. The preventive effect of human interferon-alpha preparation on upper respiratory disease, *J. Interferon Res., 1*: 169 (1980).

241. Phillpotts, R. J., Scott, G. M., Higgins, P. G., Wallace, J., Tyrrell, D. A., and Gauci, C. L. An effective dosage regimen for prophylaxis against rhinovirus infection by intranasal administration of HuIFN-alpha 2, *Antiviral Res., 3*:121 (1983).

242. Davies, H. W., Scott, G. M., Robinson, J. A., Higgins, P. G., Wootton, R., and Tyrrell, D. A. Comparative intransaal pharmacokinetics of interferon using two spray systems, *J. Interferon Res., 3*:443 (1983).

243. Herzog, C., Just, M., Berger, R., Havas, L., and Fernex, M. Intranasal interferon for contact prophylaxis against common cold in families, *Lancet, 1*:962 (1983).

244. Hayden, F. G., and Gwaltney, J. M. Intranasal interferon-α2 for pre-vention of rhinovirus infection and illness, *J. Infect. Disease, 148*: 543 (1983).

245. Hayden, F. G., and Gwaltney, J. M. Intranasal interferon-α2 treatment of experimental rhinoviral colds, *J. Infect. Dis., 150*:175 (1984).
246. Farr, B. M., Gwaltney, J. M., Adams, K. F., and Hayden, F. G. Intranasal interferon-α2 for prevention of natural rhinovirus colds, *Antimicorb. Agents Chemother., 26*:31 (1984).
247. Samo, T. C., Greenberg, S. B., Palmer, J. M., Couch, R. B., Hazmon, M. W., and Johnson, P. E. Intranasally applied recombinant leukocyte A interferon in normal volunteers. II. Determination of minimal effective and tolerable dose, *J. Infect. Dis., 150*:181 (1984).
248. Saito, H., Takenaka, H., Yoshida, S., Tsubokawa, T., Ogata, A., Imanishi, F., and Imanishi, J. Prevention from naturally acquired viral respiratory infection by interferon nasal spray, *Rhinology, 23*:291 (1985).
249. Scott, G. M., Onwabalili, J. K., Robinson, J. A., Dore, C., Secher, D. S., and Cantell, K. Tolerance of one-month intranasal interferon, *J. Med. Virol., 172*:99 (1985).
250. Douglas, R. M., Albrecht, J. K., Miles, H. B., Moore, B. W., Read, R., Worswick, D. A., and Woodward, A. J. Intranasal interferon-α2 prophylaxis of natural respiratory virus infection, *J. Infect. Dis., 151*:731 (1985).
251. Douglas, R. M., Moore, B. W., Miles, H. B., Davies, L. M., Graham, N. M., Ryan, P., Worswick, D. A., and Albrecht, J. K. Prophylactic efficacy of intranasal alpha2-interferon against rhinovirus infections in the family setting, *N. Engl. J. Med., 314*:65 (1986).
252. Hayden, F. G., Albrecht, J. K., Kaiser, D. L., and Gwaltney, J. M. Prevention of natural colds by contact prophylaxis with intranasal alpha 2-interferon, *N. Engl. J. Med., 314*:71 (1986).
253. Monto, A. S., Shope, T. C., Schwartz, S. A., and Albrecht, J. K. Intranasal interferon-α2b for seasonal prophylaxis of respiratory infection, *J. Infect. Dis., 154*:128 (1986).
254. Herzog, C., Berger, R., Fernex, M., Friesecke, K., Havas, L., Just, M., and Dubach, U. C. Intranasal interferon (γIFN-αA, Ro 22-8181) for contact prophylaxis against common cold: A randomized double-blind and placebo-controlled field study, *Antiviral Res., 6*:171 (1986).
255. Higgins, P. G., Phillpotts, R. J., Scott, G. M., Wallace, J., Bernhardt, L. L., and Tyrrell, D. A. J. Intranasal interferon as protection against experimental respiratory coronavirus infection in volunteers, *Antimicrob. Agents Chemother., 24*:713 (1983).
256. Turner, R. B., Felton, A., Kosak, K., Kelsey, D. K., and Meschievitz, C. K. Prevention of experimental coronovirus colds with intranasal α-2b interferon, *J. Infect. Dis., 154*:443 (1986).
257. Sun, C.-S., Wyde, P. R., Wilson, S. Z., and Knight, V. Efficacy of aerosolized recombinant interferons against vesicular stomatitis virus–induced lung infection in cotton rats, *J. Interferon Res., 4*:449 (1984).

258. Tyrrell, D. A. J. The efficacy and tolerance of intranasal interferons: Studies at the common cold unit, *J. Antimicrob. Chemother., 18*:153 (1986).

259. Hayden, F. G., Winther, B., Donowitz, G. R., Mills, S. E., and Innes, D. J. Human nasal mucosal responses to topically applied recombinant leukocyte A interferon, *J. Infect. Dis., 156*:64 (1987).

260. Hill, D. A., Baron, S., and Chanock, R. M. Sensitivity of common respiratory viruses to an interferon inducer in human cells, *Lancet, 2*:187 (1969).

261. Hilleman, M. R Double-stranded RNAs (poly I:C) in the prevention of viral infections, *Arch. Intern. Med., 126*:109 (1970).

262. Heberling, R. L., and Kalter, S. S. Persistence and spread of influenza virus (A2/Hong Kong) in normal and poly I:C-treated baboons (Papio cynocephalus), *Proc. Soc. Exp. Biol. Med., 135*:717 (1970).

263. Mills, J., Kapikian, A. Z., and Chanock, R. M. Evaluation of an interferon inducer in viral respiratory disease, *J.A.M.A., 219*:1179 (1972).

264. Todd, J. D., Volenec, F. J., and Paton, I. M. Interferon in nasal secretions and sera of calves after intranasal administration of avirulent infectious bovine rhinotracheitis virus: Association of interferon in nasal secretions with early resistance to challenge with virulent virus, *Infect. Immun., 5*:699 (1972).

265. Gatmaitan, B. G., Stanley, E. D., and Jackson, G. G. The limited effect of nasal interferon induced by rhinovirus and a topical chemical inducer on the course of infection, *J. Infect. Dis., 127*:401 (1973).

266. Douglas, R. G., and Betts, R. F. Effect of induced interferon in experimental rhinovirus infections in volunteers, *Infect. Immun., 9*:506 (1974).

267. Panusarn, C., Stanley, E. D., Dirda, V., Rubenis, M., and Jackson, G. G. Prevention of rhinovirus illness by a typical interferon inducer, *N. Engl. J. Med., 219*:57 (1974).

268. Francis, T. Intranasal inoculation of human individuals with the virus of epidemic influenza, *Proc. Soc. Exp. Biol. Med., 43*:337 (1940).

269. Burnet, F. M. Immunization against influenza with living attenuated virus, *Med. J. Aust., 1*:385 (1943).

270. Mawson, J., and Swan, C. Intranasal vaccination of humans with living attenuated influenza virus strains, *Med. J. Aust., 1*:394 (1943).

271. Henle, W., Henle, G., Stokes, J., and Maris, E. P. Experimental exposure of human subjects to viruses of influenza, *J. Immunonol., 52*: 145 (1946).

272. Ouilligan, J. J., and Francis, T. Serological response to intranasal administration of inactive influenza virus in children, *J. Clin. Invest., 26*: 1-79 (1947).

273. Beare, A. S., Hobson, D., Reed, S. E., and Tyrrell, D. A. A comparison of live and killed influenza-virus vaccines, *Lancet, 2*:418 (1968).

274. Waldman, R. H., Mann, J. A., and Small, P. A. Immunization against influenza: Prevention of illness in man by aerosolized inactivated vaccine, *J.A.M.A., 207*:520 (1969).

275. Wigley, F. M., Fruchtman, M. H., and Waldman, R. H. Aerosol immunization of humans with inactivated para-influenza type 2 vaccine, *N. Engl. J. Med., 283*:1250 (1970).

276. Black, F. L., and Sheridan, S. R. Studies on an attenuated measles-virus vaccine. IV. Administration of vaccine by several routes, *N. Engl J. Med., 263*:165 (1960).

277. Okuno, Y., Takahashi, M., Toyoshima, K., Yamamura, T., Sugai, T., Nakamura, K., and Kunita, N. Studies on the prophylaxis of measles with attenuated living virus. III. Inoculation tests in man and monkey with chick embryo passage measles virus, *Biken J., 3*:115 (1960).

278. McCrumb, F. R., Kress, S., Saunders, E., Snyder, M. J., and Schluederberg, A. E. Studies with live attenuated measles-virus vaccine. I. Clinical and immunologic responses in institutionalized children, *Am. J. Dis. Child., 101*:689 (1961).

279. Kress, S., Schluederberg, A. E., Hornick, R. B., Morse, L. J., Cole, J. L., Slater, E. A., and McCrumb, F. R. Studies with live attenuated measles-virus vaccine. II. Clinical and immunologic response of children in an open community, *Am. J. Dis. Child., 101*:701 (1961).

280. Okuno, Y. Vaccination with egg passage measles virus by inhalation, *Am. J. Dis. Child., 103*:381 (1962).

281. Minamitani, M., Nakamura, K., Nagahama, H., Fujii, R., Saburi, Y., and Matumoto, M. Vaccination by respiratory route with live attenuated measles virus sugiyama adapted to bovine renal cells, *Jpn. J. Exp. Med., 34*:81 (1964).

282. Okuno, Y., Ueda, S., Hosai, H., Kitawaki, T., Nakamura, K., Chiang, T. P., Okabe, A., and Onaka, M. Studies on the combined use of killed and live measles vaccine: Advantages of the inhalation method, *Biken J., 8*:81 (1965).

283. Terskikh, I. I., Danilov, A. I., and Sheltchlov, G. I. Theoretical substantiation and the effectiveness of immunization with aerosols of liquid antimeasles vaccine (Russian), *Vestn. Akad. Med. Nauk. S.S.S.R., 26*:84 (1971).

284. Sabin, A. B., Arechiga, A. F., De Castro, J. F., Sever, J. L., Madden, D. L., Shekarchi, I., and Albrecht, P. Successful immunization of children with and without maternal antibody by aerosolized measles vaccine. I. Different results with undiluted humans diploid cell and chick embryo fibroblast vaccines, *J.A.M.A., 249*:2651 (1983).

285. Ogra, P. L., and Karzon, D. T. Poliovirus antibody response in serum and nasal secretions following intranasal inoculation with inactivated poliovaccine, *J. Immunol., 102*:15 (1969).

286. Perkins, J. C., Tucker, D. N., Knopf, H. L. S., Wenzel, R. P., Hornick, R. B., Kapikian, A. Z., and Chanock, R. M. Evidence for protective effect of an inactivated rhinovirus vaccine administered by the nasal route, *Am. J. Epidemiol., 90*:319 (1969).
287. Wright, P. F., Shinozaki, T., Fleet, W., Sell, S. H., Thompson, J., and Karzon, D. T. Evaluation of a live, attenuated respiratory syncytial virus vaccine in infants, *J. Pediatr., 88*:931 (1976).

5
Intranasal Delivery of Nonpeptide Molecules

5.1 ADRENAL CORTICOSTEROIDS

The adrenal corticosteroids include both the adrenocorticoids from the adrenal cortex and epinephrine and norepinephrine from the adrenal medulla. These corticosteroids play an important role in the metabolism of carbohydrates, proteins, fats, and nucleic acids as well as in the balance of electrolytes and water.

Corticosteroids have been used in the treatment of seasonal and perennial allergic rhinitis as well as vasomotor rhinitis. For these treatments, corticosteroids are administered orally, parenterally, or intranasally. Many attempts have been made to apply corticosteroids directly to the nasal mucosa to achieve a therapeutic activity without any potential risk of systemic side effects. The intranasal administration of corticosteroids has produced a greater efficacy with minimum inhibitory effect than other routes of administration on the hypothalamus-pituitary-adrenal axis, but without adrenocortical suppression.

The nasal route has been commonly used by otolaryngologists for the administration of corticosteroids, such as cortisone (1-5) and cortisone acetate (6); hydrocortisone (5,7-12), hydrocortisone alcohol (13), hydrocortisone acetate (14,15), and hydrocortisone hemisuccinate (16); prednisolone (5,17,18) and prednisolone terbutate (19-24); 9-alpha-fluoroprednisolone (25); triamcinolone acetonide (23,24,26-28); dexamethasone phosphate (29-36); betamethasone valerate (37,38); beclomethasone dipropionate (39-59); flunisolide (59,60); budesonide (59,61,62); and toxicortol pivalate

(63). Intranasal administration of these corticosteroids has been primarily for the relief of nasal obstruction associated with rhinitis, hay fever, or nasal polyps and the secondary nasal edema associated with sinusitis or the common cold.

5.2 SEX HORMONES

In addition to the function of providing sex cells, the testes and ovaries also manufacture sex hormones which control the secondary sex characteristics. When the plasma concentration of sex hormones is low, the production of follicle-stimulating hormone (FSH), luteinizing hormone (LH), and luteotropic hormone (LTH) is stimulated, whereas its production is inhibited when the concentration is high. Therefore, a complex positive and negative feedback system subserves the cyclic phenomena of ovulation and menstruation.

When the naturally occurring ovarian steroids are administered orally at a high dose or given parenterally they can block ovulation. The undesirable side effects associated with the intake of high doses have precluded the use of ovarian steroids in the conventional methods of hormonal contraception. For oral contraception, the synthetic analogs of the steroids have been used instead, since they are effective orally at lower doses as a result of their ability to resist the hepatic "first-pass" metabolism. Therefore, they can reach the target sites of action in the brain without losing their efficacy (64,65).

5.2.1 Estradiol17β (E$_2$)

The intranasal administration of estradiol has been studied to determine its relative bioavailability in the blood and in the cerebrospinal fluid (CSF), and to assess whether or not the testicular functions are impaired (64-68). The results indicated that estradiol applied intranasally can reach the brain preferentially, and in fact more steroids enter the CSF after the nasal delivery than by intravenous injection (64,65). The plasma concentration of estradiol following intranasal administration was found to be essentially equivalent to that by intravenous administration (67). In male monkeys treated intranasally with estradiol, a decrease of testicular size, arrest of spermatogenesis, and a significant reduction in serum testosterone concentration were observed.

The systemic delivery of estradiol following intranasal administration by nasal spray was investigated in monkeys (64,65) using [3H] estradiol. The results showed that estradiol is able to enter the CSF within 1 min, and the

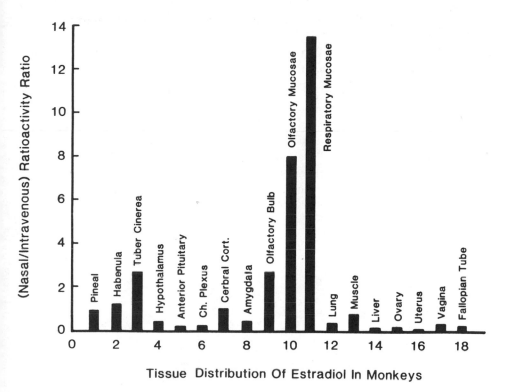

Figure 5.1 Radioactivity ratio in various tissues 1 hr following the intravenous and intranasal administration of [³H] estradiol to rhesus monkeys. The ratio was calculated from the mean DPM data obtained in two monkeys. (Calculated from data in Ref. 64.)

amount of radioactivity found in the CSF is much higher with the nasal spray than with intravenous injection. On the other hand, the amount of radioactivity in the peripheral target tissues, such as the liver, ovary, uterus, vagina, and fallopian tube, was observed to be much lower with the nasal spray than that administered intravenously. On the contrary, the olfactory bulb, olfactory mucosa, and respiratory mucosa showed much higher radioactivity in the monkeys treated with nasal spray (Figure 5.1). All the results appear to suggest that estradiol preferentially reaches the brain when administered intranasally.

There are two possible pathways for the transport of estradiol from the nasal mucosa to the brain:

1. Transfer of estradiol into the hemal compartment before entering the CSF
2. Diffusion of estradiol through the olfactory neurons by pinocytosis first into the brain and then into the CSF

The nasal absorption of estradiol in monkeys was observed to be dose dependent, and the elevation of plasma estradiol level was close to that achieved by intravenous injection. Intranasal administration also reportedly produced an increase in the estradiol levels in the CSF (66). The concentration of estradiol in the CSF was insignificantly different when estradiol was administered intranasally either as a suspension or as a solution (Figure 5.2).

The intranasal administration of estradiol to 11 female volunteers was found to induce a rapid but short-lasting increase in the circulating level of estradiol (67). A progressive increase in the mean E_1/E_2 ratio (E_1 :estrone,

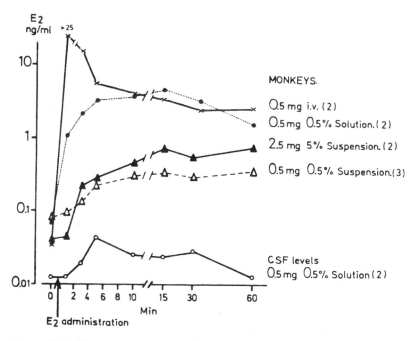

Figure 5.2 Plasma and CSF concentration profiles of estradiol following intranasal administration of estradiol (0.5 and 2.5 mg) in monkeys. (From Ref. 66, used with permission.)

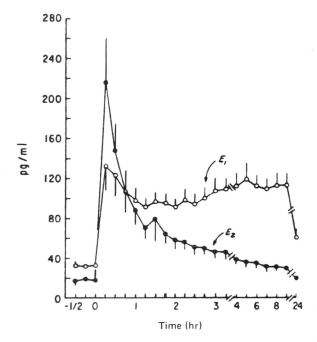

Figure 5.3 Mean (±S.E.M.) basal concentration and the incremental changes of serum E_1 and E_2 following the intranasal administration of micronized 17-beta estradiol (1 mg suspended in saline) in 11 subjects. (From Ref. 67, used with permission.)

E_2 :estradiol) was noted. Within the first hour following intranasal administration, a ratio of less than unity was observed. The ratio became greater than unity beginning at 1 hr (Figure 5.3). This increase in the ratio of E_1/E_2 might be due to the local conversion of E_2 to E_1 either by enzymatic metabolism in the nasal mucosa or by the microorganisms in the nasal cavity.

Parenteral delivery of estrogens often results in a suppression of spermatogenesis as well as a reduction of the serum level of testosterone. However, it often requires a large oral dose of estrogens in order to achieve such effects. On the other hand, the daily administration of estradiol by nasal spray in the adult male rhesus monkey for 60 days was reported to impair spermatogenesis with a significant reduction in the circulating levels of testosterone (68). The testes were noted to decrease in size after 30 days of intranasal administration and also to restract into the inguinal canal at the end of the 60-day treatment, whereas no effect was observed with the placebo. However, the plasma levels of cortisol showed no significant changes at all before, during, and at the end of treatment with estradiol or placebo. This investigation has demonstrated that estradiol administered intranasally does affect testicular functions.

5.2.2 Progesterone

Progesterone is an endogenous hormone secreted by the adrenal gland in both sexes, and also by the ovary and placenta in the female. The secretion of progesterone in the female occurs and stops during the menstrual cycle, in which the progesterone level rises throughout the luteal phase, peaks at about 7 days following ovulation, and gradually declines over the following week.

Clinically, exogenous progesterone is administered for the treatment of infertility, endometrial hyperplasia, and premenstrual syndromes. Progesterone has also been used concomitantly with estrogen for the prevention of pregnancy, which is usually in oral tablets, intramuscular implants, or intravaginal pessaries. It has been found that progesterone and its derivatives are rapidly absorbed from most routes of administration. However, a short half-life of about 4-30 min, which has been reported after oral administration, could be attributed to its extensive hepatic first-pass metabolism.

The metabolism of progesterone by the nasal mucosa was studied in mice and rats using [14C] progesterone (69,70). The nasal mucosa containing both respiratory and olfactory epithelia was incubated with [14C] progesterone in phosphate buffer at 37°C. At least three metabolites were detected after incubation for 10 min, and at least 10-12 metabolites after 30 min. After 3 hr of incubation, only 8% (in mouse) or 20% (in rat) of the total radioactivity could be attributed to the intact progesterone. Several enzymes were reportedly involved in the metabolism of progesterone by the nasal mucosa.

Intranasal administration of progesterone has been studied to determine the possible routes of transport (64,65), to evaluate testicular functions (68), to study its effect on serum testosterone levels and total sperm counts (71), and to monitor the pharmacokinetics and bioavailability of progesterone in the serum and in the CSF (74-77). The methods used for the intranasal administration of progesterone include the application of a glass atomizer for nasal spraying and a micropipette for nose drops.

[3H] Progesterone was administered intranasally as a nasal spray to rhesus monkeys to assess the feasibility of systemic absorption (64,65). The results demonstrated that progesterone is absorbed into the CSF within 1 min fol-

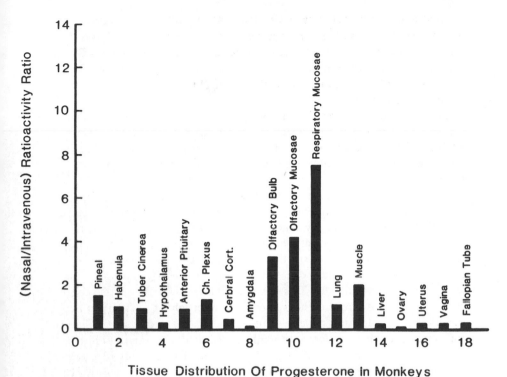

Figure 5.4 Radioactivity ratio in various tissues 1 hr after intravenous and intranasal administration of [^{3}H] progesterone to rhesus monkeys. The ratio was calculated from the mean DPM data obtained in two monkeys. (Calculated from data in Ref. 64.)

lowing administration by either nasal spray or intravenous injection. In the monkey, the amount of radioactivity in the CSF was much higher with the nasal spray than those monkeys receiving injection (Figure 5.4), whereas the plasma radioactivity following intranasal spraying was found to be negligibly small.

Intranasal administration of progesterone by nasal spray was studied in adult rhesus monkeys for over 60 days to determine whether or not testicular functions were impaired (68). The diameter of semininferous tubules was noted to be reduced, but was not as marked as that observed in the estradiol- or norethisterone-treated monkeys. A progressive decline in the mean serum concentrations of testosterone was evident. At the end of the treatment, the serum concentrations of testosterone were reduced to a level which was significantly different from the levels at the beginning of the treatment. Thus, this study suggested that intranasal administration of progesterone produces an impairment in spermatogenesis with a significant reduction in the levels of circulating testosterone.

Progesterone administered by a nasal spray was reported to cause a decrease in the night levels of testosterone and in the total sperm counts in adult monkeys (71). On the other hand, placebo spray did not produce any effect on their serum testosterone levels and sperm counts at any period tested.

Effects of progesterone on ovulation at different nasal spraying doses were also investigated in rhesus monkeys (72,73). The studies clearly showed that ovulation in rhesus monkeys can be 100% inhibited by the intranasal administration of progesterone at 2 μg/day for 10 days, in which the plasma levels of progesterone do not rise beyond 1.5 mg/ml at any stage of the cycle. However, when a higher daily dose (10-300 μg/day) was given progesterone could not prevent ovulation. This observation is not surprising if one considers the fact that progesterone is known to either inhibit or facilitate the secretion of gonadotropin depending upon the circumstances. In monkeys, for example, when progesterone is administered right after estradiol it exhibits the estrogen-induced LH surge. On the other hand, when progesterone is given in conjunction with estradiol, the estrogen-induced LH surge is significantly advanced. These studies indicate that a dosimetric dissection of the facilitatory and inhibitory effects of progesterone can be attained by administering it through the nasal route.

The pharmacokinetics of progesterone in the CSF and in the systemic circulation after intranasal and intramuscular administration was evaluated in monkeys. The effects of nasal sprays or progesterone on ovulation in rhesus monkeys was also studied (74). Most of the particles sprayed had a size ranging between 7 and 10 μm, at which most of the particles would be deposited in the olfactory region of the nasal mucosa and then transported across the olfactory dendrites into the nervous system. These particles were also found to diffuse into the submucosal blood vascular system through the supporting cells in the olfactory mucosa. Intranasal administration of progesterone (2 μg) to two adult ovariectomized monkeys was observed to attain the peak serum progesterone level of about 600 pg/ml within 10 min, whereas the peak serum level of similar magnitude was reached in 15 min after intramuscular injection. On the other hand, the peak CSF level of progesterone (about 300 pg/ml) was obtained as early as 5 min following the nasal spraying as compared to a lower peak CSF level (about 100 pg/ml) was reached at 30 min after intramuscular administration. These findings suggest that intranasal administration results in a rapid systemic absorption of progesterone as well as a preferential transfer of progesterone into the CSF as compared to intramuscular injection. The most effective dose for the inhibition of ovulation was found to be 3 μg progesterone per day, at which ovulation was inhibited in 12 out of the 20 monkeys studied. Ovulation occurred in all the animals sprayed with placebo solution only.

The bioavailability and the maximum concentration of progesterone achieved in both the CSF and systemic circulation were further evaluated in ovariectomized adult rhesus monkeys following various routes of administration (75). The maximum drug levels achieved in the serum and CSF following nasal spraying of progesterone (10 μg) with a precalibrated glass atomizer were significantly higher ($p < 0.01$) than those by intravenous and intramuscular injections, intranasal administration by nose drops, or ocular administration by eye drops. The C_{max} of progesterone in the serum and the CSF was highest following nasal spray administration, which was significantly higher than those achieved by intravenous injection, nose drops, and eye drops ($p < 0.05$) and by intramuscular administration ($p < 0.01$) (Figure 5.5). This study clearly demonstrated that the bioavailability of progesterone in both the systemic circulation and the CSF is considerably higher following the intranasal administration by nasal sprays, and that the extent of nasal absorption is dependent upon the method by which progesterone is delivered into the monkey's nostrils. The increase in bioavailability may be the result of a slow transport of progesterone to the body fluids via the nasal route as well as a slow rate of its clearance.

The systemic bioavailability and the plasma concentrations of progesterone following intranasal, intravenous, and intraduodenal administrations were also examined in rats (76,77). For intranasal administration, three different doses of radiolabeled progesterone in saline solution containing 1% polysorbate 80 were delivered into the nasal cavity by a micropipette (76). The plasma concentrations of progesterone following the intranasal administrations were observed to increase rapidly and attain peak levels within 6 min, whereas the intraduodenal administration resulted in a considerably lower plasma level (Figure 5.6). The extent of absorption, as expressed by AUC values, was noted to be directly proportional to the doses administered either intranasally or intravenously (Figure 5.7). A bioavailability of 100% was achieved with intranasal administration, whereas only 1.2% was obtained with intraduodenal administration. The pharmacokinetics and system-

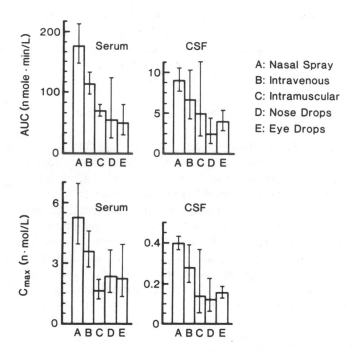

Figure 5.5 Area under concentration–time curve (AUC: 0–60 min) and maximal concentration (C_{max}) calculated in the serum and CSF following various routes of administration of progesterone (10 μg) in monkeys. Each histogram denotes the geometric mean values and the bars indicate the 95% confidence limits. (Modified from Ref. 75, used with permission.)

ic bioavailability of progesterone following the intranasal administration was also investigated in ovariectomized rabbits using nasal spray (78). The pharmacokinetic profiles indicated that following a rapid transnasal absorption the plasma concentration of progesterone is eliminated at first-order kinetics with a rate constant of 6.18 (±0.10) hr^{-1}, which is similar to that with intravenous bolus injection (6.77 ± 0.16) hr^{-1} and by oral administration (6.81 ± 0.70 hr^{-1}). However, the systemic bioavailability following the nasal spray administration was found to be much greater than that by oral solution administration (82.52 ± 13.50% vs. 7.87 ± 1.59%). The results of both studies clearly demonstrate that progesterone is rapidly absorbed into the systemic circulation from the nasal mucosa. Because of the avoidance of hepatic first-pass metabolism, the systemic bioavailability of progesterone following intranasal administration is superior to that of oral administration.

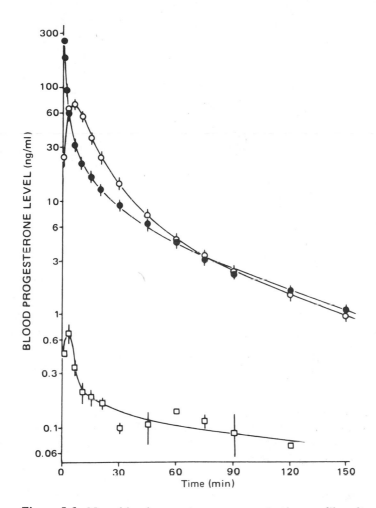

Figure 5.6 Mean blood progesterone concentration profiles after nasal (○), intravenous (●), and intraduodenal (□) administration of progesterone (50 μg) in rats. The lines were drawn through the points and the vertical bars represent standard error. (From Ref. 76, used with permission.)

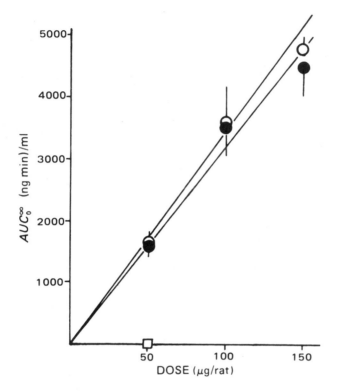

Figure 5.7 Relationship between AUC and dose after nasal (○) and intra-venous (●) administration of progesterone in rats. The square (□) represents intraduodenal administration. The vertical bars represent standard error. (From Ref. 76, used with permission.)

The pharmacokinetics of progesterone following nasal spray, intravenous injection, and intravenous infusion was studied in the ovariectomized adult rhesus monkey (79). The serum progesterone concentrations at 3 min after administration were not significantly different among these three methods of administration. Thereafter, the serum concentrations became significantly higher after both intravenous infusion and intranasal spraying as compared to the intravenous injection, whereas there was no significant difference be-tween the intravenous infusion and intranasal spraying.

Progesterone concentrations in the CSF after the intravenous injection showed a progressive decline with sampling time, whereas Progesterone

concentrations after intravenous infusion showed an increase in the first 3-
and 9-min samples, and declined progressively thereafter. When progesterone
was administered by nasal spray, its concentrations in the 9- and 15-min
samples were higher than that of the 3-min samples and then declined progressively (Table 5.1). Although progesterone concentrations in the CSF
samples taken at 3 min were not significantly different among these three
methods of administration, progesterone concentrations in all the subsequent
samples following intravenous infusion and nasal spray were significantly
higher than after intravenous injection. It is interesting to note that CSF concentrations were not different significantly between intravenous infusion and
nasal spray.

The pharmacokinetic data in terms of AUC, C_{max}, and t_{max} following
these three routes of administration clearly indicated that serum progesterone
concentrations obtained are highest following intravenous infusion followed
by intranasal spraying and intravenous injection (79). However, the pharmacokinetic profiles in the CSF suggested tht differences in the AUC, C_{max},
and t_{max} values between intravenous infusion and intranasal spraying is
statistically insignificant. The AUC, C_{max}, and t_{max} values for intravenous
injection were significantly different from intravenous infusion and intranasal spraying administration (Table 5.2).

This series of investigations have demonstrated that the concentrations
of progesterone and its bioavailability in both serum and CSF following the
nasal spray are significantly higher than those obtained after intravenous
injection, but are lower than those achieved by intravenous infusion, though
the difference is not statistically significant. These studies also suggest the
possibility of administering a physiological dose of progesterone by nasal
delivery for either replacement therapy or contraceptive purposes.

The pharmacokinetics and bioavailability of the hydroxy derivatives
of progesterone following intranasal administration using an immediate-release nasal spray and controlled-release nasal device were investigated and
compared with intravenous and oral administrations in the ovariectomized
rabbit (78). The nasal device (see Figure 3.7) was inserted into the rabbit
nasal passage, filled with 0.35 ml of progesterone suspension (60 μg/kg),
and left in place for the duration of the 6-hr study. The nasal spray achieved
peak plasma levels of progesterone within 2 min, indicating a rapid absorption of progesterone by the rabbit nasal mucosa. Nasal administration of
progesterone by the controlled-release nasal device led to a gradual increase
in the plasma levels of progesterone, which reached a plateau within 30 min,
and remained elevated throughout the 6-hr study (Figure 5.8). The systemic
bioavailabilities after the immediate-release nasal spray and controlled-release

Table 5.1 CSF Progesterone Concentration Profiles Following Administration by Diverse Methods

Time (min)	Progesterone (nM)			Analysis of variance[a]		
	i.v.	inf	n.s.	i.v. vs. inf	i.v. vs. n.s.	inf vs. n.s.
3	0.19 (0.15–0.24)	0.25 (0.17–0.35)	0.18 (0.11–0.28)	NS	NS	NS
9	0.17 (0.12–0.24)	0.42 (0.26–0.67)	0.37 (0.28–0.48)	**	**	NS
15	0.17 (0.13–0.22)	0.58 (0.38–0.88)	0.35 (0.24–0.51)	***	**	NS
30	0.10 (0.05–0.18)	0.34 (0.23–0.51)	0.23 (0.10–0.51)	*	NS	NS
60	0.04 (0.01–0.12)	0.23 (0.13–0.41)	0.18 (0.11–0.28)	*	*	NS

Data are presented as geometric mean concentrations with 95% confidence limits in parentheses (n = 9). Values have been corrected as described for Table 5.2 both here and in subsequent calculations. The 0 min values showed a range between 0.06 and 0.24 nM.
[a]One-way analysis of variance followed by multiple range test. NS, not significant; *, $p < 0.05$; **, $p < 0.01$; ***, $p < 0.001$.
Source: Modified from Ref. 79, used with permission.

Table 5.2 Pharmacokinetics of Progesterone in CSF After its Administration by Diverse Methods to Ovariectomized Monkeys

Pharmacokinetic parameter	i.v.	inf	n.s.	Analysis of variance[a]		
				i.v. vs. inf	i.v. vs. n.s.	inf vs. n.s.
AUC $\int_0^{60}$ (nM · min)	8.48 (6.51–10.95)	22.41 (15.59–32.19)	16.30 (10.28–25.84)	**	*	NS
C_{max} (nM)	0.23 (0.17–0.32)	0.66 (0.45–0.97)	0.53 (0.35–0.80)	**	**	NS
t_{max} (min)	5.91 (3.33–10.49)	13.66 (10.63–17.57)	10.20 (6.82–15.25)	*	*	NS

Data are presented as geometric mean values with 95% confidence limits in parentheses ($n = 9$).
[a]Analysis of variance followed by multiple range test. NS, not significant; *, $p < 0.05$; **, $p < 0.01$.
Source: Modified from Ref. 79, used with permission.

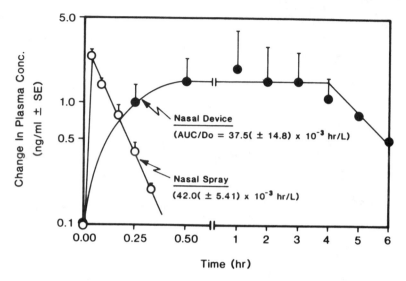

Figure 5.8 Plasma concentration profiles of progesterone on ovariectomized rabbits ($n = 4$) following intranasal administration by immediate-release nasal spray (○) and controlled-release nasal device (●). (Modifed from Ref. 78, used with permission.)

nasal device (82.5 and 72.4%, respectively) were significantly greater than those after oral administration (7.9%).

The effect of penetrant hydrophilicity on the nasal absorption of progestational steroids in ovariectomized rabbits was investigated using a progesterone derivative with one hydroxy group (17-hydroxyprogesterone), two hydroxy groups (cortexolone), and three hydroxy groups (hydrocortisone) (80). The systemic bioavailabilities of progesterone and its hydroxy derivatives after nasal administration by both immediate-release nasal spray and controlled-release nasal device were all significantly greater ($p > 0.01$) than those after oral administration (Table 5.3). The systemic bioavailability of progestins after immediate-release nasal spray showed a rank order of: 17-hydroxyprogesterone > progesterone > cortexolone > hydrocortisone, which correlated in a hyperbolic pattern with the nasal mucosa partition coefficients of the drugs (80). The systemic bioavailability of hydrocortisone following intranasal administration by a controlled-release nasal device was significantly greater ($p = 0.02$) than by immediate-release nasal spray (77.7 vs. 60.9%). It was proposed that the nasal device interfered with nasal

Table 5.3 Comparative Bioavailability of Progestins After Oral and Nasal Administration

Route	Progesterone (%)	17-OH Progesterone (%)	Cortexolone	Hydrocortisone (%)
Oral Delivery	7.9 (±1.6)	5.4 (±0.6)	5.9 (±0.7)	2.7 (±0.7)
Nasal Delivery				
spray	82.5 (±13.5)	97.1 (±12.1)	80.0 (±12.5)	60.9 (±5.8)
device	72.4 (±25.7)	88.0 (±10.8)	80.9 (±5.3)	77.7 (±4.4)

Source: D. C. Corbo, Y. C. Huang, and Y. W. Chien, unpublished data.

mucociliary clearance, which allowed a greater absorption of the more hydrophilic, slowly absorbed hydrocortisone. The results demonstrated that the extent of nasal absorption is influenced by both the mode of nasal administration and the hydrophilicity of the penetrant.

5.2.3 Norethindrone

Norethindrone (NET) has been administered intranasally in monkeys to evaluate its effect on testicular functions (68), menstrual cycle (71), and ovulation (72-74). The pharmacokinetics of NET in the CSF and blood (74) as well as the specific transport pathway for NET into the brain were also studied (81).

After intranasal administration of NET to monkeys, it was reported that a reduction in testicular size, arrest of spermatogenesis, and a significant decline of serum testosterone were observed (68).

The effects of NET on the serum testosterone level and the total sperm count in the male monkey and on the mestrual cycle in the female monkey after nasal administration have been studied by Moudgal et al. (71). The results indicated a decrease in night serum testosterone levels and in total sperm counts, whereas placebo did not produce any effects. Nasal spraying of NET in the adult cycling female monkeys between days 5 and 14 was reported to yield a shortening of the menstrual cycle with premature menstrual bleeding, which could be ascribed to the decrease in the serum levels of FSH, LH, estradiol (E_2), and progesterone (P). During the control cycle, a preovulatory increase in E_2 was observed, followed by the surge levels of LH and FSH around days 10-11 with an increase in P level during the luteal phase. In the NET-treated cycle, the characteristic preovulatory surges of E_2, LH, and FSH were inhibited. Consequently, P level did not increase during the luteal phase. These data suggested that there is a blockage in the follicular maturation and ovulatory process of the monkeys following nasal spraying of NET.

Norethindrone given intranasally has been reported to prevent ovulation in monkeys (72). Ovulation was unaffected by nasal NET at 3 μg/day, but was suppressed in all cases at a dose of 9 or 17 μg/day.

Norethindrone (NET) has been administered intranasally to female rhesus monkeys to explore the existence of specific pathways from the nose to the cerebrospinal fluid (CSF) (81). The measurable plasma level of NET was obtained at 1 min, and the peak level was reached at 30 min after intranasal administration, whereas the intravenous administration achieved its maximum plasma level 1 min after administration. However, the NET in the CSF was much lower than the corresponding plasma levels. The observations of a very rapid absorption of NET into the peripheral circulation after nasal absorption and a slow, gradual increase of the NET concentration in the CSF during the period with high blood levels do not appear to substantiate the concept of a rapid and specific transport of steroids into the CSF, as proposed by Kumar (64). The discrepancy may have resulted from a difference the preparation and in the methods of administration. In the investigation by Ohman (81), NET was formulated in a suspension form and applied to the nasal cavity as nasal drops, whereas Kumar (64) used a solution dosage form and delivered it by nasal spray instead.

The pharmacokinetics of NET in the CSF and circulation has been monitored following intranasal or intramuscular administrations in two female rhesus monkeys (74). While serum NET levels following these two routes of administration were rather similar in the order of magnitude, the peak NET concentration was reached within 5 min following intranasal administration as compared to 10 min after intramuscular injection. Following nasal spraying the peak level of NET in the CSF was much higher than that achieved by intramuscular administration. However, the peak NET level in the CSF does not precede the peak NET level in the circulation.

The most effective dose for the inhibition of ovulation was determined to be 9 µg/day for norethindrone (74). Among the 18 monkeys treated with 9 µg of NET by nasal spray ovulation was inhibited in 11, whereas ovulation occurred in all the 18 animals sprayed with the placebo formulation.

5.2.4 Testosterone

Testosterone is generally administered by intramuscular injection. Although testosterone is orally absorbed, it is ineffective as a result of its extensive metabolism in the liver and in the gastrointestinal tract before reaching the systemic circulation.

In order to facilitate the systemic bioavailability of testosterone, the nasal absorption of testosterone has been recently investigated and compared to intravenous and intraduodenal administrations in rats (80). Two different doses of [^{3}H] testosterone, at 25 and 50 µg/rat containing 1% polysorbate 80, were administered to the nasal cavity by means of a micropipette and the nostrils were then sealed with an adhesive. The concentrations of testosterone in the circulation after intranasal administration increased rapidly and attained the peak level within 2 min, whereas the intraduodenal administration resulted in considerably lower blood levels (Figure 5.9). The plasma testosterone concentrations achieved by intranasal administration were simi-

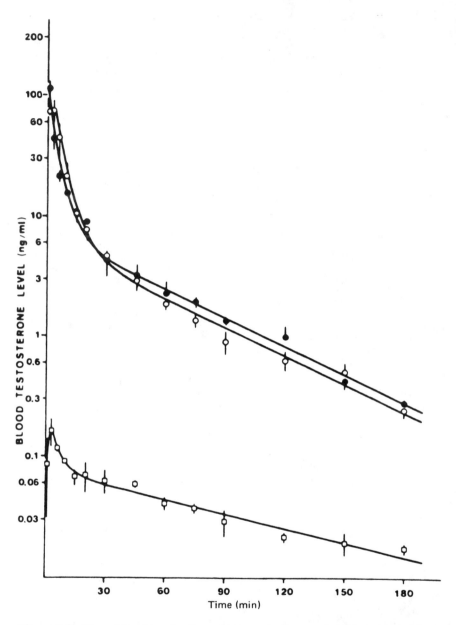

Figure 5.9 Mean blood levels of testosterone in the rats following nasal (○), intravenous (●), and intraduodenal (□) administration of testosterone (25 μg/ rat). Points represent mean values of three animals (±S.E.M.). (From Ref. 82, used with permission.)

Table 5.4 Area Under Blood Level-Time Curve (AUC) of Testosterone in Rats Following Intravenous, Nasal, and Intraduodenal Administration

Dose (μg)	Route	AUC (ng $\cdot$ h/ml)[a]	AUC (nasal, intraduodenal) / AUC (intravenous)
25	Intravenous	900.6 ($\pm$90.9)	
	Nasal	890.5 ($\pm$168.0)	0.99
	intraduodenal	8.9 ($\pm$0.2)	0.01
50	Intravenous	1716.3 ($\pm$47.2)	
	Nasal	1545.7 ($\pm$168.6)	0.90

[a]Mean ($\pm$S.E.M.) (n = 3).
Source: Modified from Ref. 82, used with permission.

lar to those after intravenous administration, with an elimination half-life of about 40 min. The intranasal bioavailability was calculated to be 99% at the 25-μg dose and 90% at the 50-μg dose, whereas the intraduodenal bioavailability was found only to be 1% at both doses studied (Table 5.4). It was concluded from these results that testosterone is rapidly absorbed from the nasal mucosa owing to avoiding the hepatic first-pass elimination.

5.3 VITAMINS

It is evident that pernicious anemia is a vitamin B_{12} deficiency state attributable to the defective absorption of this vitamin from the gastrointestinal tract. Normal absorption of B_{12} appears to require the presence of an intrinsic factor which seems to be the cause contributing to the absorption defect in pernicious anemia (83). Parenteral administration of 25 μg of vitamin B_{12} to patients with pernicious anemia in severe relapse was reported to result in a complete hematological remission. Parenteral administration of vitamin B_{12} in doses greater than 25 μg produced prompt urinary excretion of the vitamin. When 500 μg or more were administered parentereally, vitamin B_{12} was excreted approximately quantitatively in the urine. When administered orally, however, approximately 5000 μg of B_{12} was necessary to produce the same effect as the parenteral administration of 25 μg of vitamin B_{12} (83).

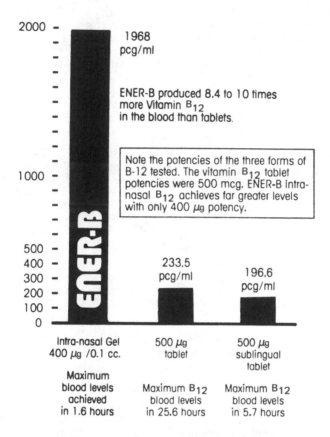

2000 —
    1968
    pcg/ml

    ENER-B produced 8.4 to 10 times
    more Vitamin B₁₂
    in the blood than tablets.

    Note the potencies of the three forms of
    B-12 tested. The vitamin B₁₂ tablet
1000 — potencies were 500 mcg. ENER-B intra-
    nasal B₁₂ achieves far greater levels
    with only 400 μg potency.

500 —
400 —   233.5
300 —   pcg/ml   196.6
200 —   pcg/ml
100 —
   0 —

  Intra-nasal Gel   500 μg   500 μg
  400 μg /0.1 cc.   tablet   sublingual
                                       tablet
  Maximum
  blood levels   Maximum B₁₂   Maximum B₁₂
  achieved   blood levels   blood levels
  in 1.6 hours   in 25.6 hours in 5.7 hours

Figure 5.10 Blood levels of vitamin B_{12} in man following intranasal and oral administration of vitamin B_{12}. The data in this chart used Nature's Bounty packaging of ENER-B. (From *Physicians' Desk Reference*, 1988, used with permission of Medical Economics Company Inc.)

Inhalation of crystalline B_{12}, which is dissolved in physiological saline or deposited on lactose powder, has resulted in adequate clinical and hematological responses in three patients with pernicious anemia (84). Vitamin B_{12} in physiological saline or lactose powder produced no objective or subjective evidence of toxicity or sensitivity at the pulmonary site. After the inhalation of 200 μg of vitamin B_{12} in saline, the urine concentration of B_{12} reached the level of 0.26 μg/ml, whereas the inhalation of approximately 500 μg of vitamin B_{12} on lactose powder increased the urinary B_{12} to 0.134 μg/ml.

Direct pulmonary instillation of 100 μg crystalline vitamin B_{12} by means of a bronchoscope resulted in urinary excretion of 9.76 μg/ml of vitamin B_{12}, which is equivalent to the intramuscular injection of 60-80 μg of vitamin B_{12}. These results suggest a definite increase in vitamin B_{12}-like growth substance in the urine of those subjects receiving vitamin B_{12} by inhalation.

Inhalation and intranasal instillation of crystalline vitamin B_{12} in either isotonic saline solution or lactose powder were observed to result in an adequate clinical and hematological response in 12 patients with pernicious anemia in relapse (85). Intranasal instillation of vitamin B_{12} has resulted in a significant B_{12} concentration in the urine. The results appear to suggest that intrinsic substance is not essential for the absorption of vitamin B_{12} from the mucosa in the respiratory tract. Furthermore, no objective or subjective evidence of toxicity or sensitivity at the local site was found in these patients.

More recently, the intranasal administration of vitamin B_{12} in gel formulations has been investigated in patients with pernicious anemia (86) and has led to the commercialization of ENER-B (Nature's Bounty) in a nasal dosage form. The nasal absorption of 400 μg of vitamin B_{12} has been compared with that of 500 μg of vitamin B_{12} given in oral or sublingual tablets. The peak blood level of vitamin B_{12} after nasal administration was found to be eight to 10 times higher, and the peak time was found to be four to 16 times shorter than those of given by tablet (Figure 5.10).

5.4 CARDIOVASCULAR DRUGS

5.4.1 Hydralazine

Hydralazine is a vasodilator and has always been used in conjunction with other antihypertensive drugs for the treatment of malignant hypertension and hypertensive emergencies. Following oral administration, hydralazine is rapidly and almost completely absorbed (87,88). However, its oral bioavailability has been found to be relatively low as a result of extensive hepatic first pass metabolism.

The nasal absorption of hydralazine as well as the effect of surfactant and solution pH has been studied in rats using the in situ nasal perfusion technique and in vivo nasal abosrption methods (89,90). The results of in situ nasal perfusion studies indicated that hydralazine disappears from the nasal cavity and from the perfusate both at a first-order kinetics. The disappearance of the drug is apparently due to the absorption through the nasal mucosa. A good linear relationship was found to exist between the absorp-

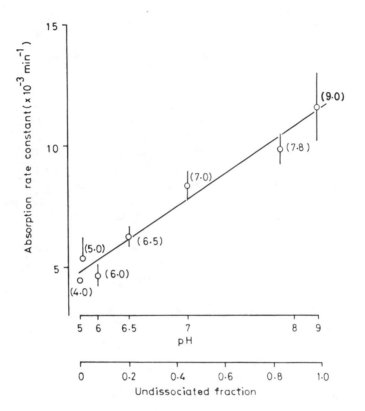

Figure 5.11 Relationship between the absorption rate constant of hydralazine (1 mM) and its undissociated fraction at various pHs. Each value represents the mean (±S.E.M.) for three rats. The number in parentheses indicates
the pH value. (From Ref. 89, used with permission.)

tion rate constant of hydralazine and the fraction of its undissociated species
calculated from the pKa value (Figure 5.11). The nasal absorption of hydralazine was markedly enhanced by surfactants, such as sodium glycocholate
and polyoxyethylene-9-lauryl ether.

In vivo nasal absorption studies conducted in rats showed that hydralazine
in saline solution (at pH 3) is well absorbed through the nasal mucosa with
the peak plasma level attained within 30 min. The nasal absorption of hydralazine was found to be facilitated, with the peak plasma level achieved earlier
(within 10 min), when the pH of the drug solution was increased from pH 3.0

Table 5.5 Area Under Blood Level-Time Curve (AUC) After Administration of Hydralazine in Rats

Route	Dose (mg/rat)	$AUC_{0 \to \infty}$ ($\mu g \cdot min \cdot ml^{-1}$)[a]	$\dfrac{AUC_{nasal,i.d.} \cdot dose_{i.v.}}{AUC_{i.v.} \cdot dose_{nasal,i.d.}}$
Intravenous (i.v.)	1.25	135.3 ($\pm$22.1)	
Intraduodenum (i.d.)	1.25	105.6 ($\pm$18.0)	0.78
Nasal:			
in saline (pH 3)	1.33	182.9 ($\pm$17.7)	1.27
in phosphate buffer (pH 6.5)	1.33	118.7 ($\pm$17.0)	0.83
in saline + 0.5% polyoxyethylene 9-lauryl ether (pH 3)	1.33	162.3 ($^+$18.7)	1.13

[a]Mean ($\pm$S.D.) for three to five rats.
Source: Modified from Ref. 89, used with permission.

to 6.5, or with the addition of 0.5% polyoxyethylene-9-lauryl ether. The intranasal bioavailability of hydralazine was found to be 127, 83, and 113%, respectively, depending upon the formulation (Table 5.5).

5.4.2 Angiotensin II Antagonist

Angiotensin II is an octapeptide that is capable of inducing the constriction of blood vessels and stimulating the production of aldosterone. Aldosterone, in turn, stimulates the retention of sodium and water by the distal convoluted tubule and the excretion of potassium. Among the derivatives of angiotensin II, the 1,8-disubstituted analogs are the most potent competitive antagonists (91-93).

Intranasal administration of (1-N-Suc-5-Val-8-phg)-angiotensin II, a specific angiotensin II antagonist, has been investigated in anesthetized rats with different degrees of experimentally elevated blood pressure (94). Each dose, in a volume of 20 μl, was given to one nostril using a Hamilton microsyringe with a polyethylene tube. The results showed that intranasal administration of 1 mg/kg of (1-N-Suc-5-Val-8-phg)-angiotensin II produces a significant, immediate decrease of blood pressure (-29 mm Hg, $p < 0.05$) for 1 hr (Figure 5.12). Following intranasal application of 0.1, 0.3, and 0.9 mg/kg

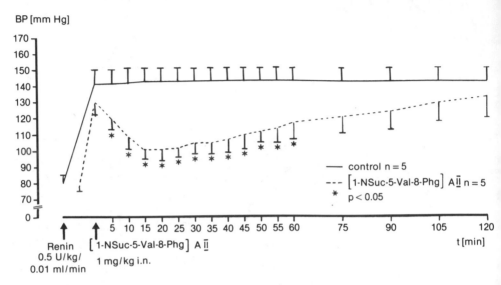

Figure 5.12 Decrease of blood pressure (BP; mean ± S.E.M.) following the intranasal administration of an angiotensin II antagonist during renin-induced pressure increase in the anesthetized rats. (From Ref. 94, used with permission.)

of this 1,8-disubstituted angiotensin II analog, a dose-dependent hypotensive response was observed (Figure 5.13).

In the acute, accelerated hypertensive model, intranasal administration of angiotensin II antagonist produced an immediate drop in blood pressure by about 33% (−39 mm Hg), whereas the control group showed a gradual decline in blood pressure (−18%) after 15 min. The fall in blood pressure observed in the treated group was highly significant ($p < 0.05$-0.001). On the other hand, intranasal administration of (1-N-Suc-5-Val-8-phg)-angiotensin II in rats did not cause any significant change in chronic renal hypertension or counteract the pressor effect of norepinephrine.

It was concluded from the studies outlined above that the angiotensin II antagonists, such as (1-N-Suc-5-Val-8-phg)-angiotensin II, have specific hypotensive effects in the different forms of experimental blood pressure elevation and produce no undesirable initial pressor response when given intranasally.

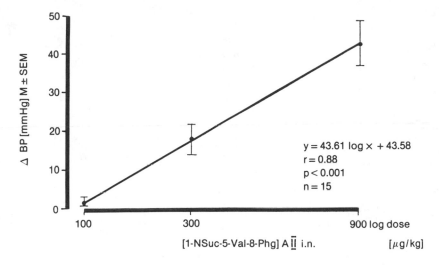

Figure 5.13 Exponential relationship between the reduction in blood pressure (BP) following intranasal administration of angiotensin II antagonist during angiotensin II–induced pressure increase in the anesthetized rats. (From Ref. 94, used with permission.)

5.4.3 Nitroglycerin

Nitroglycerin has been widely used to abort and to prevent anginal attacks. While it has a quick onset of action, its duration of activity is rather short. The primary action of nitroglycerin is to induce a relaxation of both peripheral and coronary vascular smooth muscles. As a result, it reduces the central venous pressure, and decreases both left ventricular size and cardiac stroke volume. The net effect is the reduction of myocardial oxygen consumption (95).

When taken orally, nitroglycerin is inactivated by the heaptic first-pass metabolism (96). In order to bypass the hepatic first-pass elimination (95), nitroglycerin is currently being administered orally in sublingual tablets, topically in ointments, or in transdermal patches. Intravenous administration is also useful for its rapid action, but its preparation, standardization, and stabilization have several potential problems, and this can be rather costly.

The feasibility of intranasal administration of nitroglycerin has been studied by instilling a saline solution of the drug (0.8 mg/ml) into patients

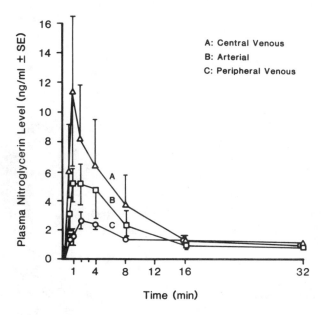

Figure 5.14 Plasma concentration profiles of nitroglycerin in various compartments following intranasal administration of nitroglycerin (0.8 mg). (Replotted from Ref. 97, used with permission.)

with coronary artery bypass surgery and the time course, vascular distribution, and the dose-related uptake of nitroglycerin examined (97). The highest nitroglycerin concentration was detected in the central venous blood followed by the arterial and peripheral venous blood (Figure 5.14). The nitroglycerin concentration in the central venous blood was observed to peak at 1 min and remained above the therapeutic level for 8 min, whereas the peripheral venous levels peaked at 2 min. In all patients, the desirable clinical effects, as indicated by the lowering of pulmonary artery pressure and/or the improvement in the S-T segment changes, were observed within 2 min. The results concluded that the intranasal administration of nitroglycerin in saline solution is a rapid and convenient alternative to intravenous injection.

The clinical effects and pharmacokinetics of nitroglycerin reported above were confirmed subsequently in five patients undergoing elective coronary artery bypass surgery (98). Apparently, nitroglycerin is rapidly absorbed into the vascular space following intranasal instillation, and the profile of nasal absorption is similar to a bolus intravenous injection. Blood levels were noted to decline rapidly as a monoexponential function and became barely detectable after 16 min. The apparent volume of distribution, clearance rate, and plasma half-life of nitroglycerin were 123.5-312.5 L, 15.8-37.2 L/min, and 5.41-5.82 min, respectively.

Intranasal administration of nitroglycerin was reported to relieve the cardiovascular stress associated with the aortic cross-clamp by decreasing the arterial blood pressure and pulmonary capillary wedge pressure (99), which occur rapidly within only 2 min. The results indicated that systolic blood pressure was reduced to a near preclamp level, with only a little change in the heart rate. If the blood pressure was still high after 2-3 min, another dose (0.4 mg) of nitroglycerin could be given and the effect can last for another 10 to 15 min.

Intranasal nitroglycerin can also be used in many other clinical situations, such as at the end of a coronary bypass operation. If the blood pressure is noted to rise just before or during the transfer from the operating room to the special care unit, a small squirt of nitroglycerin solution into the nose could solve the problem.

A metered-dose nasal nitroglycerin spray has been investigated in comparison with a soft gelatin capsule or sublingual tablet dosage form of nitroglycerin (100). The results indicated that all the treatments produce a significantly greater digital plethysmographic activity than that of the placebo. In addition, the treatments with spray and soft gelatin capsule were found to be as effective or more effective than the respective sublingual medication in generating a digital plethysmographic response.

5.4.4 Isosorbide Dinitrate

Sublingual preparations of isosorbide dinitrate have been widely used to abort and prevent anginal attacks. Isosorbide dinitrate in nasal spray (Iso-Mack Spray) has been recently compared with nitroglycerin (NTG) and isosorbide dinitrate (ISDN) in sublingual form for their central hemodynamic effect (101). The results indicated that ISDN spray has a quick onset of action (2.67 ± 2.4 min), which is comparable to that of NTG (2.67 ± 1.00 min), whereas ISDN spray yields a long duration of action (57.5 ± 42.1 min), which is comparable to that of sublingual ISDN (85.6 ± 39.5 min), and is significantly longer than that of NTG (11.4 ± 6.4 min, $p < 0.05$). Intranasal spraying of 2.5 mg ISDN appeared to produce the same level of hemodynamic changes as was induced by 0.3 mg NTG or 5 mg ISDN by sublingual administration. It was concluded that ISDN spray is a useful antianginal preparation which is capable of inducing the abortion of anginal attacks by its quick onset and long duration of action.

5.4.5 Propranolol

Propranolol, an adrenergic beta-receptor-blocking agent, is widely used for the management of hypertension and the treatment of angina pectoris. It is capable of suppressing the heart rate, contractibility, and bronchodilation as well as increasing the vasoconstriction of vascular beds (102). It is usually given orally, but may also be given intravenously for the treatment of arrhythmias. Oral administration of propranolol in five human subjects has been reported to yield a great variation in plasma level with peak concentration varying as widely as sevenfold and in systemic bioavailability ranging from 16 to 60% (103). The observed variability in blood levels and the low bioavailability could be the result of extensive hepatic first-pass metabolism (104).

Intranasal administration of propranolol has been investigated in rats as a new delivery system to enhance the bioavailability and to minimize the variation in blood levels (105). The results demonstrated that the blood propranolol concentration following intranasal administration is identical to that by intravenous injection (Figure 5.15). On the basis of this investigation it was concluded tht propranolol is rapidly absorbed by the nasal mucosa and the peak plasma level can be achieved within 5 min. Furthermore, the nasal route appears to be superior to the oral route and is as effective as the intravenous route. The area under the concentration vs. time curve (AUC) of propranolol is directly proportional to the dose administered intranasally.

The advantages of intranasal administration of propranolol were further confirmed in rats and dogs (106). Moreover, intranasal administration of propranolol in sustained-release formulations, with the addition of methylcellulose, was found to produce a low C_{max} and a longer T_{max}. The blood level of propranolol following intranasal administration with sustained-release formulations was prolonged with the bioavailability identical to that after intravenous administration.

The nasal absorption of propranolol has also been evaluated and compared with intravenous and oral administrations in humans (107). The results demonstrated that intranasal administration of propranolol HCl in 2% methylcellulose gel, with the subjects in a sitting position, produces a serum level which is identical to that by intravenous infusion. On the other hand, the oral bioavailability of propranolol HCl in tablets was found to be only 25% (Table 5.6). The results appeared to confirm the previous findings obtained in rats and dogs that propranolol is absorbed rapidly and completely from the nasal mucosa.

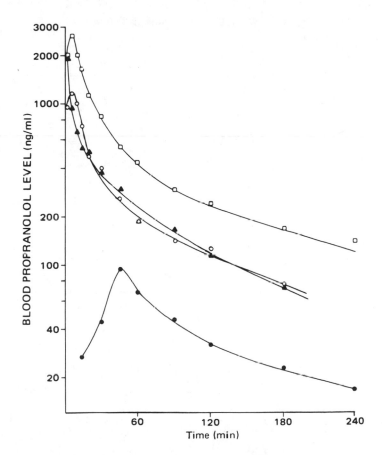

Figure 5.15 Time course of the average blood propranolol levels in the rats after intranasal administration of 1 mg/rat (○) and 2 mg/rat (□), intravenous administration of 1 mg/rat (▲), oral administration of 1 mg/rat (●). (From Ref. 105, used with permission.)

Table 5.6 Mean Area Under Serum Level-Time Curve For Propranolol Administered by Three Routes

Route	Dose (mg)	Mean $AUC_{0 \to \infty}$ (ng $\times$ hr)/ml ($\pm$S.E.)	$\dfrac{AUC_{oral,nasal} \cdot dose_{i.v.}}{AUC_{i.v.} \cdot dose_{oral,nasal}}$
Intravenous	10	175.4 ($\pm$20.4)	
Nasal	10	190.3 ($\pm$17.6)	1.09
Oral	80	349.5 ($\pm$35.2)	0.25

Source: Modified from Ref. 107, used with permission.

The chronic effect on the ciliary beat frequency after the long-term intranasal administration of propranolol has been investigated in chicken embryo and human adenoid tissue (108). The results showed that propranolol in nose drops inadversibly arrests the ciliary movement of chicken and human cilia within 20 min at a dose level of 1.0 or 0.1%, respectively.

Table 5.7 Comparison in Blood Levels[a] of [^{14}C] Clofilium Ion in Rats[b] After Various Routes of Administration

Route of administration	Dose (mg/kg)[c]	AUC (μg $\cdot$ min $\cdot$ g)[d]	Absorption (%)[e]	p[f]
Intravenous	1.2	39.5 ($\pm$4.98)		
Oral	1.2	0.53 ($\pm$0.10)[g]	1.3	0.001
Nasal	1.2	27.5 ($\pm$1.30)[h]	69.6	0.08

[a]Expressed as microgram equivalents of carbon-14 per gram of blood.
[b]Harlan Sprague-Dawley male rats ($n = 3$).
[c]Formulated in solution form.
[d]Mean ($\pm$S.E.M.) of three rats.
[e]Percentage of intravenous dose.
[f]Probability value (Student's t test) compared with intravenous administration route data.
[g]$p < 0.05$ (compared with nasal administration route data).
[h]$p > 0.05$ (compared with intravenous administration route data).
Source: Modified from Ref. 112, used with permission.

5.4.6 Clofilium Tosylate

Clofilium tosylate is a synthetic quarternary ammonium compound with anti-fibrillatory activity (109,110). The oral absorption of clofilium tosylate in rats was found to be rather poor (111). The intranasal administration of clofilium tosylate has been studied in rats as a possible means to improve its systemic bioavailability (112,113). The drug solution was delivered to the nasal cavity through esophageal cannulation tubing (see the details in Chapter 2, Section 2.1.1).

The results suggested that the difference in the blood levels of clofilium tosylate between the intranasal and intravenous administrations is statistically insignificant ($p > 0.05$). The systemic bioavailability after intranasal administration was estimated to be 69.6% as compared to only 1.3% for oral administration (Table 5.7). The AUC values were observed to increase in a linear manner in the lower dose range, but in a nonlinear manner in the higher dose range. This observation is in agreement with the data that the absorption of quaternary ammonium compound is via a diffusion mechanism (114). At the dose level of 0.3 mg/kg, the nasal bioavailability of clofilium tosylate was found to be 21-fold greater than the oral bioavailability, with the peak blood level obtained within 10 min. The data of tissue distribution of drug showed that 1 hr after the intranasal administration of radiolabeled clofilium tosylate, high levels of radioactivity were observed in the heart, lung, liver, and kidney as compared to that in the blood (Table 5.8). The results demonstrated a gradual accumulation of the drug in the heart, with the peak level attained within 4-6 hr. After 6 hr, the total radioactivity in the heart appeared to be about 18 times greater than that in the blood. The observations suggest that the clofilium tosylate ion and/or its metabolites favorably concentrate in the heart tissues, and the blood levels of radioactivity may not be an accurate index of the cardiac levels or biological responses.

5.5 AUTONOMIC NERVOUS SYSTEM DRUGS

5.5.1 Sympathomimetics

5.5.1.1 Ephedrine

The nasal absorption of ephedrine across the frontal sinus membranes in the dog has been investigated by Childrey and Essex (115). Intranasal administration of ephedrine at a dosage of 50 mg was found to produce no appreciable effect on blood pressure, whereas by parenteral administration (intravenous, intramuscular, subcutaneous) at doses ranging from 25 to 50 mg, ephedrine

Table 5.8 Tissue Distribution of [^{14}C] Clofilium Tosylate in Rats[a] After Intranasal Administration

Tissue	Distribution profiles (ng · equivalent of ^{14}C/gm Tissue)[b]				
	0.5 hr[c]	1 hr	2 hr	4 hr	6 hr
Blood	12.06 (±1.80)	9.30 (±0.34)	14.88 (±1.44)	11.80 (±1.20)	14.40 (±3.80)
Heart	82.12 (±12.54)	88.09 (±4.10)	175.16 (±23.10)	227.80 (±22.50)	263.70 (±27.00)
Lung	58.95 (±8.42)	49.47 (±4.69)	83.88 (±8.90)	97.06 (±15.20)	112.10 (±15.00)
Liver	221.31 (±29.19)	218.24 (±12.20)	328.60 (±36.30)	482.90 (±39.80)	271.90 (±36.00)
Kidney	475.13 (±87.60)	609.42 (±20.59)	944.40 (±85.50)	1116.00 (±106.80)	813.00 (±110.00)

[a]Species: Harlan Sprague-Dawley, males ($n = 3$).
[b]Each value represents the mean (±S.E.M.) of three animals.
[c]The time after intranasal administration of 0.3 mg/kg dose.
Source: Modified from Ref. 112, used with permission.

was reported to cause almost immediately a marked rise in the blood pressure which lasted for 60 min. Apparently, ephedrine is incapable of permeating the frontal sinus mucosa in sufficient quantities to cause appreciable systemic activity. However, this conclusion was reached based upon just one experiment in the dog.

5.5.1.2 Epinephrine

As the major sympathomimetic constituent in the adrenal medulla, epinephrine possesses all the strong $alpha_1$-, $beta_1$-, and $beta_2$-agonistic activities. It has been used for the management of allergic disorders, such as anaphylaxis, angioneurotic edema, giant urticaria, serum sickness, status asthmaticus; as a topical nasal decongestant; and in cardiac arrest as well as in primary open-angle glaucoma.

Intravenous administration of epinephrine in a cat was noted to cause a typical vasopressor response, whereas subcutaneous injection of the same solution gave negative results as did intranasal administration to the right frontal sinus (115). The negative results led the investigators to conclude that epinephrine is incapable of penetrating through the mucosa of the frontal sinus in sufficient quantity to produce an appreciable systemic effect.

5.5.1.3 Phenylephrine

Phenylephrine is a sympathomimetic drug with a strong alpha-agonistic, negligible beta-agonisitic, and CNS activities, it is absorbed orally without being attacked by monoamine oxidase (MAO). Phenylephrine has been used in the treatment of paroxysmal atrial tachycardia and wide-angle glaucoma. It is also used as a nasal decongestant and mydriatic.

An investigation has been carried out to determine the effects of phenylephrine HCl solution by intranasal administration in patients with various chronic illnesses: 11 with hypertension, 16 with cardiac disorders, nine with thyroid disorders, and 14 with diabetes (116). The results showed that there were no detectable untoward effects, and that the absorption from the nasal membrane is too retarded to produce any side effects.

In another study, phenylephrine (1.25-6.0 mg) was administered intranasally to 46 patients with rhinological conditions and concurrent hypertension, diabetes, cardiac, or thyroid disease. The results suggested that no alteration in blood pressure is produced (117). Furthermore, the feasibility of intranasal administration of phenylephrine HCl solution to induce systemic vasoconstriction and to increased blood pressure has been recently investigated in two groups of high-risk patients. Among these patients were 12 patients with chronic nasal congestion, whose blood pressure was normal; and 14 patients with hypertension, who were being medicated with the beta-blocker metoprolol (118). On two separate days, increasing doses of phenylephrine (0.5-4 mg) or placebo were instilled into the nostrils at hourly intervals, using a 50-μL Eppendorf pipette while the patients were in a semisupine position. Immediately afterward, the patients turned their heads to the side of the nostril that received the medication to maximize the absorption of the drug. The results showed no significant increase in blood pressure in either group of patients. Furthermore, the repeated instillations of phenylephrine also failed to yield a cumulative rise in the mean values of blood pressure in either group. Alteration in the heart rates between the groups administered with phenylephrine and placebo was small, and the mean change was not significant. In particular, no phenylephrine-induced reflex bradycardia was observed. Furthermore, the intranasal administration of phenylephrine at seven to 30 times the usual dose to patients with nasal congestion and normal blood pressure produced no significant changes in blood pressure or heart rate. The same results were also observed in the 14 patients receiving metoprolol for hypertension at doses higher than the usual recommended dose. None of the patients experienced any adverse effects from the intranasal administration of either phenylephrine or placebo.

Nasal airway resistance (Rn), which is defined as the pressure required for the air to move through the nasal passages at a specific flow rate, can be determined by measuring the transnasal pressure and nasal airflow during each breath. The intranasal administration of a nasal decongestant will change the nasal airway resistance. Phenylephrine in aqueous solution (0.25 or 0.5%) has been found to be an effective decongestant when applied intranasally in the patients with an acute nasal obstruction problem like the common cold or sinusitis (119).

The effectiveness and duration of activity of five nasal decongestants and a placebo solution has been evaluated in 21 subjects with nasal congestion (120). Following the intranasal administration of the placebo solution, nasal airway resistance was observed first to increase transiently within 2 min, and then return toward preadministration levels. Intranasal administration of formulation W-37 (which contains 0.25% phenylephrine HCl and 1.0% thonzylamine HCl) was observed to produce a transient, but impressive change in the nasal airway resistance; and a statistically significant decrease in the Rn value was obtained within 10-20 min after intranasal administration. Incorporation of 0.25% phenylpropanolamine HCl into formulation W-37 (formulation W-66) was found to yield a prolonged response, with a statistical difference in Rn values from the controls for up to 150 min. Formulation W-58, which was prepared by the addition of 0.1% volatile oil to formulation W-66, was noted to produce a slightly more consistent response, but with a shorter duration of effectiveness. On the other hand, formulation 83 (which contains 0.25% phenylephrine HCl, 0.12% methapyrilene HCl, and 0.06% volatile oil) was noted to result in an impressive and prompt decrease in Rn values, whereas the response to formulation W-72 (which contains 0.05% metizoline) was not prompt. The results outlined above demonstrated that: (a) the combination of phenylephrine and thonzylamine is least effective as a topical nasal decongestant, (b) the addition of phenylpropanolamine prolongs the duration of effectiveness for the combination of phenylephrine and thonzylamine, (c) volatile oils provide no effect as the vehicle for the combination, and (d) methapyrilene has a greater effect than thonzylamine as an antihistaminic agent in the combination.

A case of addiction and psychosis has been reported following the intranasal administration of phenylephrine by nasal spray (121). The toxic psychosis symptoms subsisded shortly after the discontinuation of medication.

5.5.1.4 Xylometazoline

Xylometazoline is a topical long-acting decongestant used for the relief of congestion due to coryza or allergic rhinitis. The ability of xylometazoline in nasal spray to reduce nasal congestion has been evaluated in 44 normal subjects with coryza resulting from upper respiratory infection (122). Rating scales were designed to measure the subjective responses, whereas the nasal airway resistance, expressed as nasal conductance (Gn), was also measured as the objective responses over a 6-hr period. The change in the Gn values following the intranasal administration of xylometazoline was found to be rapid, profound, and persistent. The increase in Gn values was statistically significant ($p < 0.05$) at all times between 10 min and up to 4 hr. The congestion was also reportedly decreased at all time periods after the intranasal administration of xylometazoline.

The nasal mucosa of 20 healthy subjects were examined before, during, and after 6 weeks of regular use of xylometazoline in nose drops (123). No diminishment in mucociliary functions was detected in all the subjects during or after the trial. In the majority of the subjects, the intranasal administration of xylometazoline over a 6-week period did not produce any major structural and/or functional change in the subjects who have a normal nasal mucosa. In the subjects with common colds, a delayed recovery in the mucociliary transport time was observed during the continued use of xylometazoline in nose drops.

Xylometazoline HCl has been compared with a synthetic prostaglandin E_2 analog (CL-116,069) in dogs for their decongestant activity following intranasal administration (124). The drugs were applied to the nasal mucosa, using a DeVilbis atomizer, in both the in vivo and in vitro studies. In the in vivo investigations, the nasal resistance to airflow, i.e., nasal patency, was measured; whereas in the in vitro evaluations, the contraction and the relaxation of the smooth muscle of the nasal blood vessels (which was isolated from the dog's nasal mucosa) were monitored. The in vivo data demonstrated that xylometazoline HCl and CL-116,069 are similar in their decongestion responses, which showed a near-maximum value to the doses close to the threshold level. The in vitro results also indicated a close similarity between the response characteristics of these two drugs in regard to their threshold and potency.

Excessive use of oxymetazoline, a hydroxyl derivative of xylometazoline, in nasal spray (Afrin/Schering) has been reported to cause bradycardia, hypotension, dizziness, and weakness (125).

5.5.1.5 Tramazoline

Tramazoline is a vasoconstrictor and has been formulated in a metered-dose nasal aerosol (Tobispray) with dexamethasone isonicotinate and neomycin sulfate to control the postoperative bleeding in 93 patients having nasal surgery (126). In 50 of the 93 patients, the results obtained at the 1- and 2-week follow-up visits were found to be excellent, as evidenced by a clear airway without crusting and mucosal edema; whereas the results in another 38 patients were rated as good, in whom a clear airway was observed with only traces of crusting, mucosal edema, or minor adhesions. A success rate of 94.6% was achieved with no cases of primary or secondary hemorrhage reported.

5.5.1.6 Dopamine

Dopamine is a natural catecholamine produced from the decarboxylation of 3,4-dihydroxyphenylalanine (DOPA). Dopamine is a precursor to norepinephrine in the noraderenergic nerves as well as a neurotransmitter in certain areas of the CNS and a few peripheral sympathetic nerves. It has been used in the treatment of shock and heart diseases.

Dopamine was found incapable of penetrating the blood-brain barrier. In monkeys who were given [^{3}H] dopamine intravenously, the radioactivity could only be detected in the blood, but not in the CSF. On the other hand, after the intranasal administration of [^{3}H] dopamine, radioactivity could be

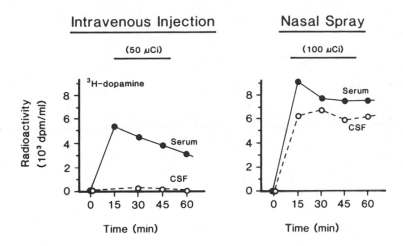

Figure 5.16 The CSF and serum levels of radioactivity in adult rhesus monkeys after intravenous (50 μCi/0.2 ml) and intranasal (100 μCi/0.2 ml) administration of [³H] dopamine. (Modified from Ref. 127, used with permission.)

detected both in the CSF and in the blood within 15 min after nasal spraying (Figure 5.16) (127). These results suggested that it is not necessary for a substance, like dopamine, to enter the hemal compartment before getting into the CSF.

5.5.1.7 Dobutamine

Dobutamine is a synthetic catecholamine which can induce a strong stimulation of the beta₁-adrenergic receptor and a mild stimulation of the beta₂- and alpha₁-receptors (128). It is a relatively selective positive inotropic drug that increases ventricular contractility and cardiac output without substantially increasing the heart rate and systemic blood pressure (129) The influence of the route of administration on the absorption of dobutamine in rats has been reported (130). The average plasma dobutamine concentrations produced by the same dose after intravenous bolus, intravenous infusion, and intranasal route are compared in Figure 5.17. The extent of absorption (AUC) following these three routes of administration are dramatically different.

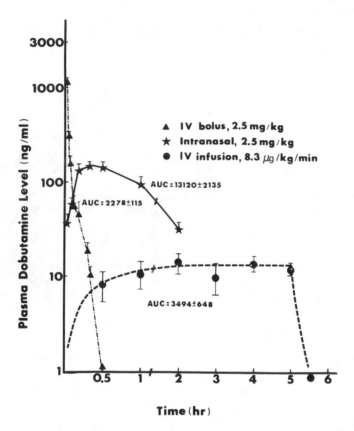

Figure 5.17 Plasma concentration profiles of dobutamine after various routes of administration (2.5 mg/kg) in rats (n = 3-4). (From Ref. 130, used with permission.)

The duration of pharmacological activity of dobutamine has been compared in dogs following the intranasal administration by a nasal regular formulation, a nasal sustained-release formulation, and an intravenous infusion (Figure 5.18). Because of the short half-life of dobutamine (about 2 min), the duration of responses achieved by the nasal regular formulation lasted for only 1 hr. However, a 4-hr duration was observed with the nasal sustained-release

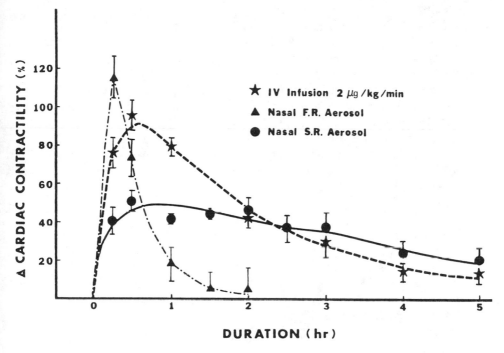

Figure 5.18 Duration of cardiac contractility in dogs after intravenous infusion of intranasal administration of dobutamine from various nasal formulations (733 μg/kg; $n = 4$). (From Ref. 130, used with permission.)

formulation. In addition, the cardiac contractility produced by the nasal sustained-release formulation was comparable to that by intravenous infusion.

5.5.2 Parasympathomimetics

5.5.2.1 Nicotine

The action of nicotine is characterized by a primary transient stimulation followed by a persistent depression of all sympathetic and parasympathetic ganglia. The mechanism of action is associated with the depolarization of the postsynaptic membrane by producing a block of synaptic transmission. The synaptic stimulatory and depressant effects of nicotine are not overcome by atropine. Nicotine is also more active on the ganglia than on the skeletal muscles, and it first stimulates and then paralyzes the central nervous system.

The absorptivity of nicotine by the sinus membrane has been studied in dogs in comparison with intravenous and subcutaneous injections (131). Intravenous administration of nicotine (1 mg) was found to cause an immediate and marked pressor response which lasted for 2 min, whereas subcutaneous injection of nicotine (20 mg) yielded only a slight rise in the blood pressure which lasted for 7 min. Intranasal administration of nicotine at the same subcutaneous dose into the left frontal sinus was also observed to produce no effect over the observation period of 35 min. Similar negative results were obtained following the injection of 4 mg of nicotine into the sunus of a cat.

5.5.2.2 Methacholine

Intranasal application of methacholine has been noted to produce a more pronounced nasal blockage in patients with rhinitis than in controls (132). Investigation of the changes in the nasal airway resistance following nasal metahcholine challenge concluded that outside the pollen season patients with hay fever have a normal nasal reactivity, but with somewhat increased bronchial reactivity (133). Topical methacholine challenge has been found to be useful as a simple and reproducible test for the measurement of nasal reactivity (134,135).

Intranasal administration of methacholine in aerosol dosage form was observed to achieve an efficient distribution of methacholine in the nasal cavity. The nasal secretory responses to the intranasal administration of methacholine was evaluated in 20 healthy subjects and a consistent, straight-line dose-response relationship was observed in each sex group studied. The responses at each level of stimulation were significantly stronger in women than in men ($p < 0.001$). Pretreatment with ipratropium (Atrovent/B-I) was noted to yield a significant reduction in the amount of secretion ($p < 0.001$) as well as a parallel displacement of the log dose-response curve.

A single challenge with 6 mg of methacholine caused significantly more secretion in perennial rhinitis patients than in normal subjects ($p < 0.001$). Intranasal methacholine challenge has been found to produce a measureable nasal hypersecretion in both normal subjects and patients with perennial rhinitis. The intranasal application of methacholine in 15 healthy subjects has been reported to trigger rhinorrhea (136). On the other hand, pretreatment with ipratropium has been found to effectively inhibit methacholine-induced hypersecretion for up to 6 hr.

Methacholine was reported to rapidly penetrate into the nasal mucous membrane when administered in an aqueous solution or diethylene glycol monoethyl ether vehicle (137). At nasal doses of 25-250 mg, methacholine was found to cause a definite local and systemic response, e.g., a transitory drop in blood pressure. Intravenous or subcutaneous administration of methacholine also produced somewhat the same effects as observed with the intranasal application. On the other hand, oral and iontophoretic administrations of methacholine were observed to produce a predominating vasodilatory effect with lower intensity, but for a longer duration.

5.5.3 Parasympatholytics

The role of parasympatholytics is to contract the blood vessels underlying the nasal mucosa, which results in stopping nasal secretions and in shrinking the nasal mucosa. Atropine and scopolamine are parasympatholytic (or antimuscarinic) drugs, and have been commonly used for the treatment of coryza and rhinorrhea caused by allergic rhinitis.

5.5.3.1 Scopolamine

The activity of scopolamine (hyoscine) following intranasal administration has been compared with oral and subcutaneous administrations by measuring salivary secretion at 50- to 30-min intervals for 2 hr (138). The control group received either a saline solution intranasally or a placebo capsule by mouth. Following the subcutaneous injection, the absorption of scopolamine was found to be rapid. A diminution of saliva occurred within 15 min (p < 0.001) with the peak effect reached after 30 min, which was followed by a gradual return toward normal production. The salivary flow was found to be markedly lower than the control value (p < 0.01). On the other hand, capsules taken orally gave the slowest response followed by oral liquid ingestion. Intranasal instillation of scopolamine was noted to induce a significant reduction in salivary production, whereas intranasal administration of 0.1-0.4 mg of scopolamine could not produce a differentiated effect. A clear dose-dependent response was observed for the dose ranging from 0.4 to 1.0 mg.

Concomitant administration with 0.25% phenylephrine HCl in nose drops was noted to hinder considerably the action of scopolamine (0.6 mg) when given immediately before scopolamine (p < 0.01), but it merely delayed the action when given 15 min beforehand.

The subjects treated with scopolamine (0.85 mg) in nasal spray produced a more delayed response than those receiving scopolamine (0.6 mg) in nose drops. The slightly more rapid absorption of scopolamine could be attributed to the fact that the nose drops contain sodium lauryl sulfate. However, the incorporation of sodium lauryl sulfate in the nasal spray has also yielded a striking increase in the absorption of scopolamine, which is as effective as nose drops. These studies also demonstrated that by intranasal administration, scopolamine achieves a more rapid, complete, and uniform absorption than by other routes of administration.

Nasal absorption of scopolamine was found to be intermediate between oral and the subcutaneous administrations as judged by the rate and the degree of antisialogigic action (138). Additional studies were carried out to compare with sublingual absorption and the effect of hyaluronidase (139). While administration of sublingual tablets of scopolamine were noted to be absorbed somewhat more rapidly and completely than did oral capsules, sublingual administration was found to be inferior to both intranasal and subcutaneous administrations (Figure 5.19). Incorporation of hyaluronidase in

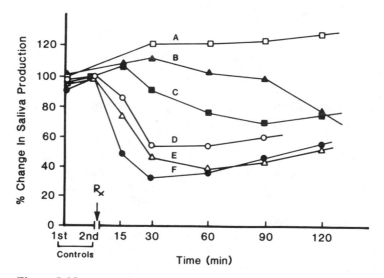

Figure 5.19 Effect of the route of administration of scopolamine on the time course for the change in saliva production (expressed as percent of second control specimen). A, oral placebo; B, oral capsule of scopolamine; C, sublingual scopolamine tablets; D, scopolamine (0.60 mg) with hyaluronidase (1 U/0.4 ml); E, scopolamine nose dropts (floor of nose); F, subcutaneous scopolamine. (Modified from Hyde et al., 1953, reproduced with permission of the copright owner—Ann. Otol. Rhinol. Laryngol.)

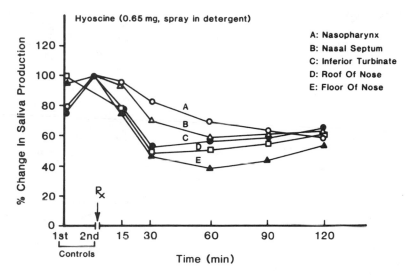

Figure 5.20 Comparison of scopolamine absorption, expressed as % change in saliva production, from different areas of the nose. Keys: (A), naso-pharynx; (B), nasal septum; (C), inferior turbinate; (D), roof of nose (Proetz position); (E), floor of nose. (Modified from Ref. 139, used with permission.)

nose drops (1 U/0.4 ml) was found to produce no significant effect either in speeding up the initial absorption of scopolamine or in the degree of absorption attained during a 90-min observation period.

In the initial 15-30 min period after the intranasal administration of scopolamine in nose drops there was significantly less absorption through the nasal septal mucosa than through the mucous membrane in the floor of the nose, in the inferior turbinate, and in the upper portion of the nose (Figure 5.20). The thin mucous membrane in the nasopharynx did not absorb the scopolamine either as rapidly or as completely as did the more vascular mucosa in the inferior turbinates and in other portions of the nose. After the 30-min period, the extent of absorption from the nasal septum and from the nasopharynx was statistically no different from other areas of the nose. It was concluded tht there is no significant difference in the systemic effect of scopolamine whether the nose drops are administered to the roof of the nose, the floor of the nose, or directly onto the inferior turbinate.

5.5.3.2 Atropine

Atropine is commonly used for nasal coryza and rhinorrhea caused by allergic rhinitis. It has also been widely recognized as an effective antidote in cases of poisoning by organophosphate compounds.

The systemic effects of atropine following intranasal administration have been evaluated in human subjects (139). Atropine was administered as nose drops (in saline) and as a nasal spray (in Duponol solution containing sodium lauryl sulfate). The nose drops were found to yield about the same effect as the nasal spray, even though they contained no sodium lauryl sulfate. Sublingual tablets were observed to be significantly less effective at the 30-min point than either the nasal spray or the nose drops, but after that the same effectiveness was achieved. On the other hand, subcutaneous administration of atropine at a 1-mg dose was noted to be definitely more effective at the 15-min point than the intranasal and sublingual administration of atropine at a 1.5-mg dose Two hours after intranasal administration, no significant improvement was observed in the nasal absorption of atropine from the nose drops with either sodium lauryl sulfate or hyaluronidase.

The nasal absorption of atropine has also been compared with scopolamine. It was noted that following intranasal administration at a 0.65-mg dose, scopolamine produced a systemic effect similar to that from atropine at a 2-mg dose. On the other hand, subcutaneous injection of 0.65 mg of scopolamine yielded a more rapid and a greater degree of salivary depression than did 1 mg of atropine at 15-, 30-, and 60-min intervals ($p < 0.05$). The observed weaker derpession of salivary secretion by atropine was due to its lower antisialogigic activity rather than to its slower absorption rate. Furthermore, more side reactions were noted with atropine than with scopolamine.

Intranasal administration of aerosolized atropine has been reported to increase the parasympathetic efferent activity and the responsiveness to the obstructive pulmonary disorders (140-142). Atropine sulfate solution was delivered intranasally by an atomizer to seven patients with rhinorrhea caused by allergic rhinitis and to 24 patients with rhinorrhea caused by viral rhinitis (143). All but one of the 31 patients demonstrated a visible reduction in secretions, with three patients showing obvious vasoconstriction of the nasal blood vessels. None of the patients reported an occurrence of dry mouth or visual disturbance. The effects of atropine was noted to last for 3-4 hr in five patients who were observed for longer periods.

5.5.3.3 Ipratropium

The topical activity of ipratropium has been used for the treatment of bronchoconstrictive diseases. However, it has no systemic effect when administered at therapeutic doses.

Intranasal administration of a parasympathomimetic compound, like methacholine, to patients with perennial rhinitis has been reported to stimulate the nasal membrane to produce a larger amount of secretion than in normal subjects (144). Pretreatment of normal subjects with ipratropium at 30 min prior to the methacholine provocation was found to result in a parallel displacement of the log dosage-response curve (144). It was noted that ipratropium reduces significantly the methacholine-induced secretion. Furthermore, considerable inhibition of nasal secretion was also observed in another study with 10 patients who were pretreated with ipratropium before methacholine provocation.

The dosage-time relationship for ipratropium has been determined in normal subjects who were pretreated with ipratropium prior to a methacholine test. The secretory response to the methacholine provocation was reduced by the pretreatment with ipratropium, which showed a 30% reduction in secretion after 5 min of pretreatment. The maximum effect of ipratropium was observed to occur at approximtely 4-6 hr, after which it slowly decreased. These investigations suggest that it is possible to effectively block the cholinergic receptors in the glands with just two puffs (40 μg) of ipratropium in each nostril at three to four times a day.

A total of 20 patients suffering from perennial rhinitis, with hypersecretion as the main symptom, have been treated with iprotropium or placebo for two 14-day periods Among these patients, 14 indicated a preference for the active formulation, whereas three preferred placebo, and the remaining five had no preference. All of the 14 patients who preferred the active formulation considered the effect to be very satisfactory and showed their willingness to continue the treatment for a longer period of time.

A study has been performed to evaluate the effect of ipratropium in nasal spray on rhinorrhea in 40 adults with naturally occurring common colds (145). All subjects received a nasal vasoconstrictor (xylometazoline, 0.1%) at 5 min before the intranasal administration of ipratropium to ensure an adequate mucosal distribution. Treatment with ipratropium in a nasal spray (q.i.d.) for 1 week was found to result in a significant reduction in the nasal discharge as compared to that of treatment with placebo (<0.001). It was noted that ipratropium is especially effective in the first 3 days of the cold during which the watery secretion is predominant. The studies concluded that ipratropium in nasal spray can be valuable in the treatment of a common cold at its onset when nasal discharge is a nuisance.

5.5.4 Prostaglandins

Prostaglandins were first isolated from the vesicular glands of sheep. Subsequently, prostaglandins were extracted from most animal tissues with good yields, and numerous prostaglandins were detected in human seminal fluid.

Various prostaglandins have many different pharmacological activities, including the stimulation of gastrointestinal and reproductive smooth muscles, and relaxation and contraction of respiratory smooth muscle, hypotensive activity, and the inhibition of lipolysis of fatty acids as well as the secretion of gastric acid and aggregation of blood platelets. Prostaglandins also act on vascular resistance and the vasoconstrictor response (146). Prostaglandins usually depress the stimulating effects of sympathetic nerve, and apparently inhibit the release of transmitter from the adrenergic nerve (147).

Four forms of prostaglandins (PGA, PGE_1, PGE_2, and PGF_1) have been known to induce constriction of the blood vessels in the dog's nasal mucosa (148). Prostaglandin E_1 and PGE_2 were found to be equipotnet to epinephrine, but the duration of their action was more than seven times as long. The topical administration of PGE_1, PGE_2, and PGF_{1a} in seven human subjects was observed to increase nasal patency in the four subjects taking PGE_1 and PGE_2, but not in those taking PGF_{1a} (149). The increase in nasal patency is a result of the constrictory effect of prostaglandins on nasal blood vessels. Prostaglandin E_1 has also been administered to 15 human subjects as a nasal vasoconstrictor (150). Good responses were observed in five subjects, no response in three subjects, and no clear response in the remaining seven subjects. When a response was observed, it lasted from 3 to 12 hr. A 100-μg dose was noted to induce uniform nasal irritation, mild burning sensation, lacrimation, and nasal throbbing.

The effect of PGE_1 and 17-phenyltrinor-PGE_2 on nasal patency has been compared to six patients with vasomotor and allergic rhinitis (151). Intranasal administration of PGE_1 at a single dose of 37.5 μg was noted to increase nasal patency in four out of six healthy subjects, whereas 17-phenyltrinor-PGE_2 increased nasal patency in all six healthy volunteers at the same dose with the effect lasting for 2-7 hr in various subjects. Additional studies with 17-phenyltrinor-PGE_2 in another 20 patients with vasomotor or allergic rhinitis has been reported to increase the patency in the treated nostril. The effect of a single dose of 17-phenyltrinor-PGE_2 was noted to last for over 7 hr in 90% of the patients. All patients were observed to experience a symptomatic relief of nasal obstruction for over 7 hr. In another group of six patients with rhinitis in whom 17-phenyltrinor-PGE$_2$ was administered to both nostrils, the increase in nasal patency was similar in both nostrils and lasted for 4-8 hr. Further studies indicated that nasal instillation of 17-phenyltrinor-PGE$_2$ increased nasal patency in all 14 patients with vasomotor rhinitis (152). The magnitude and the duration of effect were found to be dose dependent, and at a 40-μg dose the increase in nasal patency was noted to last for 6-7 hr.

A synthetic PGE$_2$ analog (CL-116,069) has been compared with xylometazoline HCl (a nasal decongestant) as well as natural PGE$_1$ and PGE$_2$ for their nasal decongestant activity in dogs (153). Using an in vivo nasal patency test and in vitro nasal blood vessel contraction tests, the synthetic PGE$_2$ analog was found to be more effective and longer lasting than other prostaglandins at the systemic or topical doses.

Prostaglandins of the E series (PGE) have been known to be synthesized and also inactivated by the nasal mucosa of the pig (154). Prostaglandin may be formed in in vitro by pieces of pig's nasal mucosa, which can be inhibited by indomethacin. The enzyme 15-hydroxyprostaglandin dehydrogenase in the nasal mucosa is known to be involved in the inactivation of PGE.

5.6 CENTRAL NERVOUS SYSTEM STIMULANTS

5.6.1 Cocaine

Because of its topical anesthetic and vasoconstricition effects, cocaine has been used in otolarynogology and in anesthesiology. The pharmacological actions of cocaine may modify the physiological responses of a patient to a surgical procedure.

Cocaine, which has gained the reputation of being the "champagne of drugs," produces an intense euphoria within 3-5 min after intranasal application, which has made it a major drug of abuse. Because cocaine is known to be hydrolyzed and rendered ineffective in the gastrointestinal tract as well as by plasma and by hepatic esterases (155,156), it is usually used intranasally.

Cocaine in solution at 4-20% has been administered intranasally by sprays, cotton pledgets, or packtails, or by rubbing a "cocaine mud" to compare the efficiency (157). It was reported tht the 10% cocaine solution causes an immediate and complete paralysis of cilia, 5% solution produces the arrest of ciliary activity within 2-3 min, and 2.5% solution stops ciliary activity after 1 hr of continuous application. Twenty-five percent cocaine paste has been found to be an effective and safe local anesthetic (158). Since the majority of cilia escaped contact with cocaine crystals, the mucous blanket was still continuously swept backwards. However, intranasal cocaine users are not exempt from addiction or other adverse consequences (159).

Using gas chromatography, plasma levels of cocaine have been measured in 20 surgical patients receiving intranasal cocaine for topical anesthesia (160). The relationship between the plasma concentrations of cocaine and its physiological effects after intranasal administration was assessed in 13 surgical patients: nine cardiovascular surgery patients and four dental patients (161,162). A 10% solution of cocaine HCl was administered topically (1.5 mg/kg) to the nasal mucosa prior to nasal intubation. Plasma cocaine was detectable within 3 min. The concentration then increased rapidly for the first 15-20 min, peaked within 15-60 min and then decreased gradually over the next 3-5 hr. The maximum plasma levels of 120-474 ng/ml were obtained with the cardiovascular patients, who appeared to have a significantly higher level of cocaine than that in the dental patients (Figures 5.21 and 5.22). Following intranasal application, cocaine was found to still remain on the nasal mucosa even after 3 hr. The plasma concentration of cocaine was per-

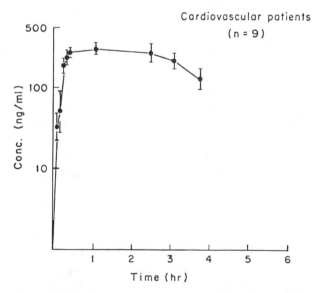

Figure 5.21 Plasma concentration profile of cocaine in cardiovascular patients. Values at 10, 15, 20, and 60 min are the mean (±S.E.M.) for nine patients. Values at other times are based on fewer patients. (From Ref. 161, used with permission.)

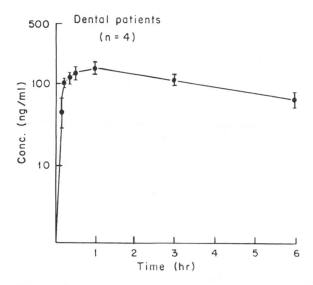

Figure 5.22 Plasma concentration profile of cocaine in dental patients. Values at 10, 15, 20 and 60 min. are the mean (±S.E.M.) for 4 patients. Values at other times are based on 3 patients. (From Ref. 161, used with permission.)

sistent for as long as 6 hr, which may be a result of its vasoconstrictive action.

The correlation between the blood concentrations of cocaine and the physiological changes induced after intranasal administration of cocaine has been further studied in four normal subjects with a moderately heavy prior use of cocaine (161). A 10% solution of cocaine was given by instillation into the nose at doses ranging from 0.19 to 1.5 mg/kg. The rate of disappearance in the plasma cocaine concentrations after the peak level was observed to be somewhat more rapid than that seen in the surgical patients. All the doses used failed to produce a discernible effect on cardiovascular functions. Pupillary size was changed at dose levels of 0.75-1.5 mg/kg, but not at the 0.19-0.38 mg/kg dosage range. Most of the subjects fell asleep at approximately 2-3 hr after intranasal administration of cocaine.

A study has been reported on the physiological and subjective effects of cocaine following the intranasal or intravenous administration of a single dose of 10 or 25 mg in 19 volunteers (163,164). Another 100 mg of cocaine was also applied intranasally to five of the subjects, once by drops and once by

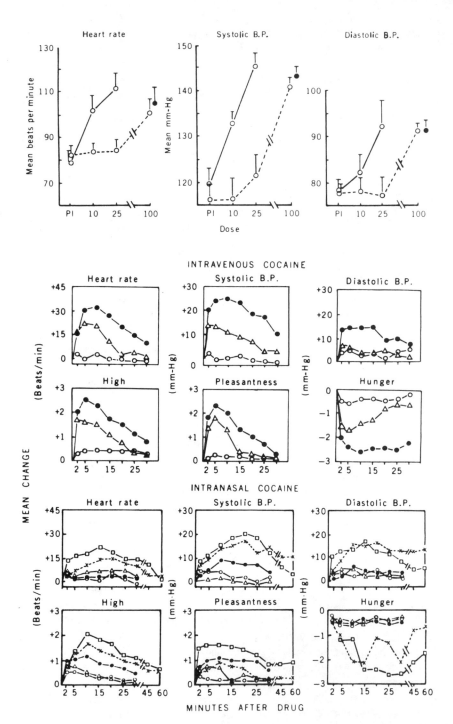

Heart rate   Systolic B.P.   Diastolic B.P.

INTRAVENOUS COCAINE

Heart rate   Systolic B.P.   Diastolic B.P.

High   Pleasantness   Hunger

INTRANASAL COCAINE

Heart rate   Systolic B.P.   Diastolic B.P.

High   Pleasantness   Hunger

MINUTES AFTER DRUG

flakes (mixed with lactose powder). A 1% lidocaine solution or 5 mg of tetracaine powder mixed with lactose powder was administered intranasally as the placebo. The heart rate as well as systolic and diastolic blood pressures were monitored. The results indicated that by intranasal administration, cocaine produces physiological and subjective effects only at the 25-mg dose, whereas the intravenous injection of 10-25 mg cocaine yields a significant ($p < 0.01$) dose-related effect on the physiological and the subjective measurements. However, a significant change ($p < 0.01$) in the heart rate and also in the systolic and diastolic blood pressures was observed following the intranasal administration of 100 mg cocaine. The magnitude of mean changes after the insufflation of cocaine flakes was noted to be greater than that following the nasal instillation of cocaine solution (Figure 5.23).

Following the intravenous injection of cocaine at 10- and 25-mg doses, no significant changes in respiratory rate, oral temperature, or hand grip strength were detected. On the other hand, significant changes were observed after the intranasal and intravenous administration of 25 mg cocaine on the subjective effects: the scale of acute effects ($p < 0.02$), the scale of "high" ($p < 0.01$), and the scale of pleasantness ($p < 0.05$). These subjective effects peaked within 10 min, and 54-68% of the effects were still evident at the end of the 30-min observation period. However, no significant difference was observed after the intranasal administration of 10 mg cocaine (Figure 5.24).

Figure 5.23 (Top) Dose-response curves for the effects on heart rate, systolic blood pressure, and diastolic blood pressure of placebo (pl), 10 (10) and 25 mg (25) cocaine administered intravenously and intranasally, and 100 mg (100) administered intranasally by drops and by flakes. Each point represents the mean of the peak changes after drug administration to 12 subjects, except points for the 100-mg dose, for which five subjects were tested. Vertical bars indicate the standard error of the mean. B.P., blood pressure; (O——O), intravenous; (O- - -O), nose drops; and (●), nasal flakes. (Bottom) Time course, over a 30-min observation period for the physiological and subjective effects of placebo, 10 and 25 mg of cocaine administered intravenously and intranasally by drops and by flakes. Each point represents the mean of 12 subjects, except for the 100-mg intranasal doses where each point represents the mean of five subjects. (O), placebo, (△), 10 mg cocaine; (●), 25 mg cocaine; (X), 100 mg cocaine in nose drops; and (□), 100 mg of cocaine in nasal flakes. (From Ref. 164, used with permission.)

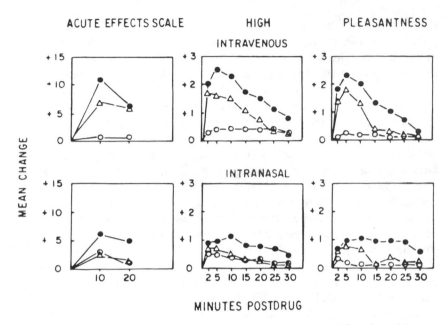

Figure 5.24 Time course, over a 30-min observation period for the subjec-tive effects of placebo (○), 10 (△) and 25 mg (●) cocaine administered intra-venously and intranasally. Each point represents the mean of 12 subjects. (From Ref. 163, used with permission.)

A study has been conducted to compare the efficacy of cocaine between oral and intranasal administrations in four human subjects (165). A 10% solution of cocaine HCl was first applied topically to the nasal mucosa with a total dose of 115-246 mg. Subsequently, the same subjects swallowed the same dosage of cocaine HCl in gelatin capsules. The results indicated that following intranasal administration, cocaine is detected in the plasma by 15 min, reaches peak levels, ranging from 61 to 408 ng/ml, within 60-120 min, and then decreases gradually over the next 2-3 hr; On the other hand, after oral administration, plasma cocaine was not detected until 30 min later, reached peak levels, ranging from 104 to 424 mg/ml, within 50-90 min, and then declined gradually over the next 4.5-5.00 hr. There was no significant difference in the peak plasma levels between oral and intranasal routes of administration. The half-life for the elimination of cocaine following oral and intranasal administrations was found to be 0.9 and 1.3 hr, respectively.

Following intranasal application of cocaine, measurable effects on the high scale were noted within 15-30 min, peaked at 15-60 min, lasted for as long as 60 min, and then decreased over the next 2-3 hr. After oral administration, on the other hand, measurable effects on the high scale occurred within 15-75 min, peaked at 45-90 min, lasted for as long as 60 min, and then declined over the next 4 hr. Peak high scales after oral administration were noted to be significantly greater than those observed following intranasal application ($p < 0.05$). Although cocaine has been reported to be ineffective when taken orally, this study showed that cocaine is well absorbed from the gastrointestinal tract to yield pharmacological effects.

A study designed to establish the correlation of physiological and subjective effects with the plasma concentrations of cocaine has been carried out in 10 subjects with a history of intravenous cocaine use (166). Cocaine was administered intravenously (cocaine HCl, 16 or 32 mg, in physiological saline) or intranasally by inhalation (100 mg of white powder consisting of 16, 64, or 96 mg of cocaine in lactose). The results demonstrated that following intravenous injection, the plasma concentrations of cocaine increased in the first 8-12 min and then began to decline. The rate of disappearance of cocaine was found in parallel with the return of the heart rate to the pretreatment levels. The maximum high occurred at approximately 3-5 min after the injection, and the effect disappeared within 30-40 min. The data suggested that both the plasma concentration of cocaine and its physiological and subjective effects are dose related. It appeared that the cardiovascular and subjective effects are highly correlated with the rapid increase in the plasma levels of cocaine, which peak early and show a parallel decrease over the first 30 min after the intravenous injection.

On the other hand, after the intranasal administration of various doses, cocaine concentrations in the plasma increased rapidly for the first 20-30 min, reached the peak plasma levels within 60 min, and then decreased gradually over the next hour. Higher nasal doses were found to achieve higher peak plasma values. Meanwhile, the onset of cardiovascular changes were observed in parallel with the increase in plasma cocaine levels with peak values being reached at approximately the same time. In addition, the subjects reported that they obtain their maximum high at 15-20 min after inhalation. However, the physiological and subjective effects were reportedly returned to the pretreatment levels within 60-90 min, which appeared to be more rapid than the decrease in the plasma levels of cocaine. The results concluded a good relationship between the changes in subjective and cardiovascular effects and the plasma concentrations of cocaine following both intravenous and intranasal administrations.

Cocaine HCl has also been compared with lidocaine HCl by intranasal administration at three different doses with normal saline as the placebo (167). This investigation was carried out to evaluate the possibility that cocaine is not unique in its psychoactivity. Peak high ratings were observed to occur within 5-15 min for cocaine, and at 15 min for the placebo. The lowest dose, 0.19 mg/kg, produced a similar peak high rating as the placebo. The 0.38 and 0.75 mg/kg dose yielded a similar mean value of peak high rating that was greater than that of the 0.19 mg/kg dose. Furthermore, the mean peak high ratings following the three lidocaine doses were very similar to those obtained after the same doses of cocaine. At the highest dose, 0.75 mg/kg, cocaine and lidocaine were observed to be associated with the self-reports of increased pleasantness, but no change in energy or involvement (on the basis of using 13-point bipolar scales of pleasantness, involvement, and energy). There was no change in both the pre- and post-ARCI (Addiction Research Center Inventory) scores following the intranasal administration of C.19 and 0.38 mg/kg of cocaine and all three doses of lidocaine. On the other hand, an increase in the number of responses on the ARCI scores was noted following the intranasal administration of 0.75 mg/kg cocaine. In summary, there was no indication of a unique euphoria or stimulation which differentiated cocaine from lidocaine.

The pharmacokinetics of cocaine following intravenous and intranasal administrations has been compared in four subjects (168). Cocaine was administered intranasally by inhaling 100 mg of the mixture of cocaine HCl (64 and 96 mg) with lactose powder. The peak plasma concentrations of cocaine after intranasal administration were found to be dependent upon the dose administered. The peak levels were 66.8 ($\pm$15.9) ng/ml at the 64-mg dose, and 133.5 ($\pm$20.9) ng/ml at the 96-mg dose, respectively. The time to reach the peak levels was 36.9 ($\pm$7.4) min after the 64-mg dose, and 41.2 ($\pm$5.5) min after the 96-mg dose (Figure 5.25). After intravenous injection, the pharmacokinetics of cocaine conformed to a one-compartment open model with first-order elimination kinetics, which had an average plasma half-life of 0.71 ($\pm$0.13) hr (Table 5.9). Following intranasal administration, on the other hand, the pharmacokinetics of cocaine conformed to a one-compartment model with first-order absorption and first-order elimination kinetics (Table 5.10). Large intra- and intersubject variations were observed in the elimination and absorption rate constants as well as the apparent volumes of distribution, etc., pharmacokinetic parameters following both routes of administration. A statistically significant difference was noted in the mean AUC values following these two modes of administration. The mean fraction of the nasal dose absorbed after administration of 64 mg co-

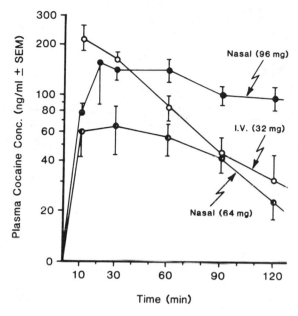

Figure 5.25 Plasma concentration profiles of cocaine in four subjects after intravenous (I.V.) and intranasal administration. Each point represents mean (±S.E.M.). (From Ref. 168, used with permission.)

Table 5.9 Pharmacokinetic Parameters After Intravenous Administration of Cocaine[a]

Subject	$AUC_{0 \to \infty}$ (ng $\cdot$ ml^{-1} $\cdot$ min)	K_e (h^{-1})	$T_{1/2}$ (h)	V (1)
1	14640	2.18	0.32	49
2	9421	0.65	1.07	276
3	16578	0.89	0.78	123
4	13944	1.01	0.69	128
Mean	13645	1.18	0.71	144
(±S.E.M.)	(±1312)	(±0.29)	(±0.13)	(±41)

[a]Dose = 32 mg.
Source: Modified from Ref. 168, used with permission.

Table 5.10 Phamacokinetic Parameters After Intranasal Administration of Cocaine

Subject	Dose (mg)	$AUC_{0\to\infty}$ (ng $\cdot$ ml^{-1} $\cdot$ min)	K_e (h^{-1})	K_a (h^{-1})	F	V (l)
1	64	8204	1.4	4.26	0.28	94
	96	29413	0.51	3.66	0.67	257
2	64	4512	0.58	1.53	0.24	354
	96	18186	0.41	3.43	0.64	492
3	64	13674	0.41	6.30	0.41	282
	96	34228	0.46	1.98	0.69	254
4	64	5262	1.43	2.08	0.19	96
	96	12456	0.56	5.68	0.30	247
Mean	64	7913	0.95	3.54	0.28	207
($\pm$S.E.M.)		(b1800)	($\pm$0.23)	($\pm$0.94)	($\pm$0.04)	($\pm$57)
	96	23570	0.48	3.68	0.57	312
		($\pm$4332)	($\pm$0.02)	($\pm$0.65)	($\pm$0.07)	($\pm$52)

Source: Modified from Ref. 168, used with permission.

caine was significantly lower than that after the 96-mg dose ($p < 0.05$), which was also reflected in the AUC values.

The pharmacokinetics of cocaine following intranasal and oral administrations has been assessed in seven human subjects (169). The results demonstrated that plasma concentrations after intranasal administration of cocaine in solution peak at a mean time of 57.6 (±5.8) min for all doses (0.19-2.0 mg/kg) as the peak lengthened in time with increase in the dose. The peak plasma levels after intranasal administration of crystalline cocaine was observed to occur slightly sooner (35 ± 13.2 min) than after the same dose of cocaine in solution (47.1 ± 6.1 min). By oral administration, however, cocaine was not detected in the plasma until 30 min after dosing and peaked at 64 (±6.7) min. Peak plasma levels by the intranasal route were found to be dose dependent.

Furthermore, the data also suggested that the pharmacokinetics of cocaine following intranasal administration can be described by a one-compartment open model with two consecutive first-order input phases and one first-order elimination phase, whereas the disposition of oral cocaine was described by a one-compartment open model with, after a lag time, a single first-order input phase and one first-order elimination phase. The mean elimination half-life for cocaine following intranasal and oral administrations was determined to be 75 (±5) and 48 (±3) min, respectively. The AUC values were linearly dependent upon the doses administered intranasally, suggesting a linear (i.e., first-order) elimination process for nasal cocaine over the dosage range studied. The AUCs after intranasal and oral administrations at the same dose level were not significantly different (23.3 ± 5.0 vs. 22.3 ± 5.4 µg/ml · min.). This agreement may be a coincidence in that incomplete absorption of cocaine from the nasal mucosa has reduced its systemic bioavailability to the same extent as the hepatic first-pass metabolism after the oral administration.

The psychological effects of cocaine at three nasal doses and their relationship with the plasma cocaine concentrations has been examined in four volunteers (170). Lidocaine HCl (0.2 mg/kg) was administered intranasally as a topically active placebo. The results demonstrated that the mean peak plasma concentrations of cocaine are dose dependent. For the 0.75- and 1.5-mg/kg doses, plasma levels peaked at 60 min, and then decreased in a log-linear fashion with an apparent elimination half-life of 1.3 hr. For the doses administered following the Latin square design, the mean peak high ratings were also found to be dose dependent. The high scale was observed to increase within 15 min, peak at 15 to 20 min, and then decrease with an apparent half-life of 0.8 hr for the 0.75- and 1.5-mg/kg doses. Although the peak high ratings were related to the peak plasma cocaine concentrations, a closer examination of the data suggests that there is no simple relationship between the highs and the plasma levels. The maximum subjective effects tended to occur prior to reaching the maximal plasma levels. The plasma level in the earlier phase of the experiment was associated with a more intense high than that during the later phase. The high sensation resulting from the administration of cocaine was a pleasant feeling, but was not a distinctive sensation.

On the other hand, all the subjects experienced peak highs at 30 min after the lidocaine administration, which decreased to baseline values within the second and fourth hour. The peak highs were also observed to be related to the dose and the peak plasma concentrations.

Because of its local anesthetic effect, intranasal administration of cocaine has been reported to relieve the symptoms and the signs associated with the syndrome of nasal ganglion neurosis (sphenopalatine Mickel's) (171). Patients with this syndrome suffered from pain at the root of their nose radiating to the occiput. In severe attacks, pain could spread to the neck, shoulder, and hands.

Using the intranasal application of cocaine, other treatments for headache and the pains of the neck and shoulder on the sphenopalatine ganglion has been reportedly successful (172). A study designed to determine whether intranasal application of cocaine exerts an analgesic effect on the experimentally induced pain has been initiated in 16 healthy male volunteers (173). Cotton-covered applicators were impregnated with either cocaine HCl solution or normal saline solution (as the placebo) and then administered intranasally on different days in a double-blind study. The results demonstrated that with little change in psychological status, cocaine applied intranasally had an analgesic effect on the experimental ischemic pain.

5.6.2 Lidocaine

As discussed above, cocaine is often applied to the nasal mucosa before a nasotracheal intubation for its combined anesthetic and vasoconstricting properties. A double-blind study designed to assess the potential replacement of cocaine with lidocaine as a topical anesthetic in nasal intubation has been performed in 75 patients (174). Each patient received one of three nasal sprays: 4% cocaine (C), an admixture of 3% lidocaine and 0.25% phenylephrine (L-P), and 0.25% phenylephrine alone (P). In the patients receiving L-P, the mean MAP (mean arterial pressure) value in the initial 5 min after the intubation was decreased by 2.3 (±2.2) mm Hg, which was significantly lower than the increase in the MAP values of 6.2 (±1.7) and 8.5

(± 2.0) mm Hg, respectively, in the patients receiving C and P (p < 0.005). The changes in heart rate and MAP were similar in patients receiving C and P. It was thus concluded that for nasotracheal intubation, intranasal application of 3% lidocaine with 0.25% phenylephrine is a viable substitute for cocaine. Because of the toxicity and the abuse potential of cocaine, the use of lidocaine-phenylephrine admixture should be encouraged.

Furthermore, an immediate reversal of acute severe laryngospasm has been reportedly accomplished in two patients by instilling intranasally 1% lidocaine in 5 ml of 0.001% epinephrine (175). Its effectiveness could be a result of the topical action of either lidocaine or epinephrine, or the simultaneous activities of both drugs. The topical decongestant activity of epinephrine may reverse mucosal edema at the level of the glottis, thereby removing the stimulus for laryngeal irritation, whereas the topical anesthetic effect of lidocaine may block the afferent or efferent neural pathways which mediates the laryngospasm.

5.7 NARCOTICS AND ANTAGONISTS

5.7.1 Buprenorphine

Buprenorphine is a synthetic opiate analgesic with combined angonist/antagonist properties and a low abuse potential (176). By parenteral administration, the duration of its action is twice as long and its analgesic potency is approximately 30 times stronger than morphine (177). By oral administration, however, buprenorphine has been shown to produce a low analgesic potency owing to the extensive first-pass metabolism (178).

The systemic bioavailability of buprenorphine via various routes of administration has been studied in female rats, using a single dose of 100 μg/kg (179). Relative to the 100% bioavailability from intraarterial administration, the mean bioavailabilities for various routes of administration were found to be: intravenous 98%, intrarectal 54%, intrahepatoportal 49%, sublingual 13%, and intraduodenal 9.7%.

In another study, intranasal administration of buprenorphine has been compared with intravenous and intraduodenal administration in rats following a single dose of 135 μg/rat (180). The buprenorphine was administered to the nasal cavity via a micropipette and the nostrils were then closed with an adhesive agent. A transnasal bioavailability of 9% was calculated. The data indicate that by intranasal administration buprenorphine is as effective as the intravenous injection.

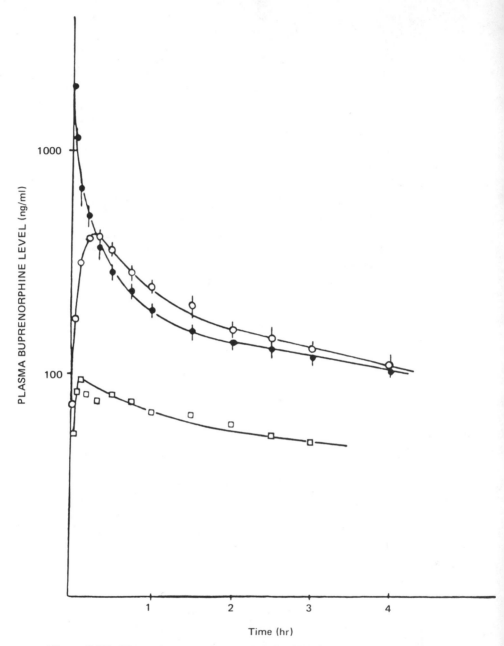

Figure 5.26 Mean plasma concentration profiles of buprenorphine after nasal (○), intravenous (●), and intraduodenal (□) administration of 30 μg of naxolone. Points represent mean (±S.E.M.) of three animals. (From Ref. 180, used with permission.)

Table 5.11 Area Under the Plasma Concentration-Time Curve of Naloxone Following Intravenous, Nasal, and Intraduodenal Administration

Route	Area under plasma concentration-time curve ($AUC_{0\rightarrow\infty}$) ($ng \cdot ml^{-1} \cdot min$)	Relative systemic availability (%)
Intravenous	1498.7 (±121.9)	100
Nasal	1517.5 (±193.5)	101
Intraduodenal	22.0 (±7.1)	1.5

Values represent the man (±S.E.M.) of three animals.
Source: Modified from Ref. 180, used with permission.

5.7.2 Naloxone

Naloxone, a narcotic antagonist without agonistic activities, has become the antinarcotic drug of choice in the treatment of narcotic overdose and in the management of postanesthesia depression induced by narcotics (181). By oral administration, naloxone is well absorbed. However, it is metabolized rapidly in the liver, which reduces its potency to only one-fifth of that by intravenous administration.

The intranasal administration of naloxone has been studied in 25 rats and compared with intravenous and intraduodenal administration (Figure 5.26) (180). The drug was administered into the nasal cavity via a micropipette and the nostrils were then closed with an adhesive agent. The nasal bioavailability calculated from the ratio of AUCs was 101%, whereas the intraduodenal administration has yielded a bioavailability of only 1.5% (Table 5.11). The half-life of naloxone following intravenous and intranasal administration was found to be 40-45 min, suggesting that nalonxone is rapidly and completely absorbed from the nasal cavity of rats.

5.8 HISTAMINES AND ANTIHISTAMINES

5.8.1 Histamine

Histamine is an important mediator for the development of the symptoms of allergic rhinitis. The release of histamine into the nasal mucosa causes irritation and sneezing, vascular engorgement and congestion, and edema of the mucosa as well as the production of excessive nasal secretions. Histamine may also be relevant in the development of the symptoms of vasomotor rhinitis and the common cold.

Histamine causes a marked fall in the blood pressure after intravenous or subcutaneous administration in the dog (182). For instance, the injection of 1 mg of histamine by intravenous and subcutaneous routes into a dog has been found to cause a distinct depressor response. However, repeated administration of the same dose into the nasal cavity or the sinus produced no effect on the blood pressure. In another dog, administration of histamine, 1 mg first and then 10 mg, into the frontal sinus also yielded no effect on the blood pressure. Apparently, histamine is absorbed so slowly from the sinus mucosa that no appreciable changes in blood pressure have been noted.

5.8.2 Antihistamines

Antihistamines block the effects of histamine on H_1-receptors. Clinical trials have demonstrated that oral H_1-antihistamines have a greater effect on sneezing and nasal discharge than on the blockage in allergic rhinitis (183, 184). However, the effect of antihistamines given alone on the symptoms of the common cold or vasomotor rhinitis is probably slight and is often unpredictable (185).

The effect of antihistamine drugs in nasal solution on the mucous membranes has been investigated in rabbits (186). It was found that Antistine-Privine (Antistine HCl, 0.5% and Privine HCl, 0.025%) is most harmful and causes almost a complete necrosis throughout the entire rabbit's nasal mucosa, while Pyribenzamine (0.5%) is the least harmful to nasal membranes. On the other hand, Allergan (pyranisamine maleate, 0.1% and phenylephrine HCl, 0.25%) was found to cause more damage than does Pyribenzamine, but considerably less than Antistine-Privine.

The potential of intranasal administration of two antihistamines, prophenpyridamine maleate and chlorprophenpyridamine maleate, has been evaluated in patients with allergic rhinits (187). In the 83 patients receiving the prophenpyridamine maleate solution, 68 patients (82.0%) exhibited a moderate to complete nasal vasoconstriction which lasted 4-6 hr or longer. In the 61 patients receiving chlorprophenpyridamine maleate solution, 48 patients (78.8%) exhibited a moderate to complete vasoconstriction, also lasting from 4 to 6 hours on the average (Table 5.12). No systemic or latent irritation of the nasal mucosa was reported.

The combination of phenylephrine and thonzylamine was found to be least effective as a topical nasal decongestant. The effectiveness of this combination was markedly enhanced by the addition of phenylpropanolamine (188).

Table 5.12 Summary of the Degree of Vasoconstriction Observed and Subjective Report

Antihistamine preparation	No. Cases	No. Relieved (% cases)			Total relief (%)
		None	Fair	Good to excellent	
Prophenpyridamine maleate solution (1.5%)	83	10 (12.0)	5 (6.0)	68 (82.0)	73 (88.0)
Chlorprophenpyridamine maleate solution (1.25%)	61	6 (9.8)	7 (11.5)	48 (78.7)	55 (90.2)

Source: Modified from Ref. 187, used with permission.

Twenty-five healthy human subjects have been provoked with histamine following local pretreatment with a H_1-receptor antagonist, chlorpheniramine maleate, and a H_2-receptor antagonist, ranitidine HCL, or a combination of these two antihistamines (189). The histamine-induced increase in the nasal airway resistance was noted to be inhibited in 52% of the subjects by the nasal spray containing the combination of these two antihistamines ($p < 0.05$), 22% by chlorpheniramine, and 29% by ranitidine, respectively. Apparently, the combination was significantly more effective than the H_1-receptor antagonist, chlorpheniramine maleate alone ($p < 0.05$). The results suggested the equal importance of H_1- and H_2-receptors on nasal blood vessels as well as an additive effect of H_1- and H_2-antihistamine.

5.8.3 Disodium Cromoglycate

Disodium cromoglycate is known to prevent the release of histmaine from mast cells which have been sensitized by specific antigens. However, it has no intrinsic antihistaminic, anticholinergic, bronchodilating, and antiserotoninic characteristics or corticosteroidlike properties. It is poorly absorbed by oral administration and is administered only by inhalation.

A double-blind crossover study comparing disodium cromoglycate (DC) and betamethasone valerate (BV), both given by the nasal route, has been carried out in 40 patients with seasonal allergic rhinitis (190). Sixteen of the patients receiving BV in aerosol recorded success in the treatment, whereas the other two were failed. By contrast, only two of the patients receiving intranasal DC, using an insufflator, at a dose of 10 mg in each nostril (q.i.d.) reported success.

Another double-blind crossover study was conducted to compare intranasal disodium cromoglycate (DC) with beclomethasone diporpionate (BDP) in 52 chronic perennial rhinitis patients (191). The results indicated that BDP is significantly more effective in relieving symptoms than DC ($p < 0.01$), whereas DC is only marginally better than placebo ($p < 0.05$).

The protective effects of disodium cromoglycate (DC) and beclomethasone dipropionate (BDP) on the immediate and delayed nasal mucosa response to allergen challenge have been investigated in human subjects with allergic rhinitis (192,193). Significant protective effects on the immediate and the delayed nasal mucosa responses were seen following the intranasal administration of DC.

The efficacy of disodium cromoglycate (DC) in powder and solution formulations in the treatment of seasonal and perennial rhinitis has been assessed in a group of 39 patients with allergic rhinitis over a period of 4 weeks (194). A crossover trial has been further carried out in 20 patients whose main symptom was nasal obstruction to compare the efficacy of DC in powder and 2% solution. The results showed that both DC powder and solution are effective, although the former appears to be somewhat more effective than the latter in those patients with rhinorrhea. However, in those patients with nasal blockage, the solution formulation appeared to be more effective because of its effective nasal distribution.

Disodium cromoglycate (DC) is a highly water-soluble compound with low oral bioavailability but good pulmonary and subcutaneous absorption. This compound is excreted unchanged in the urine and in the bile by most species, including the rat. The nasal absorption of DC has been investigated in the rat (195). Animals were dosed intranasally, using a microsyringe, with ^{14}C labeled sodium cromoglycate in saline solution. For comparison, animals were also similarly dosed intravenously or sublingually. After intravenous administration, an AUC of 32 (±9) μg/ml · min, a plasma clearance of 13 (±4) ml/min, and an elimination rate constant of 0.049 (±0.002) min^{-1} were obtained. The plasma concentrations of DC after intranasal administration rose to a mean peak of 0.3 μg/ml at approximately 20 min after dosing and fell to 0.03 μg/ml at 3 hr. The AUC value for over the 3-hr period was 19 (±6) μg/ml · min, which corresponds to a bioavailability of 60%. The intranasal absorption rate constant (K_a) was determined to be 0.059 min^{-1}.

The total amount of disodium cromoglycate (DC) excreted in the bile after intravenous administration was found to be 56% (±13%). The peak concentration in the bile appeared in the 15- or 30-min sample, which equaled approximately 10% of the dose, and declined to 1% within 2.5–3.0 hr. The amount of DC excreted in the bile over the 3-hr period was 30% (±8%), corresponding to an absorption of 53%. After sublingual administration, 3.1% (±2.2%) of the dose was excreted in the bile, corresponding to an absorption of 5.6%. The mean rates of excretion in the bile after intranasal and sublingual administration were calculated and the results indicated that the plasma data (with 60% dose absorbed) and the bile data (with 53% absorbed) following intranasal administration are in good agreement. The rapid absorption of DC suggested that the permeability of the nasal membrane is also governed by similar factors as those controlling the absorption from the lung or subcutaneous sites.

Low concentrations of the preservatives benzalkonium chloride and phenylethanol used in a 2% disodium cromoglycate nasal spray were found not to be harmful to the nasal mucosa of 16 patients with perennial rhinitis and 16 healthy volunteers (196). Disodium cromoglycate plus preservatives is clinically more effective than disodium cromoglycate alone.

Table 5.13 Pharmacokinetic Data of Meclizine in Rats After Various Routes of Administration

Parameter	Intravenous (0.64 mg)	Intranasal (0.64 mg)	Oral (6.4 mg)
	Route of administration[a]		
$t_{1/2} \, \beta$ (min)	71 (±26)	59 (±26)	57 (±13)
β (h^{-1})	0.66 (±0.20)	0.72 (±0.25)	0.78 (±0.22)
C_{max} (ng/ml)		627 (±167)	545 (±208)
T_{max} (min)		8.5 (±4.2)	49.0 (±12.7)
AUC (μg · h · ml)[b]	1.73 (±1.46)	0.88 (±0.38)	1.41 (±0.58)
Fraction absorbed[c]		0.51	0.08

[a]Data shown is the mean (±S.D.) from the following number of rats: intravenous, $n = 3$; intranasal, $n = 7$; oral, $n = 4$.
[b]AUC = Area under the concentration-time curve (from time 0 to infinity). This is estimated by the formula $A = \Sigma_{1/2}(C_i + C_{i+1})(t_{i+1} + 1 - t_i) + C^*/\beta$, which is the sum of successive trapazoids between each data point plus an estimate of the "tail" area from the last concentration-time point (C^*) to infinity.
[c] Calculated from the average AUC: $(AUC_{nasal,oral}) \times (Dose_{iv})/(AUC_{iv}) \times (Dose_{nasal,oral})$.
Source: Modified from Ref. 198, used with permission.

Table 5.14 Pharmacokinetic Data of Meclizine in Dogs After Various Routes of Administration

Parameter	Intravenous (2.5 mg)	Intranasal (5.0 mg)	Oral (12.5 mg)
	Route of administration[a]		
$t_{1/2}$ (h)	5.51 (±0.76)	5.04 (±0.26)	5.58 (±0.31)
β (h^{-1})	0.13 (±0.02)	0.14 (±0.01)	0.13 (±0.01)
C_{max} (ng/ml)		292 (±107)	211 (±94)
T_{max} (min)		11.9 (±3.2)	70.0 (±37.4)
AUC (μg · h/ml)[b]	1.07 (±0.36)	1.86 (±0.64)	1.11 (±0.31)
Fraction absorbed[c]		0.89 (±0.17)	0.22 (±0.06)

[a]All data shown is the mean (±S.D.) of results from three dogs.
[b]AUC is as defined in Table 5.13.
[c]The fraction absorbed was calculated for each dog and then averaged: $(AUC_{nasal,oral}) \times (Dose_{iv})/(AUC_{iv}) \times (Dose_{nasal,oral})$.
Source: Modifed from Ref. 198, used with permission.

A 2% aqueous solution of disodium cromoglycate (DC) has been evaluated as nasal spray in 15 adult patients with perennial rhinitis (197). In this open trial, nine patients reported an effect of the medicament. In a double-blind crossover trial in 25 patients, eight preferred DC, three preferred placebo, and 14 patients had no subjective effect from either DC or placebo. The results appear to suggest that DC has the best effect on patients with eosinophilia in the nasal smear and with a short duration of symptoms.

5.8.4 Meclizine

Meclizine is a long-acting antihistaminic agent effective in the prevention of treatment of nausea, vomiting, and dizziness associated with motion sickness.

A preclinical study of the pharmacokinetics and bioavailability of meclizine by intranasal administration has been conducted in rats and dogs (198). The results were compared to the parameters determined from the intravenous and oral administration of meclizine at comparable doses. A nasal formulation of the drug (Mecnazone) was prepared at a concentration of 50 mg/ml in 85% propylene glycol and 10% glycerol. By intranasal administration in rats, meclizine HCl yielded an absorption of about 50%, which was as effective as intravenous injection, but was about six times more effective than oral administration (8%). The mean times to peak plasma levels were found to be about 8.5 min for the nasal dose and 49.0 min after oral delivery (Table 5.13).

Furthermore, the administration of a nasal formulation (Mecnazone) to dogs also achieved similar results to those in rats (198). The fraction absorbed intranasally was about 0.89 that of an equivalent intravenous dose, but about four times that of oral absorption ($F_{oral} = 0.22$). In dogs, the mean times to peak plasma levels was 11.9 min for the nasal dose as compared to 70.0 min after an oral dose. It is thus concluded that intranasal administration of meclizine has rapidly achieved a significant plasma level of the drug, which is comparable to that seen following an equivalent intravenous dose, whereas there is four to six times more absorption than after the oral administration (Table 5.14).

5.9 ANTIMIGRAINE DRUGS

The nasal absorption of antimigraine drugs, such as ergotamine tartrate, has been reported (199-201). Ergotamine tartrate is used for the symptomatic treatment of migraine because of its vasoconstrictive action mediated by serotoninergic receptors (199,200).

Table 5.15 AUC and Relative Bioavailability of Ergotamine Tartrate in Rats Following Intravenous, Nasal, Oral, and Intraduodenal Administration With and Without Caffeine

Dose	Route	AUC 0 → 240 min $(ng \cdot min \cdot ml^{-1})^a$ mean ±S.E. for 4 rats	Relative bioavailability (0-240 min [%])
Ergotamine	Intravenous	32,900 (±3200)	
(0.5 mg/rat)	Nasal	20,400 (±4600)	62.0
	Intraduodenal	4200 (±1200)	12.7
	Oral	1700 (±1700)	5.1
Ergotamine (p.t mg/rat)	Intravenous	25,300 (±6700)	
plus caffeine (2.5 mg/rat)	Nasal	16,500 (±3200)[b]	65.4

[a]Mean (±S.E.) for 4 rats.
[b]5 rats.
Source: Modified from Ref. 201, used with permission.

Intranasal administration of ergotamine tartrate has been studied in rats in comparison with intravenous, intraduodenal, and oral administrations (201). A considerable amount of the drug was detected within 3-10 min following intranasal administration. The relative bioavailability after the dosing of 0.5 mg/rat via the oral and intraduodenal routes was only 5.1 and 12.7%, respectively, whereas the nasal bioavailability in the absence or presence of caffeine (2.5 mg/rat) was 62.0 and 65.4%, respectively (Table 5.15). The results suggest that the intranasal route of administration offers a viable alternative to parenteral injection for administering ergotamine tartrate from the standpoint of the convenience as well as the rate and the extent of absorption following intranasal administration.

5.10 ANTIBIOTICS

5.10.1 Penicillins

Penicillin has been studied for its effect on the ciliary activity in the upper respiratory tract of the rabbit (202). The results indicated that penicillin in isotonic saline solution produces no apparent deleterious effect on the ciliary action of the nasal mucosa of normal healthy rabbits. Investigations have been initiated on the administration of penicillin in aerosol form to the

nasal accessory sinuses for the treatment of chronic sinusitis (203,204).
The results concluded that aerosolized penicillin is a safe, rational and effective mode of treatment for acute infections in the upper respiratory tract and
also for infections of paranasal sinuses.

Sulbenicillin is known to be poorly absorbed from the gastrointestinal
tract as a result of its high water solubility and lack of lipophilic properties
(205). In vivo absorption studies of sulbenicillin have been performed in
rats to compare its bioavailability following intranasal, oral, and intramuscular administrations (206). After oral administration, poor absorption was
again confirmed. However, following intranasal administration, the dose recovered in the urine was nearly one-half of that seen with intramuscular administration (Figure 5.27). This result suggests that even the poorly orally
absorbed drugs may be easily absorbed by the intranasal route of administration, which could be useful as a new route of administration to enhance the
systemic bioavailability of a poorly absorbed drug.

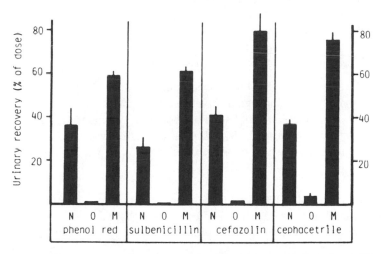

Figure 5.27 Urinary recovery of phenol red (2 mg/rat), sulbenicillin (3 mg/
rat), cefazolin (2 mg/rat), and cephacetrile (1 mg/rat) within 4 hr after various routes of administration. Each value is the mean (±S.E.M.) of three animals. (From Ref. 180, used with permission.)

5.10.2 Tyrothricin

The in vivo efficacy of tyrothricin against certain virulent bacterial infections has been reported by Greenwood et al. (202). The mucociliary beating action in the rabbit was noted to cease 5-10 min following intranasal administration of an aqueous suspension of tyrothricin at various concentrations. However, this was also observed in the controls treated with plain distilled water.

5.10.3 Cephalosporins

Cephalosporins are a group of antibiotics with antibacterial activities more potent than the penicillins. The cephalosporins have a mechanism of action very similar to that of the penicillins. They inhibit the cross linking of the peptidoglycan units in the bacterial cell wall by occupying the D-alanyl-D-alanine substrate site in the transpeptidase.

Cephacetrile and cefazolin are known to be poorly absorbed from the gastrointestinal tract owing to their high water solubility and lack of lipophilic properties (207). In rats, in vivo nasal absorption studies of cephacetrile (1 mg/rat) and cefazolin (2 mg/rat) showed that following intranasal administration, the dose excreted in the urine is nearly one-half of that seen with intramuscular administration (206) (Fig. 5.27). These studies demonstrated that even the poorly absorbed oral drugs can be easily absorbed by the intranasal route of administration.

5.10.4 Aminoglycosides

Aminoglycosides are classified as broad-spectrum antibiotics. In general, they have greater activity against gram-negative than gram-positive bacteria. The aminoglycosides combine with bacterial ribosomes, which results in the inhibition of protein synthesis. The drugs also interfere with the binding of aminoacetyl-t-RNA, which prevents the elongation of peptide chains.

5.10.4.1 Streptomycin

At concentrations of 100-1000 U/ml in isotonic saline solution, streptomycin showed no inhibitory or deleterious effect on the ciliary action of either nasal mucosa or tracheal ciliated epithelium of the normal healthy rabbits (202).

5.10.4.2 Gentamicin

Gentamicin can inhibit over 90% of the strains of *Pseudomonas aeruginosa*. Absorption of gentamicin from the gastrointestinal tract can be enhanced by coadministration with a nonionic surfactant (208). A study showed that the nasal absorption of gentamicin in healthy human subjects is enhanced by sodium glycocholate (209). In this study, three subjects were administered intranasally gentamicin in a saline solution, whereas the other two received an equivalent dose in a saline solution containing 1% sodium glycocholate. In addition, four other subjects received a saline solution of gentamicin intramuscularly. After intranasal administration of gentamicin (2 mg/kg) in the solution containing 1% sodium glycocholate, peak gentamicin concentrations of 2.48 ($\pm$0.42) μg/ml were attained after 30 min in four subjects and after 60 min in the other three subjects. The serum gentamicin concentrations achieved were similar to those obtained from intramuscular administration of genatmicin at a 0.3-mg dose. On the other hand, the amount of genamicin in the serum was undetectable when it was given intranasally without glycocholate. This study suggested that the incorporation of a surfactant to the nasal preparation is required in order to obtain a significant level of gentamicin in the systemic circulation.

5.11 ANTIVIRAL AGENTS

5.11.1 Phenyl-p-Guanidino Benzoate

When antiviral drugs are administered intranasally to animals with upper respiratory viral infections, the antiviral activities are always found to be much less than expected.

The factors which may be responsible for the reduction in the effectiveness of antiviral drugs administered intranasally have been studied (210). Mice were first infected in the upper respiratory tract with the influenza A virus and then treated with phenyl-p-guanidino benzoate (PGB). The infection was carried out intranasally by instillation of a 100 $TCID_{50}$ influenza Ao (DSP) and a good growth of virus in the upper respiratory tract was attained 30 hr after the infection. If the mice were dosed intranasally with repeated doses of PGB solution (four or five times per hour) for 6 hr immediately following the infection, a reduction in the virus growth was observed. However, there appeared to be a factor or a set of factors which were operating to greatly reduce the drug's effect when it was given directly into the nose. The most obvious possible contributory factor was that the mucociliary clearance system swept the drug out of the upper airways after each dosing. In the intact mouse, with the mucociliary transport system working normally, the hourly exposure of the upper respiratory tract to the drug, with doses given five times an hour, was found to be in the range of

7.5-12.5 min, which gave a ninefold reduction in virus growth. Whereas in the in vitro situation, a 20- to 40-fold reduction in virus growth could be obtained with drug exposure of merely 1-2 min in each hour. Thus, the clearance of drug from the nose by mucociliary transport system must be regarded as only a contributory factor, not the major one, in accounting for the relatively poor performance of the drug when given intranasally.

5.11.2 Enviroxime

Enviroxime, a benzimidazole derivative, is virostatic for rhinoviruses at a concentration of 10-40 ng/ml in tissues cultures (211). The clinical prophylactic and therapeutic effects of enviroxime have been studied in 99 volunteers infected with rhinovirus type 4 (RV4) (212). A metered-dose nasal spray was used to deliver either the enviroxime or a placebo solution in a pressurized aerosol. Each spray delivered 284 μg of enviroxime to each nostril. The enviroxime concentrations in the nasal secretions measured 12 hr after dosing on days 3, 4, and 5 were found to range from an undetectable level to 4662 ng/ml. In one group of volunteers, the drug concentration was 798 ($\pm$310) ng/ml, whereas in another group the drug concentration was only 13 ($\pm$5) ng/ml. Cold symptoms were observed in 27-73% of the volunteers in the different test groups. Fewer symptoms were observed in the subjects who were treated with enviroxime before RV4 challenge and had a mean enviroxime concentration of greater than 100 ng/ml in their nasal washes. Furthermore, a total of 20 of the 38 placebo-treated volunteers and 47 of the 61 enviroxime-treated volunteers reported a transit, mild nasal stinging for the first few minutes after nasal spraying. However, no abnormalities were detected in the total or differential leukocyte counts, hemoglobin concentrations, or the test or renal and heaptic functions which could be attributed to the intranasal administration of enviroxime by nasal spray.

5.12 INORGANIC COMPOUNDS

5.12.1 Inorganic Salts

Nasal absorption of inorganic salts, such as $CsCl$, $SrCl_2$, $BaCl_2$, and $CeCl_3$, has been studied in hamsters and compared with oral absorption (213). More than 50% of the radioactive dose of cesium (Cs), strontium (Sr), and barium (Ba) deposited on the nasal membrane were absorbed directly into the systemic circulation, whereas only less than 4% of the cerium (Ce) was absorbed intranasally. For all the isotopes studied, the nasal bioavailability was at least approximately equal, if not greater, to oral bioavailability in the first 4 hr postadministration. The results suggested that the nasopharynx is not only a major site of absorption for the inhaled aerosols of a soluble nature, but may be the most important site of absorption for aerosols with a size greater than 5 μm MMAD (mass median aerodynamic diameter), at which the nasal deposition often greatly exceeds the deposition in all other area of the respiratory tract.

5.12.2 Colloidal Gold

Using radioactive gold (^{198}Au), the possibility of penetration of colloidal gold across the nasal mucous membrane in the olfactory region to the cerebrospinal fluid (CSF) in the subarachnoid space of the anterior part of the brain has been studied in the rabbit (214). A suspension of colloidal ^{198}Au was injected unilaterally into the mucous membrane on the roof of the nose in two groups of rabbits, whereas another group of animals received an intravenous injection of the colloidal ^{198}Au. Following intravenous administration, ^{198}Au was transported from the general circulation into the CSF in the cisterns of the subarachnoid space at the base of the brain within 1-2 hr. Following intranasal injection however, a high concentration of the isotope was detected in the CSF in the cribriform plate and at the base of the olfactory lobes of the brain. This experiment has shown that ^{198}Au administered intranasally penetrates directly from the nasal mucous membrane at the olfactory region into the CSF of the anterior cranial fossa. The data suggest that there is a good transport system from the mucous membrane at the olfactory region of the nose to the cerebrospinal fluid.

The pathways for the transfer of colloidal gold were further studied in rhesus monkeys by electron microscopy (215). The colloidal gold solution was administered, using a glass atomizer, to the roof of the nose. The colloidal gold particles sprayed on the olfacory mucosa were observed in the olfactory rods and in the supporting cells. The gold particles in the olfactory neurons could be traced as far as the fila olfactoria, whereas in the supporting cells the gold particles were found either as discrete, free-lying particles or in aggregated form (Figures 5.28 and 5.29). Gold particles were also detected in the endothelial cells of the blood vessels in the lamina propria, but they could not be found in the intercellular space of the olfactory mucosa. This study suggests that the nasal route can be used for delivering drugs directly into the brain as well as into the systemic circulation.

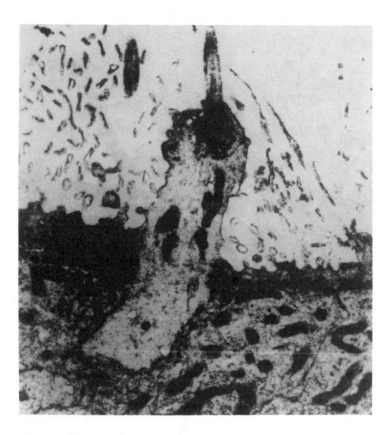

Figure 5.28 Electromicrograph of an olfactory rod and adjacent supporting cell in the rhesus monkey The apices of these two cell types are linked by tight junctions which seal off the underlying intercellular spaces in the olfactory epithelium. A pinocytotic vesicle is evident in the olfactory rod. Mag. X 27 050. (From Ref. 215 used with permission.)

5.12.3 Colloidal Carbon

Colloidal carbon has been used as a tracer to investigate the permeability of nasal vessels of the rat (216). The results indicated that colloidal carbon does not pass through the basement membrane of the capillary even at 15

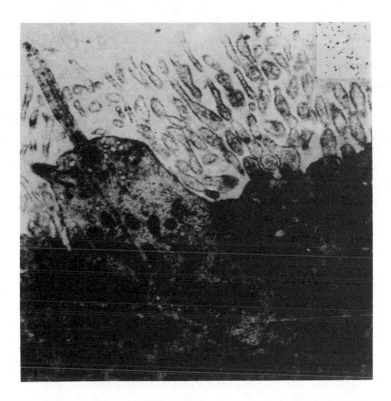

Figure 5.29 Electromicrograph of the olfactory epithelium from a rhesus monkey in which colloidal gold was sprayed. The gold particles can be visualized both in the olfactory rod and in the neighboring supporting cell. Some of the gold particles have coalesced to form electron dense masses which are associated with the mitochondria. Inset shows size of colloidal gold particles sprayed onto formvar-coated grids. Mag. X 27,000. (From Ref. 215 used with permission.)

min following intravenous infusion. On the other hand, the intercellular space among the endothelial cells was found wide open, like a liver sinusoid, and free passage of the carbon particles out of the blood vessels was observed. The carbon particles were noted to be pooled in the spacing between the endothelial cells and the basement membrane.

5.12.4 Colloidal Silver

Colloidal silver has been reported to be transported from the olfactory nerve cells into the nasopharyngeal mucous membrane and then diffuse to the systemic lymphatics (217).

5.12.5 Lead Carbonate

The powder form of lead carbonate has been found to be readily absorbed from the upper respiratory passages of cats and dogs following intranasal delivery by a nasal atomizer (218). The absorption is rapid with a magnitude far in excess of the minimal toxic dose. The possible mechanism for the nasal absorption of lead carbonate was proposed as follows (217): (a) Lead carbonate is first dissolved in the nasal mucous and then absorbed; (b) The toxic action of lead carbonate renders the mucous membrane more permeable to the passage of lead carbonate particles.

5.12.6 ^{32}P and Thorium B

When radioactive indicators, such as ^{32}P and thorium B, were administered intranasally to the middle third of the septal mucosa of rabbits or rats, maximum concentrations in the central nervous system were reached within 60 min (219). These radioactive indicators were observed to enter directly into the cerebrospinal fluid (CSF) in the anterior scala. The greatest proportion of isotope was observed in the hypothalamus, with a considerable amount being present also in the basal ganglia, olfactory lobe, and frontal lobe

REFERENCES

1. Wall, J. W., and Shure, N. Intranasal cortisone, *Arch. Otolaryngol. 56*: 172 (1952).
2. Mabry, R. L. Visual loss after intranasal corticosteroid injection: Incidence, causes, and prevention, *Arch. Otolaryngol., 107*:484 (1981).
3. Mabry R. L. Practical applications of intranasal corticosteroid injection, *Ear Nose Throat J., 60*:506 (1981).
4 Dill, J. L., and Bolstad D. S. Observation on the local use of cortisone in the nose in allergic rhinitis, *Laryngoscope, 61*:415 (1951).
5. Bagratuni, L. A comparative study of topical steroids, antihistamines and pollen vaccine in the treatment of hay fever and hay asthma, *Ann. Allergy 18*:859 (1960).
6. Seidmon, E. E. P., and Schaffer, N. Cortogen nasal suspension with chlortrimeton in the treatment of allergic rhinitis, *Ann. Allergy, 12*:85 (1954).

7. Rohen, M. B. The use of hydrocrotisone suspension in nasal allergic and infectious conditions, *Ann Allergy 113*:109 (1955).
8. Burger, J. H., and Shaffer, J. H. Controlled studies in the topical application of hydrocortisone in vasomotor rhinitis, *Ann. N.Y. Acad. Sci., 61*: 566 (1955).
9. Herzheimer, H., and McAllen M. Treatment of hay fever with hydrocortisone snuff, *Lancet, 1*:537 (1956).
10. Cotes, P. M., McLean, A., and Sayer, J. B. Absorption of inhaled hydrocortisone, *Lancet, 2*:807 (1956).
11 Mowat, G. G. Submucosal injections of hydrocortisone for allergic rhinitis and rhinitis medicamentosa, *J. Laryngol. Otol., 75*:283 (1961).
12. Lake, C. F., Logan G. B., and Peters, G. A. Treatment of ragweed hay fever with powdered hydrocortisone applied intranasally, *Staff Meet. Mayo Clin., 32*:641 (1957).
13. Tuft, H. S. Topical use of hydrocortisone alcohol in the treatment of ragweed hay fever, *Ann. Allergy, 12*:687 (1954).
14. Smith, T. T. Local use of hydrocortisone acetate in the nose, *Arch. Otolaryngol., 60*:24 (1954).
15. Taub S. J., and Hecht, R. A. Treatment of hay fever with intranasal hydrocortisone acetate powder, *Am. Pract. Digest. Treat., 10*:469 (1959).
16. Morris-Owen, R. M., and Truelove, S. C. Treatment of hay fever with local hydrocortisone hemisuccinate sodium, *Br. Med. J., 1*:969 (1958).
17. Anderson J. R., and Ogden, H. D. Topical use of prednisolone in nasal allergy, *Ann. Allergy 14*:44 (1956).
18. Godfrey M. P., and Maunsell, K. Prednisolone snuff in hay fever: A controlled trial, *Lancet, 1*:767 (1957).
19. Simmons, M. W. Intranasal injection of corticosteroids, *Calif. Med., 92*: 155 (1960).
20. Baker, D. C., and Strauss, R. B. Intranasal injections of long-acting corticosteroids, *Ann. Otol. Rhinol. Laryngol., 71*:525 (1962).
21. Mabry, R. Intranasal corticosteroid injection: Indications, technique, and complications, *Otolaryngol. Head Neck Surg., 87*:207 (1979).
22. Meyers, D. Experiences in the treatment of the allergic nasal polyp by the intrapolyp injection of prednisolone T.B.A., *Laryngoscope, 58*:1 (1958).
23. Mabry, R. L. Intranasal steroid injection during pregnancy, *South Med. J., 73*:1176 (1980).
24. Baker, D. C. Intranasal steroid injections; Indications, techniques, results and complications, *Laryngoscope, 89*:998 (1979).
25. Ghione, S., Clerico, A., Fommei, E., Cocci, F., Bartoeomei, C., and Riccioni, N. Hypertension and hypokalemia cuased by α-fluoroprednisolone in a nasal spray, *Lancet, 1*:1301 (1979).

26. Rowe, R. J., Dasler, T. W., and Kinkella, A. M. Visual changes and tri-amcinolone, *J.A.M.A.*, *201*:117 (1967).

27. McCleve, D., Goldstein, J., and Silver, S. Corticosteroid injections of the nasal turbinates: Past experience and precautions, *Otolaryngology*, *86*:851 (1978).

28. Friedman, H. T., and Hills, B. A double-blind study of triamcinolone acetonide nasal spray in allergic rhinitis, *J. Allergy*, *33*:1 (1962).

29. Norman, P. S., and Winkenwerder, W. L. Suppression of hay fever symptoms with intranasal dexamethasone aerosol, *J. Allergy*, *36*:284 (1965).

30. Smith, R. E. Dexamethasone nasal aerosol in nasal polyps and hypertrophic allergic rhinitis: A clinical and controlled evaluation, *Ann. Allergy*, *23*:273 (1968).

31. Norman, P. S., Winkenwerder, W. L., Murgatroyd, G. W., and Parsons, J. W. Evidence for the local action of intranasal dexamethasone aerosols in the suppression of hay fever symptoms, *J. Allergy*, *38*:93 (1966).

32. Michels, M. I., Smith, R. E., and Heimlich, E. M. Adrenal suppression and intranasally applied steroids, *Ann. Allergy*, *25*:569 (1967).

33. Taub, S. J. Dexamethasone nasal aerosol vs. placebo in the treatment of nasal polyposis, *Eye Ear Nose Throat Month.*, *47*:80 (1968).

34. Champion, P. K. Cushing syndrome secondary to abuse of dexamethasone nasal spray, *Arch. Intern. Med.*, *134*:750 (1974).

35. Aaron, T. H., and Muttitt, E. L. C. Intranasal dexamethasone phosphate in perennial allergic rhinitis, *Ann. Allergy*, *22*:155 (1964).

36. Aaron, T. H., and Muttitt, E. L. C. Effect of intranasal dexamethasone phosphate on the adrenal function of patients with perennial allergic rhinitis, *Ann. Allergy*, *23*:100 (1965).

37. Frankland, A. W., and Walker, S. R. A comparison of intranasal betamethasone valerate and sodium cromoglycate in seasonal allergic rhinitis, *Clin. Allergy*, *5*:295 (1975).

38. Harding, S. M., and Heath, S. Intranasal steroid aerosol in perennial rhinitis: Comparison with an antihistamine compound, *Clin. Allergy*, *6*:369 (1976).

39. Mygind, N. Local effect of intranasal beclomethasone dipropionate aerosol in hay fever, *Br. Med. J.*, *4*:464 (1973).

40. Hansen, I., and Mygind, N. Local effect of intranasal beclomethasone dipropionate aerosol in perennial rhinitis, *Acta Allergol.*, *29*:281 (1974).

41. Gibson, I., Maberly, D. J., Lal, S., Ali, M. M., and Butler, A. G. Double-blind crossover trial comparing intranasal beclomethasone diporpionate and placebo in perennial rhinitis, *Br. Med. J.*, *4*:503 (1974).

42. Mygind, N., Pedersen, C. B., Prytz, S., and Sørensen, H. Treatment of nasal polyps with intranasal beclomethasone dipropionate aerosol, *Clin. Allergy*, *5*:159 (1975).

43. Bryant, D. H., and Pepys, J. Aldecin nasal spray, *Br. Med. J.*, *1*:1319 (1977).

44. Cockcroft, D. W., MacCormack, D. W., Newhouse, M. T., and Hargreave, R. E. Beclomethasone dipropionate aerosol in allergic rhinitis, *Can. Med. Assoc. J.*, *115*:523 (1976).
45. Malm, L., and Wihl, J. A. Intranasal beclomethasone dipropionate in vasomotor rhinitis, *Acta Allergol.*, *31*:245 (1976).
46. Wheatley, D. A corticosteroid nasal spray in hay fever, *Curr. Ther. Res. Clin. Exp.*, *19*:612 (1976).
47. Editors of *British Medical Journal*. Intranasal beclomethasone: Wonder drug or hazard? *Br. Med. J.*, *2*:1522 (1976).
48. Mygind, N. Effects of beclomethasone dipropionate aerosol on nasal mucosa, *Br. J. Clin. Pharmacol.*, *4*:287S (1977).
49. Poynter, D. Beclomethasone dipropionate aerosol and nasal mucosa, *Br. J. Clin. Pharmacol.*, *4*:295S (1977).
50. Mygind, N., Johnsen, N. J., and Thomsen, J. Intranasal allergen challenge during corticosteroid treatment, *Clin. Allergy*, *7*:69 (1977).
51. Mygind, N., Sørensen, H., and Pedersen, C. B. The nasal mucosa during long-term treatment with beclomethasone dipropionate aerosol, *Acta Otolaryngol.*, *85*:437 (1978).
52. Mygind, N. Topical corticosteroids—Beclomethasone dipropionate, in *Nasal Allergy*, Blackwell, London (1978), pp. 312-332.
53. Hillas, J., Booth, R. J., Somerfield, S., Morton, R., Avery, J., and Wilson, J. P. A comparative trial of intranasal beclomethasone dipropionate and sodium cromoglycate in patients with chronic perennial rhinitis, *Clin. Allergy*, *10*:253 (1980).
54. Munch, E., Gomez, G., Harris, C., Lack, R. P., Edwards, V. A., O'Connor, P., Snowden, D. V., and Mygind, N. An open comparison of dosage frequencies of beclomethasone dipropionate in seasonal allergic rhinitis, *Clin. Allergy*, *11*:303 (1981).
55. Toft, A., Wihl, J., Toxman, J., and Mygind, N. Double-blind comparison between beclomethasone dipropionate as aerosol and as powder in patients with nasal polyposis, *Clin. Allergy*, *12*:391 (1982).
56. Mygind, N. Intranasal corticosteroid treatment of rhinitis, *Eur. J. Respir. Dis.* [*Suppl.*], *122*:192 (1982).
57. Pelikan, Z. The effects of disodium cromoglycate (DSCG) and beclomethasone dipropionate (BDA) on the delayed nasal mucosa response to allergen challenge. *Ann. Allergy*, *52*:111 (1984).
58. Harries, M. G., Anderson, P. B., Gibson, G. J., Hof, Z. E., and Baggott, P. J. A comparison of an aqueous and a pressurized nasal spray of beclomethasone dipropionate in the management of seasonal rhinitis, *Pharmatherapeutica*, *3*:623 (1984).
59. Okuda, M., Sakaguci, K., and Ohtsuka, H. Intranasal beclomethasone mode of action in nasal allergy, *Ann. Allergy*, *50*:116 (1983).
60. Turkeltaub, P. C., Norman, P. S., and Crepea, S. Treatment of ragweed

hay fever with an intranasal spray containing flunisolide, a new synthetic corticosteroid, *J. Allergy Clin. Immunol., 58*:597 (1976).

61. Henriksen, J. M., and Wenzel, A. Effect of an intranasally administered corticosteroid (budesonide) on nasal obstruction, mouth breathing and asthma, *Am. Rev. Respir. Dis., 130*:1014 (1984).

62. Pipkorn, U., and Anderson, P. Budesonide and nasal mucosal histamine content and anti-IgE induced histamine release, *Ann. Allergy, 37*:591 (1982).

63. Larochelle, P., Souich, P. D., Bolte, E., Lelorier, J., and Goyer, R. Toxicortol pivalate, a corticosteroid with no systemic glucocorticoid effect after oral, intrarectal, and intranasal application, *Clin. Pharmacol. Ther., 33*:343 (1983).

64. Anand Kumar, T. C., David, G. F. X., Unberkoman, B., and Saini, K. D. Uptake of radioactivity by body fluids and tissues in rhesus monkeys after intravenous injection or intranasal spray of tritium-labeled oestradiol and progesterone, *Curr. Sci., 43*:435 (1974).

65. Anand Kumar, T. C., David, G. F. X., Kumar, K., Umberkoman, B., and Krishnamoorthy, M. S. A new approach to fertility regulation by interfering with neuroendocrine pathway, in *Proceedings of International Symposium on Neuroendocrine Regulation of Fertility* (T. C. Anand, Ed.), Karger, Basel (1976), pp. 314-322.

66. Öhman, L., Hahnenberger, R., and Johansson, E. D. B. 17β-Estradiol levels in blood and cerebrospinal fluid after ocular and nasal administration in women and female rhesus monkeys (Macaca mulatta), *Contraception, 22*:349 (1980).

67. Rigg, L. A., Milanes, B., Villanueva, B., and Yen, S. S. C. Efficacy of intravaginal and intranasal administration of micronized estradiol-17β, *J. Clin. Endocrinol. Metab., 45*:1261 (1977).

68. Anand Kumar, T. C., Sehgal, A., David, G. F. X., Bajoj, J. S., and Prasad, M. R. N. Effects of intranasal administration of hormonal steroids on serum testosterone and spermatogenesis in rhesus monkey (Macaca mulatta), *Biol. Reprod., 22*:935 (1980).

69. Brittebo, E. B. Metabolism of progesterone by the nasal mucosa in mice and rats, *Acta Pharmacol. Toxicol., 51*:441 (1982).

70. Brittebo, E. B., and Rafter, J. J. Steroid metabolism by rat nasal mucosa: Studies on progesterone and testosterone, *J. Steroid Biochem., 20*: 1147 (1984).

71. Moudgal, R. N., Rao, A. J., Murthy, G. S. R. C., Neelakanta, R., Banavar, S. R., Kotagi, S. G., and Anand Kumar, T. C. Effect of intranasal administration of norethisterone and progesterone on pituitary and gonadal function in adult male and female bonnet monkeys (Macaca radiata), *Fertil. Steril., 44*:120 (1985).

72. Anand Kumar, T. C., David, G. F. X., and Puri, V. Ovulation in rhesus monkeys suppressed by intranasal administration of progesterone and norethisterone, *Nature, 270*:532 (1977).
73. Anand Kumar, T. C., David, G. F. X., and Puri, V. Nasal sprays for controlling ovulation in rhesus monkeys, in *Recent Advances in Primatology*, Vol. 4 (D. J. Chivers, and E. H. R. Ford, Eds.), Academic Press, New York (1978), pp. 171-175.
74. Anand Kumar, T. C., David, G. F. X., and Puri, V. Nasal spray contraceptives, in *Recent Advances in Reproduction and Regulation of Fertility* (G. P. Talwar, Ed.), Elsevier/North-Holland, Amsterdam (1979), pp. 49-56.
75. David, G. F. X., Puri, C. P., and Anand Kumar, T. C. Bioavailability of progesterone enhanced by intranasal spraying, *Experimenta, 37*:533 (1981).
76. Hussain, A. A., Hirai, S., and Bawarshi, R. Nasal absorption of natural contraception steroids in rats—Progesterone absorption, *J. Pharm. Sci., 70*.466 (1981).
77. Hussain, A. A., Hirai, S., and Bawarshi, R. Administering natural female sex hormones, *U.S. patent 4,314,925* (Feb. 16, 1981).
78. Corbo, D. C., Huang, Y. C., and Chien, Y. W. Nasal delivery of progestational steroids in ovariectomized rabbits. I. Progesterone—Comparison of pharmacokinetics with intravenous and oral administration, *Int. J. Pharm., 46*:133-140 (1988).
79. Anand Kumar, T. C., David, G. F. X., Sankaranarayanan, A., Puri, V., and Sundrani, K. R. Pharmacokinetics of progesterone after its administration to ovariectomized rhesus monkeys by injection, infusion, or nasal spraying, *Proc. Natl. Acad. Sci. USA, 79*:4185 (1982).
80. Chien, Y. W., Corbo, D. C., and Huang, Y. Nasal controlled delivery and pharmacokinetics of progestational steroids and effect of penetrant hydrophilicity, *Proceed. Intern. Symp. Control. Re. Bioact. Mater., 15*:191 (1988).
81. Öhman, I., Hahnenberger, R., and Johansson, E. D. B. Topical administration of progestational steroids in the eye and nose—A rapid absorption to the blood, *Contraception, 18*:171 (1978).
82. Hussain, A. A., Kimura, R., and Huang, C. H. Nasal absorption of testosterone in rats, *J. Pharm. Sci., 73*:1300 (1984).
83. Conley, C. L., Krevans, J. R., Chow, B. F., Barrows, C., and Lang, C. A. Observations on the absorption, utilization and excretion of vitamin B_{12}, *J. Lab. Clin. Med., 38*:84 (1951).
84. Monto, R. W., Rebuck, J. W., and Brennan, M. J. Crystalline B_{12} inhalation therapy in pernicious anemia, *Am. J. Med. Sci., 225*:113 (1953).
85. Monto, R. W., and Rebuck, J. W. Nasal instillation and inhalation of crystalline vitamin B_{12} in pernicious anemia, *Arch. Intern. Med., 93*:219 (1954).

86. Nudelman, I. Nasal delivery: A revolution in drug administration, Proceedings from 1987 Conference of the Latest Developments in Drug Delivery Systems, *Pharm. Techn.*, (1987), p. 43.

87. Lesser, J. M., Israili, Z. H., Davis, D. C., and Dayton, P. G. Metabolism and disposition of hydralazine-^{14}C in man and dog, *Drug Metab. Dispos.* *2*:351 (1974).

88. Zak, S. D., Bartlett, M. F., Wagner, W. E., Gilleran, T. G., and Lukes, G. Disposition of hydralazine in man and a specific method for its determination in biological fluids, *J. Pharm. Sci., 63*:225 (1974).

89. Kaneo, Y., Absorption from the nasal mucous membrane: I. Nasal absorption of hydralazine in rats, *Acta Pharm. Suec., 20*:379 (1983).

90. Hirai, S., Yashiki, T., Matsuzawa, T., and Mima, H. Absorption of drugs from the nasal mucosa of rat, *Int. J. Pharm., 7*:317 (1981).

91. Schölkens, B. A. Central hypotensive action of an angiotensin II-antagonist in conscious rats with experimental hypertension, *I.R.C.S., 4*:320 (1976).

92. Schökens, B. A., Wissman, H., Lindner, E., and Geiger, R. 1,8-disubstituted analogues of (IIe[5]) and (Val[5]) Angiotensin II: Difference in potency and specificity of angiotensin II-antagonistic activity, *Hoppe-Seyler Z. Physiol. Chem., 357*:825 (1976).

93. Wissman, H., Schölkens, B. A., Lindner, E., and Geiger, R. Chemie und wirkungsweise neuer angiotensin II-antagonisten. 8-C-phenylglycinanaloga des (5-isoleucin) angiotensins II, *Hoppe-Seyler Z. Physiol. Chem., 3*:1083 (1974).

94. Schökens, B. A., Lux, R., and Steinbach, R. Hypertensive action of an intranasally applied angiotensin II-antagonist, *Arch. Int. Pharmacodyn., 229*:244 (1977).

95. Mar, D. D. New topical nitroglycerin preparations. *Am. J. Nurs., 82*: 462 (1982).

96. Heinzow, B., and Ziegler, A. Comparison of the effects of nitroglycerin administered to rats by different routes, *J. Cardiovasc. Pharmacol., 3*: 573 (1981).

97. Hill, A. B., Bowley, C. J., Nahrwold, M. L., Knight, P. R., Tait, A. R., Taylor, M. D., Kirsch, M. M., and Denlinger, J. K. Intranasal administration of nitroglycerin, *Anesthesiology, 51*:S67 (1979).

98. Hill, A. B., Bowley, C. J., Nahrwold, M. L., Knight, P. R., Kirsh, M. M., and Denlinger, J. K. Intranasal administration of nitroglycerin, *Anesthesiology, 54*:346 (1981).

99. Moon, G. J., Kim, J. G., and Cookinham, F. T. Intranasal nitroglycerin (NTG) during infrarenal aortic cross-clamp, *Anesthesiology, 55*:191 (1981).

100. Erb, R., and Stoltman, W. Evaluation of two nitroglycerin dosage forms: a metered spray and a soft gelatin capsule, *J. Pharmacokinet. Biopharm., 11*:611 (1983).

101. Sito, M., Fukami, K., Sumiyoshi, T., Haze, K., and Hiramori, K. Effects of isosorbide dinitrate spray on central hemodynamics: Comparison with sublingual glyceryl trinitrate and isosorbide dinitrate, *Arzneimittelforsch./Drug Res.*, *34*:707 (1984).

102. Osol, A. *Remington's Pharmaceutical Sciences*, Mack, Easton, Pennsylvania (1986), p. 906.

103. Dollery, C. T., Davis, D. S., and Conolly, M. E. Differences in the metabolism of drugs depending upon their route of administration, *Ann. N.Y. Acad. Sci.*, *179*:108 (1971).

104. Shand, D. G., Nuckolls, E. M., and Oates, J. A. Plasma propranolol levels in adults with observation in four children, *Clin. Pharmacol. Ther.*, *11*:112 (1970).

105. Hussain, A. A., Hirai, S., and Bawarshi, R. Nasal absorption of propranolol in rats, *J. Pharm. Sci.*, *68*:1196 (1979).

106. Hussain, A. A., Hirai, S., and Bawarshi, R. Nasal absorption of propranolol from different dosage forms by rats and dogs, *J. Pharm. Sci.*, *69*:1411 (1980).

107. Hussain, A. A., Foster, T., Hirai, S., Kashihara, T., Batenhorst, R., and Jones, M. Nasal absorption of propranaolol in humans, *J. Pharm. Sci.*, *69*:1240 (1980).

108. Donk, H. J. M., and Merkus, F. W. H. M. Decreases in ciliary beat frequency due to intranasal administration of propranolol, *J. Pharm. Sci.*, *71*:595 (1982).

109. Steinberg, M. I., and Molly, B. B. Clofilium—A new antifibrillatory agent that selectively increases cellular retractoriness, *Life Sci.*, *25*: 1397 (1979).

110. Steinberg, M. I., Sullivan, M. E., Wiest, S. A., Rockhold, F. W., and Molly, B. B. Cellular electrophysiology of clofilium, a new antifibrillatory agent, in normal and ischemic canine Purkinje fibers, *J. Cardiovasc. Pharmacol.*, *3*:881 (1981).

111. Steinberg, M. I. *New Drug Annual*, Raven Press, New York (1984), p. 103.

112. Su, K. S. E., Campanale, K. M., and Gries, C. L. Nasal drug delivery system of a quaternary ammonium compound: clofilium tosylate, *J. Pharm. Sci.*, *73*:1251 (1984).

113. Su, K. S. E., and Campanale, K. M. Nasal drug delivery systems: Requirements, development and evaluations, in *Transnasal Systemic Medications* (Y. W. Chien, Ed.), Elsevier, Amsterdam (1985), pp. 139-159.

114. Hemberger, J. A., and Schanker, L. S. Mechanism of pulmonary absorption of quaternary ammonium compounds in the rat, *Drug Metab. Dispos.*, *11*:73 (1983).

115. Childrey, J. H., and Essex, H. E. Absorption from the mucosa of the frontal sinus, *Arch. Otolaryngol.*, *14*:564 (1931).

116. Van Alyea, O. E., and Donnelly, A. Intranasal medication with vaso-constrictors, *Arch. Otolaryngol., 49*:234 (1941).

117. Van Alyea, O. E., and Donnelly, W. A. Systemic effects of intranasal medication, *Eye Ear Nose Throat Month., 31*:476 (1952).

118. Myers, M. G., and Iazzetta, J. J. Intranasally administered phenyl-ephrine and blood pressure, *Can. Med. Assoc. J., 127*:365 (1982).

119. Empey, D. W., and Medder, K. T. Nasal decongestants, *Drugs, 21*:438 (1981).

120. Hamilton, L. Effect of topical decongestants on nasal airway resis-tance, *Curr. Ther. Res., 24*:261 (1978).

121. Snow, S. S., Logan, T. P., and Hollender, M. H. Nasal spray 'addiction' and psychosis: A case report, *Br. J. Psychiatr., 136*:297 (1980).

122. Hamilton, E. H. Effect of xylometazoline nasal spray on nasal conduc-tance in subjects with coryza, *J. Otolaryngol., 10*:109 (1981).

123. Petruson, B., and Hansson, H. A. Function and structure of the nasal mucosa after 6 weeks use of nose-drops, *Arch. Otolaryngol., 94*:563 (1982).

124. Jackson, R. T., and Birnbaum, J. E. A comparison of a synthetic pros-taglandin and xylometazoline hydrochloride as nasal decongestants, *Otolaryngol. Head Neck Surg., 90*:594 (1982).

125. Glazener, F., Blake, K., and Gradman, M. Bradycardia, hypotension, and near-syncope associated with afrin (oxymetazoline) nasal spray, *N. Engl. J. Med., 309*:731 (1983).

126. Lindsay, W. W. Tobispray in nasal surgery, *Med. J. Aust., 1*:751 (1977).

127. Anand Kumar, T. C., David, G. F. X., Kumar, K., Umberkoman, B., and Krishnamoorthy, M. S. A new approach with neuroendocrine path-ways, in *Neuroendocrine Regulation of Fertility* (T. C. Anand Kumar, Ed.), Karger, Basel (1976), pp. 314-322.

128. Ruffalo, R. R., Spradlin, T. A., Pollock, G. D., Waddell, J. E., and Murphy, P. J. Alpha and beta adrenergic effects of the steroeisomers of dobutamine, *J. Pharmacol. Exp. Ther., 219*:447 (1981).

129. Tuttle, R. R., and Mills, J. Dobutamine: Development of a new cate-cholamine to selectively increase cardiac contractility, *Cir. Res., 36*:185 (1975).

130. Su, K. S. E., Wilson, H. C., and Campanale, K. M. Recent advances in intranasal drug delivery systems, in *Drug Delivery Systems: Funda-mentals and Techniques* (P. Johnson and J. G. Lloyd-Jones, Eds.), Ellis Harwood, West Sussex, England (1987), pp. 224-242.

131. Childrey, J. H., and Essex, H. E. Absorption from the mucosa of the frontal sinus, *Arch. Otolaryngol., 14*:564 (1931).

132. Girard, J. P., Horvat, L., and Heimlich, E. M. Immunopathologie de la rhinite allergique tests de provocation, *Nasaux. Rev. Franc. Allerg., 14*: 175 (1974).

133. McLean, J. A., Mathews, K. P., Solomon, W. R., Brayton, P. R., and Ciarkowski, A. A. Effect of histamine and methacholine on nasal airway resistance in atopic and nonatopic subjects, *J. Allergy Clin. Immunol., 59*:165 (1977).

134. Borum, P. Nasal methacholine challenge: A test for the measurement of nasal reactivity, *J. Allergy Clin. Immunol., 63*:253 (1979).

135. Borum, P., and Mygind, N. Nasal methacholine challenge and ipratropium therapy, *Acta Otorhinolaryngol. Belg., 33*:528 (1979).

136. Temple, D. J. The absorption of nicotine from tobacco snuff through the nasal mucosa, *Arch. Pharm. (Weinheim), 308*:984 (1976).

137. Van Dellen, T. R., Bruger, M., and Wright, I. S. The absorption of acetyl-β-methylcholine chloride (mecholyl) by the nasal mucous membrane, *J. Pharmacol. Exp. Ther., 59*:413 (1937).

138. Tonndorf, J., Hyde, R. W., Chinn, H. I., and Lett, J. E. Absorption from the nasal mucous membrane: Systemic effect of hyoscine following intranasal administration, *Ann. Otol. Rhinol. Laryngol., 62*:630 (1953).

139. Hyde, R. W., Tonndorf, J., and Chinn, H. I. Absorption from the nasal mucous membrane, *Ann. Otol. Rhinol. Laryngol., 62*:957 (1953).

140. Wick, M. M., and Ingram, R. H. Bronchorrheal responsive to aerosolized atropine, *J.A.M.A., 235*:1356 (1976).

141. Cavanaugh, M. J., and Cooper, D. M. Inhaled atropine sulfate dose-response characteristics, *Am. Rev. Respir. Dis., 114*:517 (1976).

142. Hemstreet, M. P. B. Atropine nebulization-simple and safe, *Ann. Allergy, 44*:138 (1980).

143. Jackson, R. T., and Teichgraeber, J. Low-dose topical atropine for rhinorrhea, *Arch. Otolaryngol., 107*:288 (1981).

144. Borum, P., and Mygind, N. Nasal metahcholine challenge and ipratropium therapy, *Acta Otorhinolaryngol. Belg., 33*:528 (1979).

145. Borum, P., Olsen, L., Winther, B., and Mygind, N. Ipratropium nasal spray: A new treatment for rhinorrhea in the common cold, *Am. Rev. Respir. Dis., 123*:418 (1981).

146. Lippton, H. L., Chapnick, B. M., and Kadowitz, P. J. Influence of prostaglandins on vasoconstrictor responses in the hindquarters vascualr bed of the cat, *Prostaglandins Med., 6*:183 (1981).

147. Hedquist, P. Basic methods of prostaglandin action on automatic transmission, *Ann. Rev. Pharmacol. Toxicol., 17*:259 (1977).

148. Stovall, R., and Jackson, R. T. Prostaglandins and nasal blood flow, *Ann. Otol. Rhinol. Laryngol., 76*:1051 (1967).

149. Änggard, A. The effect of prostaglandins on nasal airway resistance in man, *Ann. Otol. Rhinol. Laryngol., 78*:657 (1969).

150. Jackson, R. T. Prostaglandin E_1 as a nasal constrictor in normal human volunteers, *Curr. Ther. Res., 12*:711 (1970).

151. Karim, S. M. M., Adaikan, P. G., and Kunaratnam, N. Effect of topical prostaglandins on nasal spray patency in man, *Prostaglandins, 15*:457 (1978).

152. Karim, S. M. M., Adaiken, P. G., and Kunaratnam, N. Effect of 17-phenyl-PGF$_{2\alpha}$ on nasal patency in man, *Prostaglandins Med., 3*:33 (1979).

153. Jackson, R. T., and Birnbaum, J. E. A comparison of a synthetic prostaglandin and xylometazoline hydrochloride as nasal decongestants, *Otolaryngol. Head Neck Surg., 90*:595 (1982).

154. Bedwani, J. R., Eccles, R., and Jones, A. S. A study of the synthesis and inactivation of prostaglandin E by pig nasal mucosa, *Acta Otolaryngol. (Stockh.), 98*:308 (1984).

155. Stewart, D. J., Inaba, T., Lucassen, M., and Kalow, W. Cocaine metabolism: Cocaine and norcocaine hydroloysis by liver and serum esterases, *Clin. Pharmacol. Ther., 25*:464 (1979).

156. Stewart, D. J., Inaba, T., Tang, B. K., and Kalow, W. Hydrolysis of cocaine in human plasma by cholinesterase, *Life Sci., 20*:1557 (1977).

157. Unger, M. A new method of cocainizing the nasal mucosa, *Eye Ear Nose Throat Month., 43*:60 (1964).

158. Barton, R. P. E., and Gray, R. F. E. The transport of crystalline cocaine in the nasal mucous blanket, *J. Laryngol. Otol., 93*:1201 (1979).

159. Washton, A. M., Gold, M. S., and Pottash, A. C. Intranasal cocaine addiction, *Lancet, 2*:1374 (1983).

160. Jatlow, P. I., and Bailey, D. N. Gas-chromatographic analysis for cocaine in human plasma, with use of a nitrogen detector, *Clin. Chem., 21* 1918 (1975).

161. Byck, R., Jatlow, P. I., Barash, P., and Dyke, C. V. Cocaine: Blood concentration and physiological effect after intranasal application in man, in *Cocaine and Other Stimulants* (E. H. Ellinwood, and M. M. Kilbey, Eds.), Plenum Press, New York (1976), pp. 629-646.

162. Dyke, C. V., Barash, P. G., Jatlow, P. I., and Byck, R. Cocaine: Plasma concentrations after intranasal application in man, *Science, 195*:859 (1977).

163. Resnick, R. B., Kestenbaum, R. S., and Schwartz, L. K. Acute systemic effects of cocaine in man: A controlled study of intranasal and intravenous route of administration, in *Cocaine and Other Stimulants* (E. H. Ellinwood, and M. M. Kilbey, Eds.), Plenum Press, New York (1976), pp. 615-628.

164. Resnick, R. B., Kestenbaum, R. S., and Schwartz, L. K. Acute systemic effects of cocaine in man: A controlled study by intranasal and intravenous routes, *Science, 195*:696 (1977).

165. Dyke, C. V., Jatlow, P., Ungerer, J., Barash, P. G., and Byck, R. Oral cocaine: Plasma concentrations and central effects, *Science, 200*:211 (1978).

166. Javaid, J. I., Fischman, M. W., Schuster, C. R., Dekirmenjian, H., and Davis, J. M. Cocaine plasma concentration: Relation to physiological and subjective effects in humans, *Science*, *202*:227 (1978).

167. Dyke, C. V., Jatlow, P., Ungerer, J., Barash, P., and Byck, R. Cocaine and lidocaine have similar psychological effects after intranasal application, *Life Sci.*, *24*:271 (1979).

168. Javaid, J. I., Musa, M. N., Fischman, M., Schuster, C. R., and Davis, J. M. Kinetics of cocaine in humans after intravenous and intranasal administration, *Biopharm. Drug Dispos.*, *4*:9 (1983).

169. Wilkinson, P., Dyke, C. V., Jatlow, P., Barash, P., and Byck, R. Intranasal and oral cocaine kinetics, *Clin. Pharmacol. Ther.*, *27*:386 (1980).

170. Dyke, C. V., Ungerer, J., Jatlow, P., Barash, P., and Byck, R. Intranasal cocaine: Dose relationships of psychological effects and plasma levels, *Int. J. Psychiat. Med.*, *12*:1 (1982).

171. Sluder, G. The anatomical and clinical relations of the sphenopalatine ganglion of the nose, *N. Y. Med. J.*, *90*:293 (1909).

172. Stewart, D., and Lambert, V. Further observations on sphenopalatine ganglion, *J. Laryngol. Otol.*, *49*:319 (1934).

173. Yang, J. C., Clark, W. C., Dooley, J. C., and Mignogna, F. V. Effect of intranasal cocaine on experimental pain in man, *Anesth. Analg.*, *61*:358 (1982).

174. Gross, J. B., Hartigan, M. L., and Schaffer, D. W. A suitable for 4% cocaine before blind nasotracheal intubation: 3% lidocaine-0.25% phenylephrine nasal spray, *Anesth. Analg.*, *63*:915 (1984).

175. Johnson, L. A. Immediate reversal of severe laryngospasm by intranasally instilled lidocaine with epinephrine, *Ann. Emerg. Med.*, *14*:275 (1985).

176. Heel, R. C., Brogden, R. N., Speight, T. M., and Avery, G. S. Buprenorphine: A new strong analgesic, *Curr. Ther.*, *5*:29 (1979).

177. Kay, B. A. double-blind comparison of morphine and buprenophine in the prevention of pain after operation, *Br. J. Anaesth.*, *50*:605 (1978).

178. Rance, M. J., and Shillingford, J. S. The metabolism of phenolic opiates by rat intestine, Xenobiotica, 7:529 (1977).

179. Brewster, D., Humphrey, M. J., and Mcleavy, M. A. The systemic bioavailability of buprenorphine by various routes of administration. *J. Pharm. Pharmacol.*, *33*:500 (1981).

180. Hussain, A. A., Kimura, R., Huang, C. H., and Kashihara, T. Nasal absorption of naloxone and buprenorphine in rats, *Int. J. Pharm.*, *21*:233 (1984).

181. Ngai, S. H., Berkowitz, B. A., Yang, J. C., Hempstead, J., and Spector, S. Pharmacokinetics of naloxone in rats and in man: Basis for its potency and short duration of action, *Anesthesiology*, *44*:398 (1976).

182. Childrey, J. H., and Essex, H. E. Absorption from the mucosa of the frontal sinus, *Arch. Otolaryngol., 14*:564 (1931).

183. Connell, J. T. A novel method to assess antihistamine and decongestant efficacy, *Ann. Allergy, 42*:278 (1979).

184. Wong, L, Hendeles, L., and Weinberger, M. Pharmacologic prophylaxis of allergic rhinitis: Relative efficacy of hydroxyzine and chlorpheniramine, *J. Allergy Clin. Immunol., 67*:273 (1981).

185. West, S., Brandon, B., Stolley, P., and Rumrill, R. A review of antihistamine and the common cold, *Pediatrics, 56*:100 (1975).

186. Gundrum, L. K. Experimental investigations on action of antihistaminic nasal solutions, *Calif. Med., 75*:207 (1951).

187. Schaffer, N., and Seidmon, E. The intranasal use of prophenpyridamine maleate and chloroprophenpyridamine maleate in allergic rhinitis, *Ann. Allergy, 10*:194 (1952).

188. Hamilton, L. H. Effect of topical decongestants on nasal airway resistance, *Curr. Ther. Res., 24*:261 (1978).

189. Secher, C., Kirkegaard, J., Borum, P., Maansson, A., Osterhammel, P., and Mygind, N. Significance of H_1 and H_2 receptors in the human nose: Rationale for topical use of combined antihistamine preparations, *J. Allergy Clin. Immunol., 70*:211 (1982).

190. Frankland, A. W., and Walker, S. R. A comparison of intranasal betamethasone valerate and sodium cromoglycate in seasonal allergic rhinitis, *Clin. Allergy, 5*:295 (1975).

191. Hillas, J., Booth, R. J., Somerfield, S., Morton, R., AVery, J., and Wilson, J. D. A comparative trial of intranasal beclomethasone dipropionate and sodium cromoglycate in patients with chronic perennial rhinitis, *Clin. Allergy, 10*:253 (1980).

192. Pelikan, Z. The effects of disodium cromoglycate and beclomethasone dipropionate on the late nasal mucosa response to allergen challenge, *Ann. Allergy, 49*:200 (1982).

193. Pelikan, Z. The effects of disodium cromoglycate (DSCG) and beclomethasone dipropionate (BDA) on the delayed nasal mucosa response to allergen challenge, *Ann. Allergy, 52*:111 (1984).

194. Resta, O, Barbaro, M. P. F., and Carnimeo, N. A comparison of sodium cromoglycate nasal solution and powder in the treatment of allergic rhinitis, *Br. J. Clin. Pract., 36*:94 (1982).

195. Fisher, A. N., Brown, K., Davis, S. S., Parr, G. D., and Smith, D. A. The nasal absorption of sodium cromoglycate in the albino rat, *J. Pharm. Pharmacol., 37*:38 (1985).

196. Mygin, N., Viner, A. S., and Jackman, N., The influence on nasal mucosa of unpreserved and preserved nasal sprays containing disodium cromoglycate, *Rhinology, 12*:49 (1974).

197. Mygind, N., Hansen, I. B., and Jørgensen, M., Disodium cromoglycate

nasal spray in adult patients with perennial rhinitis, *Acta. Allergol., 27*: 372 (1972).

198. Chovan, J. P., Klett, R. P., and Rakietin, N. Comparison of meclizine levels in the plasma of rats and dogs after intranasal, intravenous, and oral administration, *J. Pharm. Sci., 74*:1111 (1985).

199. Saxena, P. R. Selective carotid vasoconstriction by ergotamine as a relevant mechanism in its antimigraine action, *Arch. Neurobiol., 37*: 301 (1974).

200. Müller-Schweinitzer, E. Responsiveness of isolated canine cerebral and peripheral arteries to ergotamine, *Naunyn Schmiedebergs Arch. Pharmacol., 292*:113 (1976).

201. Hussain, A. A., Kimura, R., Huang, C. H., and Mustafa, R. Nasal absorption of ergotamine tartrate in rats, *Int. J. Pharm., 21*:289 (1984).

202. Greenwood, G., Pittenger, R. E., Constant, G. A., and Ivy, A. C. Effect of zephiran chloride, tyrothricin, penicillin and streptomycin on ciliary action, *Arch. Otolaryngol., 43*:623 (1946).

203. Barach, A., Garthwaite, B., and Anderson, F. F. An apparatus for the introduction of penicillin aerosol into the nasal accessory sinuses with a case report of a patient with chronic sinusitis, *Ann. Int. Med., 24*:97 (1946).

204. McAuliffe, G. W., and Mueller, G. C. Aerosol penicillin administered in paranasal sinusitis with balanced suction and pressure, *Arch. Otolaryngol., 46*:67 (1947).

205. Bergan, T. Penicillins, *Antibiot. Chemother., 25*:1 (1978).

206. Hirai, S., Yashiki, T., Matsuzawa, T., and Mima, H. Absorption of drugs from the nasal mucosa of rat, *Int. J. Pharm., 7*:317 (1981).

207. Brogard, J. M., Comte, F., and Pinget, M. Pharmacokinetics of cephalosporin antibiotics, *Antibiot. Chemother., 25*:123 (1978).

208. Rubinstein, A., Rubinstein, E., Toitum, E., and Donbrow, M. Increase on intestinal absorption of gentamicin and amitracin by nonionic surfactant, *Antimicrob. Agents Chemother., 19*:696 (1981).

209. Rubinstein, A. Intranasal administration of gentamicin in human subjects, *Antimicrob. Agents Chemother., 23*:778 (1983).

210. Bucknall, R. A. Why aren't antivirals effective when administered intranasally?, in *Chemotherapy and Control of Influenza* (J. S. Oxford and J. D. Williams, Eds.), Academic Press, New York (1976), pp. 77-80.

211. Delong, D. C., and Reed, S. E. Inhibition of rhinovirus replication in organ cultures by a potential antiviral drug, *J. Infect. Dis., 141*:87 (1980).

212. Levandowski, R. A., Pachucki, C. T., Rubenis, M., and Jackson, G. G. Topical enviroxime against rhinovirus infection, *Antimicrob. Agents Chemother., 22*:1004 (1982).

213. Cuddihy, R. G., and Ozog, J. A. Nasal absorption of CsCl, $SrCl_2$, $BaCl_2$ and $CeCl_3$ in syrian hamsters, *Health Phys.*, *25*:219 (1973).

214. Czerniawska, A. Experimental investigations on the penetration of [198] Au from nasal mucous membrane into cerebrospinal fluid, *Acta Otolaryng. (Stockh.)*, *70*:58 (1970).

215. Gopinath, P. G., Gopinath, G., and Kumar, T. C. A. Target site of intranasally sprayed substances and their transport across the nasal mucosa: A new insight into the intranasal route of drug delivery, *Curr. Ther. Res.*, *23*:596 (1978).

216. Watanabe, K., Watanabe, I., Saito, Y., and Mizuhira, V. Characteristics of capillary permeability in nasal mucosa, *Ann. Otol.*, *89*:377 (1980).

217. Blumgart, H. L. A study of the mechanism of absorption of substances from the nasopharynx, *Arch. Intern. Med.*, *33*:415 (1924).

218. Blumgart, H. L. Lead studies VI. Absorption of lead by the upper respiratory passages, *J. Ind. Hyg.*, *5*:153 (1923).

219. Orosz, A., Földes, I., Kósa, C. S., Tóth, G. Radioactive isotope studies of the connection between the lymph circulation of the nasal mucosa, the cranial cavity and cerebrospinal fluid, *Acta Physiol. Acad. Sci., Hung.*, *11*:75 (1957).

6
Intranasal Delivery of Diagnostic Drugs

6.1 PHENOLSULFONPHTHALEIN

Phenolsulfonphthalein (phenol red) is useful for the diagnosis of kidney functions. When injected intramuscularly or intravenously, it starts being excreted in 5–10 min and is almost totally excreted within 2 hr in the patients with normal kidney functions. However, in patients with deficient renal functions, the first appearance of the dye in the urine is delayed. As a result, the degree of functional deficiency of the kidney may be estimated from the proportionate amount of phenol red excreted within 2 hr.

The absorption of phenol red from the sinus membrane was studied in the dog (1). When phenol red was injected subcutaneously as a control, the dye began to appear in the urine within 15 min. More than 50% of the dose was excreted during the first hour, and only traces were present during the third hour. When phenol red was injected into the nasal mucosa of the dog, the dye appeared in the urine at 1 hr and 50 min after the injection, and only faint traces were present at 6 hr and 45 min later. If phenol red was injected into the right frontal sinus, the agent began to appear in the urine 105 min after the administration and continued to appear for 7.5 hr.

The intranasal administration of phenol red was also studied in the rat using an in situ recirculation method and an in vivo nasal absorption technique (2). The results of the in situ recirculation study suggested that phenol red in a pH 7.4 buffer appears to have only little nasal absorption within 2 hr. Furthermore, using the in vivo nasal absorption technique, the systemic

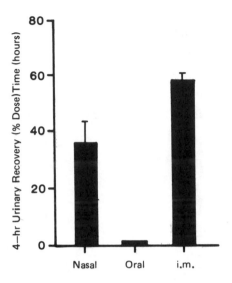

Figure 6.1 Urinary recoveries of phenol red within 4 hr after the administration through various routes in rats (2 mg/rat). Each value is the mean (±SE) for four to seven animals. (Modified from Ref. 2, used with permission.)

bioavailability of phenol red by nasal delivery was compared with those administered by the oral and intramuscular routes. The results indicated that the absorption was poor after oral administration, whereas the fraction of dose excreted in the urine following nasal administration exceeded one-half of that by intramuscular injection (Figure 6.1). The difference in the extent of nasal absorption between the in situ and the in vivo studies is probably due to the difference in the experimental conditions. For example, the volume of nasal solution (0.2-0.3 ml) is very small in the in vivo studies as compared to the recirculating solution (20 ml) used in the in situ experiments.

6.2 DYE T-1824

In monkeys, dye T-1824 was detected in the blood within only a few minutes after intranasal administration. The results suggested that dye T-1824 in solution is rapidly transported from the nasal mucosa and directly enters into the blood stream (3).

6.3 VITAL DYES

Vital dyes, like trypan blue and Evans blue, at high concentrations were observed to pass through the nasal mucosa of the cat, dog, and rabbits and to be present in the lymph for several hours (4). However, the dyes are unable to enter the cranium because they cannot pass through the sheath, or they pass through it at a rate which is much slower than the outward flux of cerebrospinal fluid.

6.4 POTASSIUM FERROCYANIDE

Transported from the olfactory nerve cells, potassium ferrocyanide delivered by an atomizer enters the lymphatic meshwork and then to the retropharyngeal lymph nodes (5).

Following intranasal instillation, the combination of potassium ferrocyanide and iron ammonium citrate was reportedly absorbed through the nasal mucosa and ascended to the cranial cavity from the perineural sheaths of the olfactory filaments (6). Both dyes can be found in the subarachnoid space and in the cervical lymph nodes. On the other hand, the nasal absorption of potassium ferrocyanide and iron ammonium citrate in the mouse occurs chiefly by way of the olfactory sensory cells, and reaches the subarachnoid space and a pia-arachnoid membrane within 2 min following intranasal instillation (7). In rabbits, potassium ferrocyanide and iron ammonium citrate were observed to pass the nasal epithelium and were found in the lymph vessels and in the connective tissue space of the nasal mucosa (8). These substances were also observed in the tissue space of perineural sheath in the filaments of th olfactory nerve and traveled to the region of olfacory bulb.

6.5 SECRETIN

Secretin, a polypeptide hormone with a molecular weight of 3055, is secreted by the duodenal mucosa and to a lesser extent also by the upper jejunal mucosa. It is known to stimulate the secretion of water and bicarbonate from the pancreas, and is often used in the diagnosis of pancreatic disorders. It is clinically used for the treatment of duodenal ulcer.

Secretin is easily degraded in the gastrointestinal tract and, therefore, is usually administered by the parenteral route. Intravenous injection of this hormone in persons with normal pancreatic secretion should yield an increase in the volume of secretion as well as the bicarbonate content from the pancreas. Reduced secretory volume and diminished bicarbonate concentration are indications of pancreatic disorders.

Table 6.1 Effect of pH on Pancreatic Juice Secretion After Intravenous and Intranasal Administration of Secretin

pH	Route	Dosage unit (CHR unit)	TSV_{90} (μL ± SEM)[a,b]	SV_{max} (μL ± SEM)[a]	t_{max}(min)	r^c
6.40	i.v.	1	15.67 ± 3.11	11.96 ± 1.36	0–15	
2.10	nasal	10	47.92 ± 6.19 (2.67 ± 2.60)	11.42 ± 1.38	15–30	0.306
2.94	nasal	10	48.33 ± 8.03 (−1.50 ± 1.18)	11.17 ± 1.91	45–60	0.308
3.81	nasal	10	39.06 ± 3.24 (1.67 ± 1.44)	7.38 ± 1.13	60–75	0.249
4.79	nasal	10	30.13 ± 5.27 (−0.67 ± 0.89)	8.13 ± 1.33	15–30	0.192
6.33	nasal	10	15.14 ± 3.55 (0.67 ± 1.66)	3.79 ± 1.22	45–60	0.097
7.00	nasal	10	6.58 ± 2.19 (−1.67 ± 3.57)	2.42 ± 0.66	15–30	0.042
8.00	nasal	10	8.25 ± 2.07 (0.33 ± 0.49)	4.50 ± 1.03	15–30	0.053

[a]The data are expressed as mean ± SEM (n = 4–8 rats); total secreted volume of pancreatic juice during 90 min (TSV_{90}) maximum secreted volume of pancreatic juice during 15 min (SV_{max}); time to SV_{max} (t_{max}).
[b]The data enclosed in parentheses are control data (n = 3 rats).
[c]r Indicates the absorption ratio of intranasal administration to intravenous administration and is expressed as n = TSV_{90} (intranasal)/TSV_{90} (intravenous) × 1/dosage unit of intranasal administration.
Source: From Ref. 9, used with permission.

Table 6.2 Effect of Osmolarity on Pancreatic Juice Secretion After Intranasal Administration of Secretin

NaCl(M)[a]	Route	Dosage unit (CHR unit)	TSV$_{90}$ (μL ± SEM)[b,c]	SV$_{max}$ (μL ± SEM)[b]	t$_{max}$(min)	r[d]
0.154	i.v.	1	15.67 ± 3.11	11.96 ± 1.39	0-15	
0.000	nasal	10	13.90 ± 6.29 (0.16 ± 0.36)	3.40 ± 1.00	45-60	0.089
0.154	nasal	10	16.46 ± 1.94 (−1.17 ± 2.75)	5.67 ± 0.41	15-30	0.105
0.462	nasal	10	22.20[e] ± 2.33 (−0.5 ± 1.55)	7.92 ± 1.43	15-30	0.142
1.078	nasal	10	15.58 ± 1.29 (2.33 ± 1.36)	6.59 ± 0.59	15-30	0.099

[a]At pH 6.4.

[b]The data are expressed as mean ± SEM (n = 5-7 rats); total secreted volume of pancreatic juice during 90 min (TSV$_{90}$); maximum secreted volume of pancreatic juice during 15 min (SV$_{max}$); time to SV$_{max}$ (t$_{max}$).

[c]The data enclosed in parentheses are control data (n = 3 rats).

[d]r Indicates the absorption ratio of intranasal administration to intravenous administration and is expressed as r = TSV$_{90}$ (intranasal)/TSV$_{90}$ (intravenous) × 1/dosage unit of intranasal administration.

[e]Significantly different (p < 0.05).

Source: From Ref. 9, used with permission.

A study was undertaken to assess the absorbability of secretin by the nasal mucosa and the effects of pH and salt concentration on its nasal absorption (9). Using a microsyringe, the solution of secretin was directly administered into the nasal cavity of the rat. The amount of secretin absorbed was measured by biological assay and the data were then compared with intravenous administration. Linear relationship between the TSV_{90} (the total volume of pancreatic juice secreted during a period of 90 min) and the logarithm of the secretin dose administered was obtained for both intravenous administration (1-5 CHR units) and nasal delivery (5-40 CHR units). From the pharmacological response, a relative bioavailability of 10% was calculated for nasal delivery.

The nasal absorption of secretin was found to increase linearly as the pH decreased from 7.0 to 2.94, whereas it was approximately the same at pH 2.1-2.94 and 7-8 (Table 6.1). In comparison with intravenous administration, the absorption ratio (r) of secretin in the weakly alkaline solution was one-third or one-seventh of that at acidic pH condition, whereas t_{max} was prolonged at pH 2.94, 3.81, and 6.33. The amount and the rate of nasa absorption of secretin were also observed to be affected by the sodium chloride content in the saline solution (Table 6.2). The maximum value of absorption ratio was obtained with a nasal solution containing 0.462 M of saline. This study reveals that development of a nasal dosage form for secretin is feasible, and that the nasal absorption of secretin could be improved by optimizing the pH and NaCl concentration in nasal solution.

6.6 PENTAGASTRIN

Pentagastrin, a synthetic gastrinlike pentapeptide, is a diagnostic drug for evaluating the secretory function of gastric acid. It has been shown to stimulate gastric secretion when given by intravenous infusion, and by subcutaneous or intramuscular injection. In most patients, the secretion of gastric acid is increased within 10 min after subcutaneous injection of pentagastrin and reaches a peak level within 20 to 30 min.

The gastric response to the intranasal administration of pentagastrin was compared with intravenous infusion or subcutaneous injection in 12 patients (10). The output of gastric acid after the repeated intranasal administrations of pentagastrin snuff (1 mg/10 min) was observed to be as great as the maximal output following the continuous intravenous infusion of pentagastrin. The acid response to a subcutaneous dose (0.1 mg) of pentagastrin was matched by the response to a nasal dose (0.3-0.5 mg) of pentagastrin. The results indicate that pentagastrin by nasal application is an effective

method to stimulate gastric acid secretion and could probably replace subcutaneous or intramuscular injection in the routine diagnosis of gastric secretion.

6.7 CERULEIN

Cerulein is an active decapeptide extracted from the skin of the Australian
frog (*Hyla caerulea*) and possesses the activities of gastrin as well as those of
cholecystokinin-pancreozymin. It induces contraction of the gallbladder,
stimulates the pancreatic secretion of exocrine and gastric acid, delays gastric
emptying, inhibits the motility of the proximal duodenum, and stimulates
the motility of the distal small intestine and to a lesser extent the colon.
Gallbladder contraction is evident in 10 min after the intramuscular injection
of cerulein and the organ reduces by more than 40% of the original size
within 15 to 20 min.

The nasal absorption of cerulein was studied in 24 subjects (11). Lyo-
philized cerulein was dissolved in an alcoholic solution and administered
nasally with an ordinary atomizer in doses of 0.1, 0.25, 0.5, and 1 μg per kg.
With the nasal dose of 0.1 μg/kg, the reduction in gallbladder size was found
never to exceed 10% and lasted for about 15-20 min. Increased evacuation
of the gallbladder was observed in parallel with the increase in the dose of
cerulein administered nasally. With a higher dose of 1 μg/kg, there was a
potent cholecystokinetic effect and the gallbladder decreased to about 40%
of its initial premedication size. Spasmogenic activity was noted to begin at
10 min after the insufflation and lasted for 2 hr. The cholecystokinetic response to the nasal dose of 0.5 μg/kg was approximately matched by the
response to the doses at 0.5 μg/kg and 0.05 μg/kg by intramuscular and
intravenous injection, respectively. At the threshold doses, the ratio of
activity between the intranasal and intravenous routes was found to be about
1/100. This study concluded that the effect of the nasally applied cerulein is
achieved by absorption through the mucous membrane. Furthermore, the
intranasal administration of cerulein seems to be of value in clinical uses for
radiological examination of the biliary tract.

REFERENCES

1. Childrey, J. H., and Essex, H. E. Absorption from the mucosa of the
   frontal sinus, *Arch. Otolaryngol., 14*:564 (1931).
2. Hirai, S., Yashiki, T., Matswzawa, T., and Mima, H. Absorption of drugs
   from the nasal mucosa of rats, *Int. J. Pharm., 7*:317 (1981).

3. Yoffey, J. M. The lymphatic pathway for absorption from the naso-pharynx, *Lancet, 1*:530 (1941).
4. Yoffey, J. M., and Drinker, C. K. The lymphatic pathway from the nose and pharynx, *J. Exp. Med., 68*:629 (1938).
5. Blumgart, H. L. A study of the mechanism of absorption of substances from the nasopharynx, *Arch. Intern. Med., 33*:415 (1924).
6. Clark, W. E. Le Gros Anatomical investigation into the routes by which infections may pass from the nasal cavities into the brain, *Rep. Publ. Hlth. Med. Subj. No. 54*, London (1929).
7. Rake, G. Absorption through the nasal mucosa of mice, *Proc. Soc. Exp. Biol. Med., 34*:369 (1936).
8. Faber, W. M. The nasal mucosa and the subarachnoid space, *Am. J. Anat., 62*:121 (1937).
9. Ohwaki, T., Ando, H., Watanabe, S., and Miyake, Y. Effect of nose, pH, and osmolarity on nasal absorption of secretin in rats, *J. Pharm. Sci., 74*:550 (1985).
10. Wormsley, K. G. Pentagastrin snuff, *Lancet, 1*:57 (1968).
11. Agosti, A., and Bertaccini, G. Nasal absorption of caerulein, *Lancet, 1*:580 (1969).

Index

299